NUCLEAR CARDIOVASCULAR IMAGING

Current Clinical Practice

NUCLEAR CARDIOVASCULAR IMAGING

Current Clinical Practice

Edited by

Milton J. Guiberteau, MD

Associate Professor
Department of Clinical Radiology
University of Texas Medical School at Houston
Director
Department of Nuclear Medicine
St. Joseph Hospital
Houston, Texas

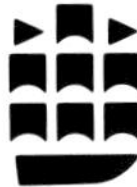

CHURCHILL LIVINGSTONE
New York, Edinburgh, London, Melbourne

Library of Congress Cataloging-in-Publication Data

Nuclear cardiovascular imaging: current clinical practice/edited by
   Milton J. Guiberteau.
       p.   cm.
     Includes bibliographical references.
     ISBN 0-443-08577-3
     1. Heart—Radionuclide imaging.   2. Coronary heart disease—
   Radionuclide imaging.   I. Guiberteau, Milton J.
     [DNLM: 1. Cardiovascular System—radionuclide imaging.
   2. Tomography, Emission Computed—methods.   WG 141.5.R2 N9653]
   RC683.5.R33N84   1990
   616.1′07575—dc20
DNLM/DLC
   for Library of Congress   89-22316
                                                                        CIP

Distributed in the United Kingdom by Churchill Livingstone,
Robert Stevenson House, 1–3 Baxter's Place, Leith Walk, Edinburgh
EH1 3AF, and by associated companies, branches, and
representatives throughout the world.

Accurate indications, adverse reactions, and dosage schedules for
drugs are provided in this book, but it is possible that they may
change. The reader is urged to review the package information data
of the manufacturers of the medications mentioned.

The publishers have made every effort to trace the copyright holders
for borrowed material. If they have inadvertently overlooked any,
they will be pleased to make the necessary arrangements at the first
opportunity.

Acquisitions Editor: *Linda Panzarella*
Copy Editor: *Kimberly Quinlan*
Production Designer: *Marci Jordan*
Production Supervisor: *Jocelyn Eckstein*

Printed in the United States of America

First published in 1990

Contributors

Nathaniel M. Alpert, PhD
Associate Professor, Department of Radiology, Harvard Medical School; Associate Applied Physicist, Division of Nuclear Medicine, Massachusetts General Hospital, Boston, Massachusetts

Anthony R. Benedetto, PhD
Associate Professor, Division of Nuclear Medicine, Department of Radiology, University of Texas Medical School at Galveston, Galveston, Texas

Ralph Blumhardt, MD
Associate Professor, Department of Radiology and Chief, Department of Nuclear Medicine, University of Texas Medical School at San Antonio, Texas

Ronald J. Callahan, PhD
Assistant Professor, Department of Radiology, Harvard Medical School; Director of Nuclear Pharmacy, Massachusetts General Hospital, Boston, Massachusetts

John C. Cedarholm, MD
Fellow, Department of Medicine (Cardiology), Emory University School of Medicine; Research Fellow, Carlyle Fraser Heart Center, Crawford Long Hospital, Atlanta, Georgia

Henry M. Chilton, PharmD
Associate Professor, Department of Radiology, Bowman Gray School of Medicine of Wake Forest University, Winston Salem, North Carolina

Ian P. Clements, MD
Assistant Professor, Department of Medicine, Mayo Medical School; Consultant, Division of Cardiovascular Diseases and Internal Medicine, Mayo Clinic and Mayo Foundation, Rochester, Minnesota

John A. Correia, PhD

Associate Professor, Department of Radiology, Harvard Medical School; Associate Applied Physicist, Division of Radiological Science and Technology, Massachusetts General Hospital, Boston, Massachusetts

E. Gordon DePuey, MD

Associate Professor, Department of Radiology, Emory University School of Medicine, Atlanta, Georgia

Keith C. Fischer, MD

Assistant Professor, Department of Clinical Radiology, Washington University Medical School; Chief, Division of Nuclear Medicine, Jewish Hospital of Saint Louis, Saint Louis, Missouri

Ernest V. Garcia, PhD

Associate Professor, Department of Radiology, Emory University School of Medicine; Director, Department of Nuclear Medicine Physics, Emory University Hospital, Atlanta, Georgia

K. Lance Gould, MD

Professor, Department of Medicine, University of Texas Medical School at Houston; Director, Positron Diagnostic and Research Center, Houston, Texas

Milton J. Guiberteau, MD

Associate Professor, Department of Clinical Radiology, University of Texas Medical School at Houston; Director, Department of Nuclear Medicine, St. Joseph Hospital, Houston, Texas

Ban-An Khaw, PhD

Associate Professor, Department of Radiology, Harvard Medical School; Associate Biochemist, Cardiac Unit, and Assistant Radiochemist, Nuclear Medicine Division, Department of Radiology, Massachusetts General Hospital, Boston, Massachusetts

E. Edmund Kim, MD

Professor of Radiology and Medicine, University of Texas Medical School at Houston; Chief, Section of Experimental Nuclear Medicine, Division of Diagnostic Imaging, and Director, Center for Metabolic and Experimental Imaging, M.D. Anderson Cancer Center, Houston, Texas

Peter P. Liu, MD

Assistant Professor, Department of Medicine, University of Toronto Faculty of Medicine; Co-Director, Nuclear Cardiology Laboratory, Toronto General Hospital, Ontario, Canada

Sharon E. Martin, PhD

Assistant Professor, Department of Medicine (Cardiology) and Department of Physiology, Emory University School of Medicine; Research Physiologist, Carlyle Fraser Heart Center, Crawford Long Hospital, Atlanta, Georgia

Warren H. Moore, MD

Assistant Professor, Department of Radiology (Nuclear Medicine), Baylor College of Medicine; Chief, Nuclear Medicine Service, St. Luke's Episcopal Hospital/Texas Children's Hospital, Houston, Texas

Martin L. Nusynowitz, MD

Professor and Director, Division of Nuclear Medicine, Department of Radiology, University of Texas Medical School at Galveston, Galveston, Texas

Randolph E. Patterson, MD

Associate Professor, Department of Medicine (Cardiology) and Department of Radiology, Emory University School of Medicine; Medical Director, Department of Nuclear Cardiology, Carlyle Fraser Heart Center, Crawford Long Hospital, Atlanta, Georgia

Mark R. Starling, MD

Associate Professor, Department of Internal Medicine, University of Michigan Medical School, Ann Arbor, Michigan

Tsunehiro Yasuda, MD

Assistant Professor, Department of Radiology, Harvard Medical School; Assistant in Radiology, Nuclear Medicine Division, Department of Radiology and Clinical Assistant in Medicine, Cardiac Unit, Massachusetts General Hospital, Boston, Massachusetts

Preface

In the past two decades, cardiovascular nuclear medicine has grown from a gleam in the researcher's eye to a full-fledged imaging subspecialty that is still actively evolving. In any such evolution, there is an attendant need to periodically assess and/or reassess the technological armamentarium in order to gain insight into the state of the art of clinical practice. This volume engages this task through a review and update of major aspects of current nuclear cardiovascular imaging from the perspectives of experienced clinicians with hands-on experience as well as through introduction of new technologies and radiopharmaceuticals by those in the forefront of the field. The book is intended primarily to meet the needs of the imaging physician in clinical practice. As such and in the interest of length, the book is not meant to be a complete compendium of nuclear cardiology. It is designed to provide in-depth discussions of areas that are or will likely become staples of nuclear cardiovascular imaging as well as to view from practical standpoints the horizons of new technology.

The book begins with a detailed review of pathophysiologic concepts that are essential to understanding fundamental cardiovascular nuclear imaging and its applications in the diagnosis and management of coronary artery disease. A survey of the radiopharmaceuticals currently in diagnostic use and those under development—including isonitriles, BATO compounds, and labeled antimyosin—provides the reader with a concise review and update of the field. A chapter on the assessment of myocardial injury using labeled antimyosin antibodies provides further discussion of this very promising agent and allows a comparison with pyrophosphate imaging procedures which have remained in contrast relatively static over the past decade.

Appropriately, a large portion of the book is devoted to the procedures which comprise the core of nuclear cardiovascular imaging: perfusion and functional imaging. Emphasis is given to the performance, quality control, data interpretation, and clinical application of stress-thallium SPECT imaging with a detailed discussion of practical, technical, and interpretative considerations. Both qualitative and quantitative methods are presented, and special attention is given to the "bullseye" approach by clinicians intimate with its development and application. A chapter on dipyridamole thallium imaging as a stress-thallium alternative is an appreciation of its growing popularity.

The current status of the imaging of left and right ventricular function at rest in the diagnosis and evaluation of both coronary and noncoronary disease states is addressed from the clinical point of view including both equilibrium and first-pass techniques. A very clear and concise presentation of the often underutilized, but clinically valuable first-pass technique is given additional treatment. Of particular interest to most imaging physicians is the current position of exercise ventriculography in the diagnostic setting, especially since this test has undergone new scrutiny in its application to broader patient segments. This technique and issues related to its place in the diagnostic environment are discussed, with emphasis on relevance to the clinical laboratory.

Appreciation of the widened applications of nuclear techniques from those of diagnosis alone requires the inclusion of an encompassing review of experience in the application of nuclear testing to prognostication and risk stratification in both acute and chronic coronary artery disease. This includes their use in therapeutic decision-making and post-treatment evaluation.

Although clinical positron emission tomography (PET) is still in its infancy, the book would not be complete without an introduction to the positron camera and a brief exposure to at least early experience in a practical clinical setting. Finally, because the literature has few current reviews addressing the vascular applications of nuclear techniques, a short chapter on the widespread procedure known as nuclear venography has been included.

I am very grateful to the contributing authors for their excellent work. This group represents some of the most knowledgeable specialists in their areas. Additionally, my thanks to the editorial staff of Churchill Livingstone, especially Ms. Linda Panzarella and Ms. Kim Loretucci, and to Ms. Joyce Bennett for their assistance in the preparation of this volume.

Milton J. Guiberteau, MD

Contents

1

Pathophysiology of Coronary Artery Disease as Applied to Nuclear Imaging

Randolph E. Patterson
Sharon E. Martin
John C. Cedarholm

Several recent basic science advances are important to understanding diagnostic imaging for coronary artery disease (CAD). Advances can be grouped into two major areas: (1) causes of coronary arterial lumen obstruction, and (2) consequences of coronary arterial lumen obstruction. There are three primary causes of coronary arterial lumen obstruction: (1) atherosclerotic plaque, (2) platelet aggregates (plugs) and thrombosis, and (3) vascular spasm. In recent years, it has become clear that these three processes interact to further reduce the lumen in many patients with CAD.

The consequences for the heart of coronary arterial lumen obstruction include abnormalities that can be imaged by various modalities:

1. *Reduction of coronary blood flow:* The first and most important consequence of coronary arterial lumen obstruction is to reduce coronary blood flow. A crucial issue in cardiovascular imaging is to define a coronary arterial lesion that is significant in that it reduces maximum coronary blood flow below a critical level.

2. *Development of collaterals:* Reduced antegrade coronary blood flow through the obstructed artery stimulates the development of coronary arterial collateral branches which help restore flow to the myocardium supplied by the stenotic artery. This important process compensates somewhat for the reduced flow.

3. *Ischemia:* When coronary blood flow cannot meet the myocardial metabolic de-

mands, ischemia occurs and produces contractile dysfunction, metabolic abnormalities, and electrophysiologic abnormalities.

4. *Myocardial Infarction:* When the blood flow deficit and ischemia persist long enough (20 to 30 minutes), myocardial infarction results, producing a region of tissue with inflammation and edema, followed by fibrosis. This mass of infarcted tissue composes a certain size or percentage of the left ventricle. The infarcted tissue does not contract, so the overall function of the left ventricle is reduced. The infarcted region also constitutes an electrically dead zone that alters the resting electrocardiogram (ECG) and can promote cardiac dysrhythmias.

The distinction between ischemic and infarcted myocardium is crucial to clinical decisions about revascularization therapy, but this distinction remains an important challenge to cardiac imaging.

CAUSES OF CORONARY LUMEN OBSTRUCTION

The coronary artery lumen can be obstructed by one or more of three pathologic processes: atherosclerotic plaque, platelet aggregation and thrombosis, and vascular spasm.

Atherosclerotic Plaque

Atherosclerotic plaque is formed from cholesterol and other blood lipid products.[1] The cholesterol is carried from the bloodstream into the plaque by low-density lipoproteins (LDLs). It is possible that high-density lipoproteins (HDLs) may act as a reverse cholesterol transport process to remove cholesterol from the arterial wall, although this has not been proved.[2] The process of depositing cholesterol and plaque into the arterial wall involves a transformation of muscular cells in the media to help form the plaque. The entire process appears to be initiated by injury to the delicate endothelial lining of the artery,[3] which can be produced by arterial hypertension, diabetes, smoking, possibly spasm, and possibly platelet plugging. It is of interest that iodine-labeled LDL cholesterol has been imaged in human carotid arterial plaques. Although the exact process of coronary atherosclerosis remains unknown, the importance of cholesterol has been emphasized during the past 5 years by the demonstration that reducing cholesterol in the blood either by diet or by drugs can retard the development of atherosclerosis in coronary arteries visualized by angiography in the NHLBI Type II Hyperlipidemia Study.[4] More importantly, reduction of cholesterol prolonged life in patients who survived their first myocardial infarction, as demonstrated in the NHLBI Lipid Clinic Study.[5,6]

Platelet Aggregates and Thrombosis

As a general response to tissue injury, such as a laceration, the local blood vessels develop spasm to minimize blood loss. In the next step, platelets aggregate from the blood at the site of the cut in the vessel wall to plug the hole in the vessel.[7] Eventually, the cascade of clotting factors is activated to lay down a thrombus to seal the hole in the blood vessel.[7] During its production, the clot is in a dynamic state for some time, with more clot being synthesized but more offsetting processes being activated to lyse the blood clot. Second, endothelial injury appears to be an important stimulus for platelet aggregation and clotting, but the mechanisms that cause a coronary artery that is partially occluded by atherosclerotic plaque to become totally occluded by plaque as well as platelets and thrombus remain unknown.[8]

It is quite clear, however, that the process of clot formation in the coronary artery is indeed the pivotal event that produces myocardial infarction in the vast majority of patients with that condition. This has been proved by coronary angiography performed in the acute phase of myocardial infarction showing totally obstructed vessels that do not open with intracoronary nitroglycerin.[9] In other studies, radiolabeled platelets have been imaged in the coronary arteries of dogs[10] and humans.[11]

Finally, the best proof that blood clotting plays an important role in lumen obstruction during myocardial infarction is the fact that several thrombolytic agents, such as streptokinase[12] and recombinant tissue plasminogen activator (rTPA),[13] can be injected to break down the clot and reopen the coronary artery in patients during the acute phase of a myocardial infarction. This remains a crucial issue for investigation, and both platelets and clotting factors have been labeled by isotopic tracers to help investigate this important issue. Our institution participated in a study of the ability of rTPA to attack coronary clots in the acute stage of myocardial infarction.[14] Our preliminary work suggests that reperfusion within 4 to 6 hours of onset of chest pain in an acute myocardial infarction can reduce signs of myocardial injury on dynamic magnetic resonance imaging (MRI), producing, for example, less severely impaired systolic wall thickening and less increase in signal intensity, probably related to tissue edema.[15] Reperfusion was accomplished by rTPA and, in some patients by acute percutaneous transluminal coronary angioplasty (PTCA) as well. A major unanswered question is whether it is wise to perform PTCA during acute myocardial infarction when thrombolytic therapy has restored flow but left a high-grade coronary stenosis.

Vascular Spasm

During the past decade, there has been abundant proof that a large coronary artery can develop spasm to stop flow and produce symptoms of angina at rest.[16] The proof has consisted of coronary arteriograms performed during spontaneous episodes of angina at rest to demonstrate that one large coronary artery is totally occluded during pain and can be reopened with nitroglycerin, which also relieves symptoms.[16] In order to avoid spasm provoked by the presence of a catheter in the coronary artery, there have also been studies of patients with intravenous (IV) thallium injections during spontaneous episodes of angina at rest.[17] These scans have shown perfusion defects during pain and normal scans in the same patient in the absence of pain. In patients with episodes of chest pain at rest, the symptoms and electrocardiographic (ECG) findings can usually be reproduced by an IV injection of ergonovine in the cardiac catheterization laboratory to provoke spasm of a coronary artery.[18] This spasm is well seen on the arteriogram.[18] This diagnostic test appears to be useful in identifying the cause of chest pain in patients with angina at rest, especially those who have normal large coronary arteries as visualized by an angiogram. It must be pointed out, however, that ergonovine can also provoke esophageal spasm and result in chest discomfort. This test is probably not safe to perform outside a cardiac catheterization laboratory, as the patient might require an intracoronary injection of nitroglycerin or calcium channel-blocking drug to abolish spasm.

For many years, there has been speculation that some patients with chest pain syndromes have a disease involving coronary arteries smaller than those visualized by the coronary arteriogram (100-μm diameter).[19] During the past few years, interesting evidence has been developed on this point.[20] A group of patients with chest pain at rest were studied who had relatively normal large coronary arteries and no evidence of large vessel spasm during ergonovine testing. In some of these patients, chest pain, ECG changes, and abnormal lactate production developed, indicating myocardial ischemia after ergonovine injection.[20] Measurements of coronary sinus blood flow by the thermodilution technique demonstrated an inadequate coronary blood flow despite normal size large coronary arteries visualized by the arteriogram. These studies indicate that small vessels, not observed by coronary angiography, can contribute to a critical reduction in blood flow in patients with chest pain at rest.[20] These patients have responded well to intensive treatment with nitrates and calcium-entry blocking drugs. Thus, it appears that spasm of small coronary arteries may be an important clinical entity.

None of these studies has yet been able to indicate the mechanisms that cause coronary arterial spasm. The most obvious mechanism for investigation was to determine whether the activation of α-adrenergic receptors in the coronary arteries could produce spasm. Indeed, many patients show a reduction in coronary blood flow (measured as coronary sinus blood flow, by the thermodilution method) during the cold pressor test, in which the patient immersed the hand in ice water, provoking a set of reflexes that raises blood pressure and causes vasoconstriction elsewhere.[21] Since the patients tested in this group had large vessel coronary disease, the results are not specific for coronary spasm. In fact, the atherosclerotic blockage of the coronary arteries might have limited the expected increase in blood flow in that group as blood pressure increased.[21] The metabolites of norepinephrine metabolism and norepinephrine itself have been measured in blood and urine and found to be no different in patients with coronary spasm than in those patients who do not have coronary spasm.[22] Furthermore, Chierchia et al.[23] used α-adrenergic blocking drugs and found that patients with coronary spasm show no reduction in the frequency of episodes of spontaneous chest pain or ST-T-wave changes on the ECG monitor. Furthermore, there were no other signs of increased sympathetic neural discharge to the heart, such as changes in QT interval, in patients with preceding episodes of coronary spasm.[23] For these reasons, stimulation of α-adrenergic receptors, per se, has not been considered an adequate explanation for coronary spasm.

An exciting body of evidence has developed during the past decade concerning prostaglandin products and their possible role in blood vessel constriction and dilation.[24] In particular, thromboxane A_2 has been found to be the most potent coronary vasoconstrictor known. However, two groups have used blocking drugs that have virtually abolished the production of thromboxane A_2 (measured by its breakdown product in urine, thromboxane B_2) and yet have shown no change in the frequency of attacks of spontaneous chest pain and ST-T-wave abnormalities on the 24-hour ECG monitor.[25,26] Thus, within the limits of currently available measurement techniques for prostaglandin products, it would appear that thromboxane, per se, cannot be proposed as the chemical mediator of coronary spasm.

It is interesting that one of the initial barriers to acceptance of the idea of coronary spasm by cardiologists was the large body of evidence developed by coronary physiologists over the past 50 years that indicates that coronary blood flow is regulated to meet myocardial oxygen demand very precisely under normal conditions.[27,28] It has seemed hard to believe that infusion of a vasoconstrictor into the coronary circulation could overcome this powerful endogenous regulatory system to reduce blood flow enough to cause myocardial ischemia. Interest in the issue of possible chemical mediators of coronary spasm has involved the study of a group of compounds called neuropeptides.[29,30] These peptide hormones are usually produced in the brain and other nerve cells, where they can either be released locally from nerves or into the blood. Whether some of these neuropeptides, such as vasopressin[29] and neuropeptide-Y,[30] can cause vasoconstriction severe enough to overcome normal regulation of blood flow and result in myocardial ischemia has been investigated by using dogs with normal coronary arteries and measuring coronary blood flow by an electromagnetic flow probe placed around the artery. A small cannula was employed to infuse the peptides directly into the circumflex coronary artery. It was discovered that doses of vasopressin and neuropeptide-Y caused a reduction in coronary blood flow with no change in aortic pressure or heart rate.

The more important issue in these studies was to determine whether the reduction in coronary blood flow under the circumstances would be sufficient to cause myocardial ischemia. One can conceive of a regulatory system that would permit some minor reduction in flow but that would, by a relesase of vasodilator metabolites, overcome the constrictor process before it had caused ischemia. To test for the presence of ischemia, ECG and left ventricular ejection fractions (LVEF) by gated blood-pool scans were performed.[31] ST-T-wave changes were noted on the ECG, which were consistent with, but certainly not proof of, ischemia. One would have to rule out a possible direct electrophysiologic effect of the peptides in order to prove that this was due to ischemia. Also noted were reductions in LVEF, but a reduction in ejection fraction under these circumstances might possibly be explained by a negative inotropic effect of the peptides. Even though no such effect of these peptides has been demonstrated, one could debate about this type of evidence from gated blood-pool scans. For these reasons, a special fiberoptic intramyocardial pH probe was also used.[32] This probe was inserted directly into the myocardium, where it measured predominantly extracellular fluid pH. It was found that both vasopressin and neuropeptide-Y caused a decrease in intramyocardial pH in the left ventricle. Especially when combined with the abnormalities .in the ECG and gated blood-pool scan, these results prove that these neuropeptides are capable of reducing blood flow severely

enough to produce myocardial ischemia in animals without arterial disease.[29,30] The evidence to date does not provide any information concerning whether these peptides are the cause of coronary flow reductions or coronary spasm in humans. It is of interest, however, that neuropeptide-Y has been isolated by immunohistochemical techniques in the nerves surrounding the coronary arteries in human autopsy samples.[33] Thus, there appears to be ample reason to pursue active investigation of this particular peptide as a possible chemical mediator of human coronary spasm.

Combined Factors

Finally, a very important concept has emerged during the past several years—that in many patients, a combination of mechanisms accounts for reduction in coronary blood flow.[16] For example, many patients have coronary atherosclerotic narrowing of the large coronary arteries demonstrated by coronary arteriography, yet also have what is called variable threshold angina. In this syndrome, the patient is able to perform only limited activity before developing chest pain early in the morning, yet may be able to perform much greater levels of physical activity before experiencing chest discomfort in the afternoon. It is also known that such patients may have major differences in exercise tolerance on different days, accounting for "good days and bad days" for the patient which often confuse and frustrate the patient, the family, and the employer. During the past few years, indirect evidence has developed that this pattern of variable threshold angina is frequently explained by spasm of large or small coronary arteries to limit coronary blood flow during certain periods.[16] Objective exercise testing confirms the clinical impression that evidence of ischemia occurs at markedly different exercise workloads at different times of day in these people. An important consequence of this type of angina is that many of the symptoms can be relieved by effective coronary vasodilators.[34] It appears that some people with coronary artery spasm can, indeed, develop acute myocardial infarction,[35] but this is certainly the minority of people with myocardial infarction. However, it is easy to see how a patient with a 40% narrowing of the major coronary artery due to atherosclerotic plaque could develop mild constriction of the same vessel and increase the severity of the lumen obstruction to 70 percent. Thus, a lesion observed on angiography and thought to be insignificant could become significant in a matter of seconds due to mild coronary spasm.

In summary, radionuclide imaging of cardiovascular diseases has been well served by imaging of cardiac perfusion and function. In the future, however, even greater advances may be possible by emphasis on imaging of labeled components of the atherosclerotic plaque, platelets, clotting factors and, perhaps, receptors in the arteries, per se.

CONSEQUENCES OF CORONARY ARTERIAL LUMEN OBSTRUCTION

Coronary arterial lumen obstruction by any mechanism leads to several consequences: limitation of coronary blood flow, development of coronary collaterals, the potential for coronary steal, myocardial ischemia (with its abnormalities of contraction, metabolism and electrophysiology), and, finally, myocardial infarction.

Limitation of Coronary Blood Flow

The primary problem with CAD is that coronary blood flow is reduced, manifested as a reduction in the maximum coronary blood flow that can be carried by an artery when the lumen obstruction is moderate.[36] The ability of coronary blood flow to increase from its baseline to its maximum value is

called coronary blood flow reserve capacity. About half the lumen diameter can be obstructed before there is any reduction in coronary blood flow reserve, that is, in the maximum blood flow that can be carried by coronary artery.[36] The artery must be obstructed by 80 to 90 percent before there is any reduction in the flow available at rest.[36] These findings have emerged from studies in animals in which coronary blood flow can be measured precisely by an electromagnetic flow probe and coronary lumen diameter can be measured by mechanical calipers. Such precise measurements are not available in humans.

A major issue in contemporary cardiology and a major indication for radionuclide studies during stress is to determine the functional significance of coronary arterial narrowing observed on angiography. The angiographer calls a lesion significant when it reduces lumen diameter by 50 to 70 percent.[37] However, it is well known that the angiographic appearance of coronary arterial narrowing, especially when interpreted subjectively, is not a precise predictor of reductions in coronary blood flow.[37] One study compared coronary arteriography with postmortem analysis of the coronary arteries and found a very poor correlation between experienced angiographers' readings of the coronary arteriogram and the postmortem appearance of the coronary artery.[38] More importantly, White et al.[39] correlated coronary arteriographic findings with the peak coronary blood flow velocity during stress measured in the coronary artery at the time of open-heart surgery by a minimally invasive ultrasonic doppler flowmeter. These workers found a very poor correlation between peak flow velocity and angiographic estimates of percentage of coronary arterial narrowing ($r = 0.2$).[39] There are other promising ways to improve the arteriographic estimates, such as a computer program to characterize the coronary arterial lumen size and shape more accurately,[40] as well as videodensitometric methods to estimate coronary blood flow from dye injections during coronary angiography.[41]

In clinical practice, however, the job of estimating the functional significance of a coronary lesion usually falls to the nuclear medicine department. The angiographer most often seeks help in assessing the significance of borderline lesions that reduce lumen diameter by 30 to 70 percent. The idea is to impose a stress on the circulation so that coronary blood flow is increased to nearly maximum values. This can be done by exercise in most circumstances but may occasionally be better performed by IV administration of dipyridamole, a coronary vasodilator drug.[42] When coronary blood flow is increased to a maximum value in normal arteries, it is easier to detect a difference in flow between a normal artery and an artery that is blocked by atherosclerotic plaque. In this way, it is easier to appreciate the contrast between the blood flow rates in normal versus partially occluded coronary arteries. The common interpretation is that if a patient shows a defect on exercise thallium imaging or a wall-motion abnormality or drop in ejection fraction on exercise measurement of left ventricular function that the anatomic lesion observed by angiography is functionally significant.

In work by Hamilton et al.[42,43] with qualitative planar ^{201}Tl imaging and in a preliminary study with qualitative single photon emission computed tomographic (SPECT) imaging of ^{201}Tl by Shonkoff et al.,[44] there was a significant increase in the number of positive tests as the severity of coronary narrowing measured by calipers on arteriograms increased. In another preliminary study of SPECT ^{201}Tl imaging, in animals, Cedarholm et al.[45] found that a quantitative analysis by the bull's-eye ischemic score correlated well with the severity of reduction in maximum coronary blood flow during isoproterenol infusion and could distinguish between coronary stenoses that did or did not impair regional myocardial contraction as measured by ultra-

sonic crystals. These data suggest that a defect on SPECT ^{201}Tl during catecholamine stress in an animal with a coronary stenosis implies ischemia, not merely a difference in perfusion.

It must be emphasized, however, that using ^{201}Tl or other radionuclide imaging procedures to define a functionally significant coronary stenosis in humans assumes that the nuclear medicine test is the gold standard and that the coronary arteriogram has become the variable to be assessed. This approach is the opposite of the standard approach, whereby nuclear cardiology procedures are validated against the coronary arteriographic gold standard. For example, there have been several indications during the past few years that patients with mild 20 to 60 percent narrowing of lumen diameter will often be those who exhibit positive exercise thallium scans, consistent with the idea that the thallium scan may provide a better "gold standard" than does the coronary arteriogram, under some circumstances. The issue of whether coronary angiography or stress radionuclide imaging provides the better reference method is not yet settled.[46] Clinical practice in many centers, however, allows for the referral of patients for angioplasty or coronary bypass surgery on the basis of abnormalities demonstrated on stress radionuclide imaging when coronary arteriography shows a borderline significant lesion. There is no physiologic mystery about assessing the functional significance of a coronary lesion. Rather, the problem lies in the inadequacies of the techniques available to assess coronary blood flow in humans.

Development of Coronary Collaterals

Another consequence of (and compensation for) coronary arterial lumen obstruction when antegrade flow is reduced by an atherosclerotic plaque is the development of coronary arterial collateral vessels.[47] The collateral coronary arteries are present in rudimentary form from birth onward and are called upon to enlarge and carry larger volumes of flow when there is an obstruction developing in the normal channels. The collaterals can then take flow from a normal coronary artery around an obstruction in another coronary branch to perfuse the distal vascular bed. Thus, the collaterals are relatively large channels that supply blood to a major coronary arterial branch and distribute it within the same vascular distribution as that major arterial branch with the occlusion. Coronary collaterals are not small arteries the size of capillaries but rather are larger.[48]

It appears clear that there is a high degree of variability in the development of collaterals in members of any one species as well as differences among species (e.g., dogs, pigs, sheep, primates, and humans). The variability among different individuals of the same species may outweigh the variability among different species. Any comparison of different species with humans must first take note of the major methodologic problem of measuring collateral blood flow in humans.[47] Thus, the most obvious species difference between humans and animals is the ability to measure collateral coronary blood flow accurately in animals by radioactive plastic microspheres and other techniques, used in controlled conditions, in contrast to the very limited methods and conditions available for estimating collateral perfusion in humans.[47]

It has clearly been demonstrated in animals that when the collateral circulation is well developed, it can restore resting coronary blood flow to normal after a gradual total occlusion of a coronary artery.[47–49] Thus, if an artery is gradually occluded by controlled coronary constriction, the myocardium supplied by that vessel will not undergo infarction, and collaterals will be well developed. With stress, however, many of these animals

that show adequate protection of the myocardium at rest demonstrate blood flow that does not increase as much through collaterals as it does through native vessels supplying normal myocardium.[48,49] This has been most clearly demonstrated by exercise tests in dogs measuring collateral coronary blood flow by the radioactive plastic microsphere method with in vitro postmortem counting, which measures flow per gram of tissue supplied by normal arteries compared with flow per gram of tissue supplied by collaterals.[48,49]

In humans, problems with techniques to estimate collateral function limit such studies. Any human study that attempts to assess the functional significance of large collaterals seen on angiography in patients with partial occlusion of a coronary artery is subject to serious misinterpretation.[47,50] First, the partial occlusion permits a variable amount of antegrade flow, which is not measured. Thus, the contractile function of the myocardium distal to the stenosis will depend not only on collaterals but on a variable amount of antegrade flow as well. Second, the criteria to identify functionally adequate collaterals on angiography are poor. Several such criteria of the adequacy of collateral filling include the size of the vessel beyond the point of stenosis, subjective grading of the intensity of visualization of contrast material in the artery beyond the occlusion,[37,50,51] and the time required for a dye to pass from the normal artery to the obstructed artery (which appears to be inversely related to collateral perfusion measured by intracoronary xenon).[50,51] Finally, one way to determine whether the myocardium supplied by collaterals functions adequately is to assess its regional contraction from a contrast angiogram.[37]

In general, studies that have reported that coronary collaterals are not adequate to supply the demands of the myocardium in humans[37] have generally been flawed by trying to assess collaterals in the presence of some antegrade flow, difficulty assessing the degree of collateral development, and difficulty determining whether the myocardium supplied by the collaterals is necrotic (and therefore does not need collateral flow) or viable (and therefore does need collateral flow).[47,50] For example, one study found that in a group of 22 patients with totally occluded coronary arteries, 6 patients showed normal planar thallium scans in the distribution of the occluded coronary artery during exercise.[50] This normal exercise ^{201}Tl image correlated with shorter dye appearance times on coronary arteriography as another index of the adequacy of their collateral development. An interesting finding in that study was that people with totally occluded left anterior descending (LAD) coronary arteries rarely had adequate collaterals defined by exercise thallium scanning, whereas patients with totally occluded right or circumflex coronary arteries usually had adequate protection by collaterals measured by exercise thallium scans.[50] There did not appear to be a differential sensitivity of the planar thallium imaging technique for the anterior versus inferior walls of the heart in a group of patients with myocardial infarctions represented by Q waves and akinetic segments of the contrast ventriculogram. In those patients, there was an equal sensitivity of planar thallium imaging to detect the infarct in the anterior wall (92 percent) versus the inferior or posterolateral walls (88 percent). Thus, it appears that the LAD coronary artery cannot be protected as well by collaterals as can the right or circumflex coronary arteries.[50] The most likely explanation for this difference is that the mass of myocardium supplied by the LAD coronary artery is larger than that supplied by the right or circumflex coronary artery in humans. This would correlate with animal studies that have shown that the collateral flow per gram of tissue is lower when the mass of the left ventricle supplied by the occluded coronary artery is larger.[52]

Coronary Steal

The phenomenon of coronary steal is often raised by clinicians, and especially by those performing imaging techniques. The experiment defining coronary steal was first performed by Fam and MacGregor,[53] who showed that when one artery was totally occluded and dependent for its blood flow on collaterals from an adjacent artery, they could demonstrate a reduction in collateral flow, under certain circumstances. In their experiments, they produced a severe partial occlusion in the artery that was supplying collaterals to an artery with total occlusion. During administration of the vasodilator, dipyridamole, these investigators were able to show a reduction in collateral flow measured directly as retrograde flow from the cut end of the occluded artery distal to the site of ligation.[53]

The mechanism of this reduced collateral flow was proposed to be as follows: dipyridamole *increased flow velocity* through the partially occluded coronary artery, and this increase in flow velocity would be expected to cause a *decrease in pressure* in that partially occluded artery. If one recalls from physics that total energy in such a system must remain constant and is the sum of kinetic energy (roughly equivalent to flow velocity) and potential energy (roughly equivalent to the pressure gradient), this is easy to understand. As dipyridamole dilates the small arterioles in the myocardium supplied by the partially occluded artery, it can have no further effect on the arterioles in the ischemic region, which are already maximally dilated by the process of ischemia itself. With the dilation of these arterioles, more blood rushes through the artery; therefore, flow velocity must increase as flow crosses the partial coronary stenosis. In that partially occluded artery, there is a further drop in pressure distal to the stenosis. This drop in pressure distal to the partial stenosis means that the pressure at the origin of the collateral vessels will now be decreased. Collateral vessels are quite dependent on the pressure gradient across them to drive blood flow into the ischemic myocardium; thus, collateral flow will drop when pressure in the artery from which the collaterals originate drops.

In subsequent studies, Becker[54] indicated that coronary steal could not occur when only one artery was occluded and other arteries were normal. His experiments were based on microsphere studies designed to identify the ischemic zone and to measure collateral blood flow during administration of dipyridamole plus methoxamine to hold aortic pressure constant.[54] Patterson and Kirk[55] performed studies using adenosine as a vasodilator while holding left main coronary artery pressure constant with a special cannula and perfusion pump. When one artery was occluded and the left main coronary artery pressure was maintained constant, adenosine was able to induce a small coronary steal, indicating that there is some pressure gradient across the coronary circulation proximal to the origins of the coronary collaterals. This pressure drop would predict that about 10 percent of the resistance of the coronary circulation is present in the large coronary arteries proximal to the origin of the collaterals.

The significance of this finding is that the magnitude of coronary steal is small when one artery is totally occluded and other arteries are normal. The magnitude of coronary steal is amplified greatly when there is a partial stenosis in the coronary circulation in another artery proximal to the origin of collateral vessels. There is a roughly linear relationship between the magnitude of coronary steal and the severity of stenosis of the left main coronary artery proximal to the origin of the collaterals.[55] This phenomenon helps explain why multivessel coronary disease, and especially left main coronary disease, has such a serious impact on the coronary circulation and the life expectancy of the patient. Multivessel disease jeopardizes the origin of

collateral vessels and thus further decreases perfusion of the myocardium.

In contrast to exercise or catecholamine stress, during thallium imaging with dipyridamole, it appears that myocardium does not need to be ischemic in order to produce a thallium defect.[42] Dipyridamole dilates normal vessels, delivers more flow through normal arteries, and gives a brighter image on thallium imaging in those regions. By contrast, myocardium supplied by a stenotic coronary artery will not show as great an increase in blood flow or thallium distribution so that it will appear as a defect. Furthermore, in the occasional patient in whom evidence of ischemia such as chest pain and/or ECG changes does develop during dipyridamole imaging, one mechanism could be arterial hypotension. When blood pressure is reduced below the level that sustains coronary blood flow across the stenotic coronary lesions, the patient may well experience ischemia. Coronary steal cannot be differentiated in these circumstances. When arterial pressure is reduced, the reduced arterial pressure is transmitted down the partially occluded coronary artery, further reducing collateral perfusion of the area supplied by the collateral vessels. Thus, one cannot distinguish coronary steal when arterial pressure has also decreased. This mechanism, however, of increased flow velocity reducing the pressure at the origin of collaterals probably contributes to ischemia under these conditions. In fact, recent studies have demonstrated development of transient abnormalities of LV regional contraction during dipyridamole infusion to confirm ischemia in a few patients.

Border Zone

The concept of a border zone between normal and infarcted or ischemic myocardium is critical to understanding the mechanisms of ischemia and infarction, antianginal therapy, reduction of infarct size and how to interpret myocardial images in patients with CAD.[52]

When a coronary artery is occluded in an animal, there is a gradation of flow from the most severe deficit in the center of the zone supplied by the occluded artery, to normal flow in the zone supplied by an adjacent patent coronary artery. This transition or gradient region in animals is small (about 0.5 to 1.0 cm). The explanation of this gradient has been supplied in recent years by differential labeling methods developed by Kirk and colleagues.[52,56–60] This gradient is explained by an overlap between myocardium supplied by the occluded artery (ischemic) and the normal myocardium supplied by the adjacent patent arteries. In this zone, where myocardium supplied by the the two arteries overlaps, there is an algebraic mixture of the two types of tissue to account for the value of flow that is intermediate between normal and ischemic myocardium. When the two different tissue types are separated by experimental procedures for labeling normal versus ischemic myocardium, there is virtually no residual gradient, or it is only a few cell thicknesses thick.[56–61] Thus, the lateral border zone surrounding the central core of severely ischemic myocardium is explained by a mixture of normal and ischemic myocardium rather than by a region of myocardium with intermediate injury.

This concept is pivotal to understanding salvage of acutely ischemic myocardium. The salvage occurs across a transmural border zone within the ischemic region.[52,56–61] Thus, myocardium that is supplied totally by the occluded artery shows a gradient of blood flow from most severe reduction at the endocardial surface to least severe reduction at the epicardial surface. Across this transmural border zone, there is a gradient of blood flow, ischemic metabolites such as lactate, adenosine triphosphate (ATP) and creatine phosphate (CK),[52,62] and pH.[32] The more severe the flow reduction, the lower the flow in the endocardium.[63] These findings have important corollaries, in that myocardial infarctions are virtually always more severe at the endocardial surface and less severe at the epicardial surface.[64] The definition of a transmural infarct recorded by Q waves on the ECG correlates with about a half-thickness of the myocardium infarcted at autopsy.[64] Thus, as we perform interventions to salvage acutely ischemic myocardium, we are attempting to arrest the progress of infarction, which moves like a wavefront from endocardium toward the epicardium within the zones supplied by the occluded artery.[65] By contrast, clinicians are not attempting to stop the spread of infarction laterally, unless there is a second severely occluded artery that may lead to infarction. This is why imaging techniques serve best to determine whether there are additional coronary arteries involved by severe narrowings in addition to the infarcted vessel[66] because the images demonstrate lateral relationships. Imaging techniques are less reliable for determining whether there is surviving tissue in the epicardium overlying the infarct in the endocardial portion of the LV wall thickness, a transmural relationship.

Myocardial Ischemia

Ischemia is defined as the situation where blood flow cannot meet myocardial oxygen demands, and this situation leads to the following abnormalities.

CONTRACTILE DYSFUNCTION

In 1933 Tennant and Wiggers[67] demonstrated in the dog an abnormality of contraction in the region supplied by an occluded coronary artery. This developed within a minute of the occlusion. The finding was confirmed by contrast left ventriculography in human CAD in 1967 by Herman and Gorlin and their colleagues.[68] In addition, they pointed out that the larger and more severe regional contractile deficits led to impaired overall function of the left ventricle.[69] The cause of the early contractile failure of ischemic myocardium has not been determined with certainty but may be related to an accumulation of hydrogen ions which displace calcium from its binding sites on contractile proteins.[70] The earliest contractile defect does not depend on a depletion of tissue ATP, when the total concentration of ATP in heart muscle is considered.[71]

This impairment of contraction affects primarily the myocardium that is dependent on the stenotic coronary artery (ischemic zone). The ischemic zone shows impaired systolic wall inward motion on gated equilibrium or first-pass blood-pool scans, echocardiography, contrast ventriculography, dynamic cine computerized tomography (CT), and dynamic magnetic resonance imaging. Corresponding changes in LV regional systolic wall thickening can be seen on echocardiography, CT, or magnetic resonance imaging (MRI). The greater the abnormality of LV regional function, the greater the impairment of LV global function.[69] Global function can be assessed by any of the above methods as the ejection fraction: LVEF = (end-diastolic volume) − (end-systolic volume) / (end-diastolic volume). LVEF is a major predictor of patient prognosis in CAD.[72] Global cardiac function can also be assessed by cardiac output and LV filling pressures after insertion of appropriate intravascular catheters, such as Swan-Ganz balloon-tipped thermodilution catheter in the pulmonary artery.[73,74] LV global function can remain nearly normal despite impaired contraction of the ischemic zone because of a compensatory increase in contraction of nonischemic myocardium. Thus, measurement of regional contraction is more sensitive than measurement of global function to assess the effects of CAD on the heart.[75,76] In patients with CAD, regional contraction is often normal at rest but becomes abnormal during stresses imposed by exercise or drugs that increase the work of the heart.[77,78]

Many cardiac diseases, including CAD, also affect the diastolic function of the LV, making it functionally stiffer. It appears that the diastolic function of the heart is influenced by native, ATP-dependent, and passive elastic properties of the myocardium.[79] Acute ischemia can impair ATP availability for active relaxation during early diastole, and prior infarction can destroy elastic tissue that is needed for passive relaxation.[80,81] These abnormalities can be measured as decreased peak filling rate and delayed time from end-systole until peak filling rate.[79] In addition, one of the major abnormalities of ischemic myocardium is delayed contraction.[31] Thus, the ischemic zone may contract after the remainder of the LV has begun its early diastolic filling phase.[31] This competition between different LV regions during early diastole impairs the normal increase in LV diastolic filling volume but increases LV diastolic pressure, which may cause further inhibition of LV filling from the left atrium (LA) by making the pressure gradient (LA-LV) less favorable for LV filling.

Whatever mechanisms are involved, impaired LV diastolic and/or systolic function during acute ischemia or infarction can cause shortness of breath.[74] As the LV becomes functionally stiffer, a higher filling pressure is required to achieve the same diastolic LV volume. This higher filling pressure is transmitted from LV to LA to pulmonary veins to pulmonary capillaries. The higher pressure causes fluid to leak out into the interstitial spaces of the lung where it impinges upon alveolar air spaces and increases the work of breathing.[82] In addition, exercise-induced LV dysfunction is associated with an abnormal increase in lung uptake, during exercise, of ^{201}Tl[83] or pulmonary blood volume by gated blood-pool scanning.[84] The latter two markers during exercise are often associated with three-vessel CAD.[83,84]

Acute myocardial ischemia exerts its effect on contractile function quickly, before there are measurable metabolic effects.[71] The effects of ischemia on contractile function, however, can persist even after coronary blood flow is restored.[85] The cause of this prolonged inhibition of contraction by transient ischemia is uncertain, but it may be depletion of the precursors of ATP during ischemia.[86] This phenomenon has been referred to as *stunned myocardium* because the contractile function will improve gradually over time after restoration of coronary blood flow.[87] An important clinical consequence of this prolonged effect of ischemia on contraction is that it complicates interpretation of regional LV contraction as an index of myocardial viability shortly after a prolonged ischemic event. For example, regional LV wall motion may remain quite abnormal for a few days after a myocarcial infarction interrupted by acute reperfusion and then recover substantially by a few weeks later.[75,76] Practically, this fact limits the clinical value of regional wall-motion measurements a few hours' or days after thrombolytic therapy to decide whether the patient has viable but jeopardized myocardium that might benefit from angioplasty or bypass surgery. There have been suggestions that inotropic stimulation can overcome the prolonged effect of ischemia on regional myocardial contraction.[88,89]

In summary, one of the major roles of cardiac imaging is to assess the effects of acute and chronic CAD on global and regional cardiac function in systole and diastole.

METABOLIC ABNORMALITIES

Reduction of coronary blood flow causes two types of problems for myocardial metabolism: (1) inadequate delivery of oxygen and other nutrients (which might be viewed as inadequate delivery of food and fuel); and (2) the inadequate washout of CO_2, lactic acid, and other metabolic breakdown products (which might be viewed as inadequate removal of waste products).

Metabolic abnormalities occur rapidly in ischemic myocardium, but measurable abnormalities do lag somewhat behind contractile defects.[71] There is a depletion of high-energy phosphates such as ATP and creatine phosphate.[52,90] This presumably results because of the lack of oxygen to serve as the final electron acceptor for mitochondrial oxidative phosphorylation.[90] When oxidative phosphorylation is impaired, high-energy phosphate bonds cannot be produced, leading to depletion of ATP and creatine phosphate.[90] Ischemic metabolic abnormalities are often characterized by abnormal lactate metabolism. Normally some lactate is present in arterial blood, and is taken up by the heart muscle and used as an energy substrate.[52,90] This is because lactate can be converted in the presence of oxygen to pyruvate and metabolized.[90] By contrast, in ischemic myocardium, where little oxygen is available, the lactate cannot be taken up and used to produce pyruvate; rather, pyruvate is degraded to lactate. When pyruvate is degraded to lactate, it cannot be metabolized and is therefore released into coronary venous blood. Thus, under ischemic circumstances, more lactate is released from the heart than is taken up.[90] The accumulation of lactate leads to tissue acidosis, which may contribute to further contractile dysfunction and to inhibition of anaerobic glycolysis.[90] Thus, the accumulation of waste products of metabolism such as lactic acid inhibit anaerobic glycolysis in the further production of energy in the absence of oxygen in the heart muscle.

Finally, the main energy substrates of heart muscle are fatty acids, which supply about 70 percent of the energy requirements under normal circumstances.[90] However, during ischemia, when oxygen is not available, fatty acids cannot be metabolized to produce ATP.[90] Thus, ischemic myocardium cannot use fatty acids because of the absence of oxygen as a final electronic receptor for mitochondrial oxidative phosphorylation. For this reason, fatty acids accumulate in the heart and are not taken up when labeled exogenous fatty acids are injected into the circulation.

This has been demonstrated elegantly by positron emission tomography (PET).[91]

ELECTROPHYSIOLOGIC ABNORMALITIES

Electrophysiologic abnormalities also develop when myocardium becomes ischemic and lead to repolarization abnormalities seen in the ST-T-waves of the ECG[92] and cardiac arrhythmias.[93] Critical dysrhythmias such as ventricular tachycardia and ventricular fibrillation are by far the most common cause of sudden death.[93]

Myocardial Infarction

When the abnormalities of ischemia persist long enough (15 to 30 minutes in the subendocardium; a few hours in the subepicardium), the result is acute myocardial infarction.[52] This produces loss of cell membrane function, inflammation, edema, and later fibrosis in the region of myocardium.[52]

INFARCT SIZE

The size of a region of necrotic myocardium is of enormous importance to the individual. The mass of necrotic myocardium, expressed as a percentage of the entire left ventricle, has a major impact on the patient's prognosis because cardiac functional impairment[73–76] and electrical instability[93,94] correlate closely with infarct size. The major clinical need and use for measurements of infarct size in living humans is to estimate the impact of interventions on the mass of infarcted myocardium. The ideal method would enable one to obtain an early predicted infarct size and then to compare it 2 to 4 weeks later with a final observed infarct size. If these measurements could be made in a control group of patients to show a good prediction of final infarct size by a measurement obtained early, this group of patients could be compared with a second group treated with an intervention

administered between measurements to see whether final observed infarct size was indeed less than the infarct size that would have been predicted from the early measurement. This type methodology is sorely needed to evaluate drugs, thrombolytic therapy, acute coronary angioplasty and coronary bypass graft surgery, and other potential means of reducing infarct size in humans. For human studies during acute myocardial infarction, such a measurement would have to be safe and rapid in order to avoid interference with the care of these very sick patients.

One way to measure infarct size experimentally is by postmortem studies with or without dyes such as nitrophenyltetrazolium to stain intact mitochondria in myocardium.[52,94] In regions with no functioning mitochondria, there will be an absence of stain, while in regions with functioning myocardium, there will be a clear uptake of the stain to distinguish the two regions. This is confirmed by histologic study of tissue under the microscope to confirm that stained regions are normal and that unstained regions are, in fact, necrotic.[52,94] Using this technique, it has been possible to perform experiments in animals to assess the effects of different interventions on infarct size.

Another way to assess infarct size in animals has been to measure the content of the CK enzyme in the tissue.[56,95] This enzyme is normally present in tissue to catalyze the transfer of high-energy phosphate bonds. Because the large enzyme molecule leaks out when the cell membrane is irreversibly injured, the concentration of CK in the myocardial sample is a good indicator of its viability.[52,56,95]

The methods available to estimate infarct size in living humans are limited, however. ECG is the oldest and most widely used method. The ECG pattern of acute myocardial infarction (ST elevation, T-wave inversion, and Q waves) can qualitatively detect transmural infarcts fairly reliably.[64] The problem occurs in trying to quantitate the amount of myocardium infarcted. This has been estimated by maps of ST elevation at multiple sites over the precordium[92] or Q waves over the precordium for anterior infarcts, but the methods do not work at all for inferior infarcts.[92] Furthermore, there have been several challenges to the validity of ECG mapping to quantitate the mass of infarcted myocardium.[72] In general, it appears that ECG methods do not work well enough to be useful for clinical investigation.

Clinically, a more indirect approach is required, which involves measuring the amount of CK released into the venous blood from the necrotic myocardium and trying to reconstruct the total amount of CK washed out by performing frequent sampling at different times.[95] Other methods to identify infarcted myocardium have included the pyrophosphate staining of calcium around the border of an infarct.[96] Another approach, devised by Khaw et al,[97] is to use an antibody to the myocardial contractile protein, myosin. Normally, myosin is covered by its intact cell membrane and thus would not be available for binding by an antibody. If the cell membrane is irreversibly damaged and is leaking, the antibody molecule can enter the cell and be detected if the antibody is labeled.[97] Any of these techniques can be used experimentally to dissect out and confirm portions of the heart that appear to be necrotic.

The mass of tissue with a ^{201}Tl perfusion deficit of a certain degree of severity offers one approach that is at least measurable in vivo. Silverman et al.[98] showed that a semiquantitatively estimated defect on the ^{201}Tl scan performed during the early phase of acute myocardial infarction predicts the patient's ultimate prognosis with a fair degree of reliability. Pyrophosphate hot-spot imaging has been more difficult to quantitate, but

new tomographic methods may make it more useful. Measurement of CK and its myocardial (MB) isoenzymes in the blood as a function of time have been shown to be affected by many variables other than infarct size.[95] Most dramatically, reperfusion, by thrombolytic therapy or acute angioplasty, appears to cause a marked earlier release and/or washout of enzymes that can be misinterpreted as worsened tissue necrosis.[95] The massive release, however, appears to be a result of high-flow washing out the enzyme into blood.[95]

One of the more reliable ways to estimate infarct size has been to estimate its impact on LV function. It has been known for some time that simply the presence of acute shortness of breath with a myocardial infarction is a bad prognostic sign; this was taken advantage of in a clinical classification of infarct severity based on symptoms and signs.[99] In addition, the presence of rales and gallops on physical exam and of interstitial pulmonary edema on chest radiography are other markers of a fairly large infarct causing congestive heart failure.[99] More sophisticated measurements also confirm the same trends more reliably. Measurement of pulmonary capillary wedge pressure by the Swan-Ganz catheter and cardiac output by the thermodilution technique has been performed extensively in the coronary care unit and shown to characterize patients with different severities of myocardial infarction with different prognoses.[73,74] Indeed, there is a correlation between the elevation of pulmonary capillary wedge pressure and the amount of CK enzyme released in the blood.[74] In addition, both indexes appear to correlate with other estimates of impaired global or regional LV function 1 month after acute myocardial infarction.[100] For example, left ventricular ejection fraction (LVEF) shows a rough correlation with infarct size experimentally and with prognosis in humans.[72,100] However, the ejection fraction that correlates with infarct size must be one measured 2 weeks to 2 months after an infarct at a time when the infarcted tissue is clearly separate from ischemic or stunned myocardium.[75,87] This stunned myocardium can produce more severe initial reduction of LV function than will result from the final infarct.

Other somewhat more precise ways to assess infarct size by LV function are to estimate regional function in some quantitative way, expressed either as a perimeter of the LV outline on contrast angiography that does not contract well[100] or as the area of poorly contracting left ventricle on a radionuclide angiogram.[101] Several measurements of this type have been shown to correlate roughly with infarct size in animals and with the cruder measurements available in humans.

Further, electrophysiologic variables such as the ease of producing arrhythmias by programmed electrical stimulation have also been shown to correlate with the mass of myocardium that is infarcted experimentally. In studies in dogs, a close linear correlation ($r = 0.92$) has been found between infarct size measured by tetrazolium and histology versus a quantitative index of electrical instability measured during programmed electrical stimulation 4 days after acute myocardial infarction in the dog.[94] Califf et al.[102] found that the frequency and type of ventricular premature beats measured on Holter ECG monitoring correlated roughly with the regional abnormalities of contraction measured on contrast angiograms a few weeks after infarction. Finally, the presence and quantitative importance of infarction may be assessed by imaging a labeled antibody to myosin.[97] After an acute myocardial infarction, it is necessary to apply several of these physiologic principles to assessment of the patient for further evaluation.[103] In general, the patient's prognosis is determined by the amount of irreversible myocardial damage and by the amount of myocardium that becomes reversibly ischemic during stress.

INFARCT VERSUS ISCHEMIA

Estimating whether a region of myocardium is irreversibly infarcted, reversibly ischemic, or normal is absolutely crucial to deciding whether to perform invasive interventions such as thrombolytic therapy, angioplasty, or coronary bypass graft surgery on patients early in the course of infarction or after an infarction. A very common reason that patients are sent for stress radionuclide studies is to distinguish irreversibly infarcted from reversibly ischemic myocardium. Although changes in the severity of a defect on thallium from early to delayed rest images have some value in this regard, they are not perfect arbiters of viability. Thirty to 40 percent of fixed defects that show no redistribution from exercise to delayed rest thallium imaging can disappear entirely after a successful coronary angioplasty[104] or coronary bypass graft surgery.[105] By contrast, some redistribution can certainly occur in the myocardium overlying an infarct and cause an overestimation of reversibility. Assessment of regional contraction at rest and exercise or with nitroglycerin, postextrasystolic potentiation,[88] or catecholamines[77] may also be useful but are not entirely specific for this diagnostic dilemma.

Once again, the issue is not mysterious, but techniques for making measurements in humans are limited. Experimentally, occlusion of a coronary artery creates infarction in the endocardial third to half of the LV wall thickness supplied by that artery.[106] There will still be surviving normal tissue in the outer two-thirds to one-half. However, because the artery is still totally occluded and collaterals may not be adequate, some ischemia may develop with stress in the middle third of the ventricular wall thickness between the infarct in the endocardium and normal tissue in the epicardium.[106] In one study in which low-level exercise stress ^{201}Tl imaging studies were performed 10 days after an acute myocardial infarction, reversible ^{201}Tl defects identified patients who were at high risk of future development of unstable angina, infarction, or sudden death.[107] These results are encouraging because they suggest that ^{201}Tl imaging can, in this setting, distinguish infarct from ischemia. The clinical problem is that it is difficult to detect these fine gradations by available techniques and the mixture of infarcted, ischemic, and normal tissue may not be differentiated accurately by current radionuclide methods.

CONCLUSION

Coronary arteries can become obstructed by any one or a combination of the following mechanisms: atherosclerotic plaque, platelet aggregates, thrombosis, and vascular spasm. The consequences of coronary artery obstruction include limited antegrade coronary blood flow, enhanced coronary collateral blood flow, the potential for coronary steal, a transmural border zone between endocardium and epicardium, myocardial ischemia, (contractile dysfunction, metabolic abnormalities, and electrophysiologic abnormalities), and myocardial infarction. Cardiovascular imaging has enjoyed its greatest success in identifying abnormalities of blood flow and contraction but it has remained difficult to distinguish myocardial ischemia from infarction. In this latter respect, PET and MRI may offer some advances.

Positron emission tomographic imaging, by Schelbert's group, of fluorine-10-deoxyglucose (FDG) in animals with experimental myocardial ischemia or infarction suggests that FDG activity is high relative to blood flow tracers in regions with potentially reversible ischemia.[105,108,109] By contrast, regions with infarction show similar severe reductions in both FDG and blood flow tracers, presumably due to the absence of anaerobic metabolism in permanently infarcted myocardium.[108] Preliminary human studies also suggest that PET imaging of FDG and blood flow tracers can distinguish reversible ischemia from permanent infarction.[109] In addition, other abnormalities can be visualized by MRI in infarcted myocardium, such as changes in relaxation times, that probably correlate with tissue edema.[15,110] Because of its high spatial resolution, MRI holds promise for distinguishing irreversibly infarcted from reversibly ischemic myocardium, although it has not yet been worked out. This technique can also demonstrate regional contraction and wall thickness to further clarify the size of an infarction.

From a practical clinical viewpoint, a desirable (but not currently available) test would provide answers quickly (in minutes) to two questions: (1) In this patient, how much myocardium is reversibly ischemic as opposed to permanently infarcted? (2) If the coronary artery could be reopened by some acute intervention, how much myocardium could be salvaged relative to the damage destined to result from the infarct with no intervention?

REFERENCES

1. Ross R: The pathogenesis of atherosclerosis—An update. N Engl J Med 314:488, 1986
2. Gotto AM Jr, Jones PH, Scott LW: The diagnosis and management of hyperlipidemia. Disease-a-Month 32:252, 1986
3. McMillan GC. Overview: Nature and definitions of atherosclerosis. [In Lee KT (ed): Atherosclerosis.] Ann NY Acad Sci 454:1, 1985
4. Brensike JF, Levy RI, Kelsey SF, et al: Effects of therapy with cholestyramine on progression of coronary atherosclerosis: Results of the NHLBI Type II coronary intervention study. Circulation 69:313, 1984
5. Lipid Research Clinics: Program: The Lipid Research Clinics' coronary primary prevention trial results. I. Reduction in incidence of coronary heart disease. JAMA 251:351, 1984
6. NIH Consensus Development Conference Statement: Lowering Blood Cholesterol to Prevent Heart Disease. Vol. 5, No. 7. Na-

tional Institutes of Health, Washington, DC, 1984

7. Mustard JF, Packman MA, Kinlough-Rathbone RL: Platelets, atherosclerosis and clinical complications. p. 70. In Moore S (ed): Vascular Injury and Atheroscolerosis. Marcel Dekker, New York, 1981

8. Moore S: Thrombosis and atherogenesis—The chicken and the egg (contribution of platelets in atherogenesis). [In Lee KT (ed): Atherosclerosis.] Ann NY Acad Sci 454:146, 1985

9. DeWood MA, Spores J, Notske R, et al: Prevalence of total coronary occlusion during the early hours of transmural myocardial infarction. N Engl J Med 303:897, 1980

10. Riba AL, Thakur ML, Gottschalk A, et al: Imaging experimental coronary artery thrombosis with indium-111 platelets. Circulation 60:767, 1979

11. Stratton JR, Ritchie JL: Indium-111-labeled platelet imaging in man. p. 139. In Pohost GM, Higgins CB, Morganroth J, Ritchie JL, Schelbert HR (eds): New Concepts in Cardiac Imaging. Year Book Medical Publishers, Chicago, 1987

12. Rentrop KP, Feit F, Blanke H, et al: Effects of intracoronary streptokinase and intracoronary nitroglycerin infusion on coronary angiographic patterns in mortality in patients with acute myocardial infarction. N Engl J Med 311:1457, 1984

13. Sobel BE, Geltman EM, Ticfenbrun AJ, et al: Improvement of regional myocardial metabolism after coronary thrombolysis induced with tissue-type plasminogen activator of streptokinase. Circulation 69:983, 1984

14. Topol EJ, Morris DC, Smalling RW: A multicenter, randomized, placebo-controlled trial of a new form of intravenous recombinant tissue-type plasminogen activator (Activase) in acute myocardial infarction. J Am Coll Cardiol 9:1205, 1987

15. Pettigrew RI, Churchwell AL, Liberman HA, et al: NMR imaging to assess the effects of recombinant tissue plasminogen activator on acute myocardial infarction. J Nucl Med 28:591 1987 (abst 142)

16. Maseri A, Chierchia S: Coronary artery spasm: demonstration, definition, diagnosis and consequences. Prog Cardiovasc Dis 25:169, 1982

17. Maseri A, Parodi O, Severi S, Pesola A: Transient transmural reduction of myocardial blood flow demonstrated by thallium-201 scintigraphy, as a cause of variant angina. Circulation 54:280, 1976

18. Bertrand ME, LaBlanche JM, Tilmant PY, et al: Frequency of provoked coronary arterial spasm in 1089 consecutive patients undergoing coronary arteriography. Circulation 65:1299, 1982

19. James TH: Anatomy of the Coronary Arteries. Harper & Row, Hagerstown, MD, 1961

20. Cannon RO, Watson RM, Rosing DR, Epstein SE: Angina caused by reduced vasodilator reserve of the small coronary arteries. J Am Coll Cardiol 1:1359, 1983

21. Mudge GH, Crossman W, Mills RM, et al: Reflex increase in coronary vascular resistance in patients with ischemic heart disease. N Engl J Med 295:1333, 1976

22. Robertson D, Robertson RM, Nies AS, et al: Variant angina pectoris: Investigation of indices of sympathetic nervous system function. Am J Cardiol 43:1080, 1979

23. Chierchia S, Davies G, Berkenboom G, et al: Alpha-adrenergic receptors and coronary spasm: An elusive link. Circulation 69:8, 1984

24. Dusting GJ, Moncada S, Vane JR: Prostaglandins, their intermediates and precurrors: Cardiovascular actions and regulatory roles in normal and abnormal circulatory systems. Prog Cardiovasc Dis 21:405, 1979

25. Robertson RM, Robertson D, Roberts LJ, et al: Thromboxane A_2 and vasotonic angina pectoris: Evidence from direct measurements and inhibitory trials. N Engl J Med 304:998, 1981

26. Chierchia S, DeCanterna R, Crea P, et al: Failure of thromboxane A_2 blockade to prevent attacks of vasotonic angina. Circulation 66:702, 1982

27. Eckenhoff JE, Hafkenschiel JH, Landmesser CM, Harmel M: Cardiac oxygen metabolism and control of the coronary circulation. Am J Physiol 149:634, 1947

28. Berne RM, Rubio R: Coronary circulation. p. 873. In Berne RM, Sperlakis N (eds): Handbook of Physiology: The Cardiovascular System. Section 2, Vol. 1. American Physiology Society, Washington, DC, 1979

29. Maturi MF, Markle DR, Greene R, et al:

Can coronary vasoconstriction induced by vasopressin cause myocardial ischemia in dogs? J Am Coll Cardiol 3:642, 1984 (abst)

30. Maturi MF, Greene R, Speir E, et al: Neuropeptide Y: a peptide found in human coronary arteries constricts primarily small coronary arteries to produce myocardial ischemia in dogs. J Clin Invest 83:1217, 1989

31. Green MV, Jones-Collins BA, Bacharach SL, et al: Scintigraphic quantitation of asynchronous myocardial motion during the left ventricular isovolumic relaxation period: A study in the dog during acute ischemia. J Am Coll Cardiol 4:72, 1984

32. Watson RM, Markle DR, Ro YM, et al: Transmural pH gradient in canine myocardial ischemia. Am J Physiol 15:H232, 1984

33. Gu J, Adrain TE, Tatemoto K, et al: Neuropeptide-Y (NPY)—A major cardiac neuropeptide. Lancet 1:1008, 1983

34. Antman E, Muller J, Goldberg S, et al: Nifedipine therapy for coronary artery spasm: Experience in 127 patients. N Engl J Med 302:1269, 1980

35. Maseri A, L'Abbate A, Baroldi G, et al: Coronary vasospasm as a possible cause of myocardial infarction. A conclusion derived from the study of "preinfarction" angina. N Engl J Med 299:1271, 1978

36. Gould KL, Lipscomb K: Effects of coronary stenoses on coronary flow reserve and resistance. Am J Cardiol 34:48, 1974

37. Gorlin R: Coronary Artery Disease. WB Saunders, Philadelphia, 1976

38. Schwartz JN, Kong Y, Hackell DB, Bartel AG: Comparison of angiographic and post mortem findings in patients with coronary artery disease. Am J Cardiol 36:174, 1975

39. White CW, Wright CB, Doty DB, et al: Does visual interpretation of the coronary arteriogram predict the physiologic importance of a coronary stenosis. N Engl J Med 310:819, 1984

40. Brown BG, Bolson E, Drimer M, Dodge HT: Quantitative coronary arteriography. Estimation of dimensions, hemodynamic resistance, and atheroma mass of coronary artery lesions using the arteriogram and digital computation. Circulation 55:2, 1977

41. Ruithauser W, Bussmann W, Noseda G, et al: Blood flow measurement through single coronary arteries by roentgendensitometry.

Part I. a comparison of flow measured by a radiologic technique applicable in the intact organism by electromagnetic flowmeter. AJR 109:12, 1970

42. Gould KL, Schelbert HR, Phelps ME, Hoffman EJ: Noninvasive assessment of coronary stenosis by myocardial perfusion imaging during pharmacologic coronary vasodilation. V. Detection of 47% diameter coronary stenosis with intravenous N-13 ammonia and emission computed tomography in intact dogs. Am J Cardiol 43:200, 1979

43. Ritchie JL, Trobaugh GB, Hamilton GW, et al: Myocardial imaging with thallium-201 at rest and during exercise. Comparison with coronary arteriography and resting and stress electrocardiography. Circulation 56:66, 1977

44. Shonkoff D, Eisner RL, Gober A, et al: What quantitative criteria should be used to read defects on the SPECT T1-201 bullseye display in men? ROC analysis. J Nucl Med 28:674, 1987 (abst 493)

45. Cedarholm JC, Martin SE, Greene R, et al: Can SPECT T1-201 determine the "physiological significance" of a coronary stenosis? J Nucl Med 28:666, 1987 (abst 458)

46. Gerson MC: Test accuracy, test selection, and test result interpretation in chronic coronary artery disease. p. 309. In MC Gerson (ed): Cardiac Nuclear Mecicine. McGraw-Hill, New York, 1987

47. Gregg DE, Patterson RE: Functional importance of the collateral coronary circulation. N Engl J Med 303:1404, 1980

48. Schaper W: The Collateral Circulation of the Heart. Elsevier, New York, 1971

49. Fedor JM, Rembert JC, McIntosh DM, Greenfield JC Jr: Effects of exercise and pacing-induced tachycardia on coronary collateral flow in the awake dog. Circ Res 46:214, 1980

50. Eng C, Patterson RE, Horowitz SF, et al: Functional collateral responses to exercise assessed by myocardial perfusion imaging. Circulation 66:309, 1982

51. Smith SC, Gorlin R, Herman MV, et al: Myocardial blood flow in man: Effects of coronary collateral circulation and coronary artery bypass surgery. J Clin Invest 51:2556, 1972

52. Kirk ES, Jennings RB: Pathophysiology of myocardial ischemia. p. 979. In Hurst JW,

Logue RB, Rackley CE, et al (eds): The Heart, Arteries and Veins. 5th Ed. McGraw-Hill, New York, 1982

53. Fam WM, McGregor M: Effect of coronary vasodilator drugs on retrograde flow in areas of chronic myocardial ischemia. Circ Res 15:355, 1964

54. Becker LC: Conditions for vasodilator-induced coronary steal in experimental myocardial ischemia. Circulation 57:1103, 1978

55. Patterson RE, Kirk ES: Coronary steal mechanisms in dogs with single vessel occlusion and other arteries normal. Circulation 67:1009, 1983

56. Hirzel HO, Sonnenblick EH, Kirk ES: Absence of a lateral borderzone of intermediate creatine phosphokinase depletion surrounding a central infarct 24 hours after acute coronary occlusion in the dog. Circ Res 41:673, 1977

57. Patterson RE, Kirk ES: Analysis of coronary collateral structure, function and ischemic border zones in pigs. Am J Physiol 13:H23, 1983

58. Okun E, Factor SM, Kirk ES: End capillary loops in the heart: An explanation for discrete myocardial infarctions without borderzones. Science 206:565, 1979

59. Factor SM, Okun EM, Kirk ES: The histological lateral border of acute canine myocardial infarction. Circ Res 48:640, 1981

60. Factor SM, Okun EM, Minase T, Kirk ES: The microcirculation of the human heart: End-capillary loops with discrete perfusion fields. Circulation 66:1241, 1982

61. Patterson RE, Weintraub WS, Halgash DA, et al: Spatial distribution of 14-C-lidocaine in blood flow in transmural and lateral borderzones of ischemic canine myocardium. Am J Cardiol 50:63, 1982

62. Dunn RB, Griggs DM Jr: Transmural gradients in ventricular tissue metabolites produced by stopping coronary blood flow in the dog. Circ Res 37:438, 1975

63. Gregg DE. The natural history of coronary collateral development. Circ Res 35:335, 1974

64. Savage RM, Wagner GS, Ideker RE, et al: Correlation of post-mortem anatomic findings with electrocardiographic changes in patients with myocardial infarction. Circulation 55:279, 1977

65. Reimer KA, Jennings RB: The "wave front phenomenon" of myocardial ischemic cell death. II. Transmural progression of necrosis within the framework of ischemic bed size (myocardium at risk) and collateral flow. Lab Invest 40:633, 1979

66. Patterson RE, Horowitz SF, Eng C, et al: Can noninvasive exercise test criteria identify patients with left main or 3-vessel coronary disease after a first myocardial infarction? Am J Cardiol 51:361, 1983

67. Tennant R, Wiggers CJ: The effect of coronary occlusion on myocardial contraction. Am J Physiol 112:351, 1933

68. Herman MV, Henile RA, Klein MD, Gorlin R: Localized disorders in myocardial contraction. N Engl J Med 227:222, 1967

69. Herman MV, Gorlin R: Implications of left ventricular asynergy. Am J Cardiol 23:538, 1969

70. Katz AM: Effects of ischemia on the contractile processes of heart muscle. Am J Cardiol 32:456, 1973

71. Carmeliet E: Perspective; myocardial ischemia; reversible and irreversible changes. Circulation 70:149, 1984

72. The Multicenter Postinfarction Research Group: Risk stratification and survival after myocardial infarction. N Engl J Med 309:331, 1983

73. Forrester JS, Diamond G, Chattejee K, Swan HJC: Medical therapy of acute myocardial infarction by application of hemodynamic subsets. N Engl J Med 295:1356, 1404, 1976

74. Russel RO Jr, Mantle JA, Rogers WJ, Rackley CE: Current status of hemodynamic monitoring: Indications, diagnosis and complications. p. 1. In CE Rackley (ed): Critical Care Medicine. Cardiovascular Clinics. FA Davis, Philadelphia, 1981

75. Stack RS, Phillips HR, Grierson DS, et al: Functional improvement of jeopardized myocardium following intracoronary streptokinase infusion in acute myocardial infarction. J Clin Invest 72:824, 1983

76. Sheehan FH, Bolson EL, Dodge HT, et al: Advantages and applications of the centerline method for characterizing regional ventricular function. Circulation 74:293, 1986

77. Horn HR, Teichholz LE, Cohn PF, et al: Augmentation of left ventricular contraction

pattern in coronary artery disease by inotropic catecholamines: The epinephrine ventriculogram. Circulation 49:1063, 1974

78. Borer JS, Bacharach SL, Green MV, et al: Real-time radionuclide cineangiography in the noninvasive evaluation of global and regional left ventricular function at rest and during exercise in patients with coronary artery disease. N Engl J Med 296:839, 1977

79. Bonow RO, Bacharach SL: Left ventricular diastolic function: Evaluation by radionuclide ventriculography. p. 107. In Pohost GM, Higgins CB, Morganroth J (eds): New Concepts in Cardiac Imaging. Year Book Medical Publishers, Chicago, 1987

80. Brutsaert DL, Housmans RR, Goethals MA: Dual control of relaxation. II. Hemodynamic determinants of the left ventricular isovolumic pressure decline. Am J Physiol 239:H1, 1980

81. Mirsky I: Assessment of diastolic function: Suggested methods and future consideration. Circulation 69:836, 1984

82. Fishman AP: Pulmonary edema: The water-exchanging function of the lung. Circulation 46:390, 1972

83. Boucher CA, Zir LM, Beller GA, et al: Increased pulmonary uptake of thallium-201 during exercise myocardial imaging: Clinical hemodynamic and angiographic implications in patients with coronary artery disease. Am J Cardiol 46:189, 1980

84. Okada RD, Pohost GM, Kirshenbaum HD, et al: Radionuclide-determined change in pulmonary blood volume with exercise: Improved sensitivity of multigated blood-pool scanning in detecting coronary artery disease. N Engl J Med 301:569, 1979

85. Weiner JM, Apstein CS, Arthur JH, et al: Persistence of myocardial injury following brief periods of coronary occlusion. Cardiovasc Res 10:678, 1976

86. Swain JL, Sabina RL, McHale PA, et al: Prolonged myocarcial nucleotide depletion after brief ischemia in the open-chest dog. Am J Physiol 242:H818, 1982

87. Braunwald E, Kloner RA: The stunned myocardium: Prolonged, postischemic ventricular dysfunction. Circulation 66:1146, 1982

88. Dyke SH, Cohn PF, Gorlin R, Sonnenblick EH: Detection of residual myocardial function in coronary artery disease using postextrasystolic potentiation. Circulation 50:694, 1974

89. Theroux P, Ross J Jr, Franklin D, et al: Regional myocardial function in the conscious dog during acute coronary occlusion and responses to morhpine, propranolol, nitroglycerin and lidocaine. Circulation 53:302, 1976

90. Neely JR, Morgan HE: Relationship between carbohydrate and lipid metabolism in the energy balance of heart muscle. Annu Rev Physiol 36:413, 1974

91. Ter-Pogossian NM, Klein MS, Markham J, et al: Regional assessment of myocardial metabolic integrity in vivo by positron emission tomography with 11-C-labeled palmitate. Circulation 61:242, 1980

92. Holland RP, Brooks H: TQ-ST segment mapping: Critical review and analysis of current concepts. Am J Cardiol 40:110, 1977

93. Williams DO, Scherlag BJ, Hope RR, et al: Pathophysiology of malignant ventricular arrhythmias during acute myocardial ischemia. Circulation 50:1163, 1974

94. Jones-Collins BA, Patterson RE: Quantitative measurement of electrical instability as a function of myocardial infarction size in dogs. Am J Cardiol 48:858, 1981

95. Roberts R, Sobel BE: Creatine kinase isoenzymes in the assessment of heart disease. Am Heart J 95:521, 1978

96. Willerson JT, Parkey RW, Lewis SE, et al: Hot-spot imaging for patients with acute myocardial infarction. J Cardiovasc Med 7:291, 1982

97. Khaw BA, Beller GA, Haber E: Experimental myocardial infarct imaging following intravenous administration of iodine-131 labeled antibody (Fab')$_2$ fragment specific for cardiac myosin. Circulation 57:743, 1978

98. Silverman KJ, Becker LC, Bulkley BH, et al: Value of early thallium-201 scintigraphy for predicting mortality in patients with acute myocardial infarction. Circulation 61:996, 1980

99. Norris RM, Brandt PWT, Caughey DE, et al: A new coronary prognostic index. Lancet 1:277, 1969

100. Rackley CE: Quantitative evaluation of left ventricular function by radiographic techniques. Circulation 54:862, 1976

101. Green MV, Bacharach SL: Functional imaging of the heart: Methods, limitations and examples from gated blood pool scintigraphy. Prog Cardiovasc Dis 28:319, 1986

102. Califf RM, Burks JM, Behar VS, et al: Relationship among ventricular arrhythmias, coronary artery disease, and angiographic and electrocardiographic indicators of myocardial fibrosis. Circulation 57:275, 1978

103. Epstein SE, Palmeri ST, Patterson RE: Evaluation of patients after acute myocardial infarction: Indications for cardiac catheterization and surgical intervention. N Engl J Med 307:1487, 1982

104. Cloninger KG, DePuey EG, Garcia EV, et al: Redistribution abnormalities in exercise thallium images: Unresolved ischemia vs. infarction. J Nucl Med 27:997, 1986 (abst)

105. Tillisch J, Marshall R, Schelbert H, et al: Reversibility of wall motion abnormalities: Preoperative determination using position tomography, 18-fluorodeoxyglucose and 13-NH$_3$. Circulation 68(suppl III):387, 1983 (abst)

106. Patterson RE, Jones-Collins BA, Aamodt R: Impaired collateral blood flow reserve early after nontransmural myocardial infarction in conscious dogs. Am J Cardiol 50:1133, 1982

107. Gibson RS, Watson DD, Craddock GB, et al: Prediction of cardiac events after uncomplicated myocardial infarction: A prospective study comparing predischarge exercise thallium-201 scintigraphy and coronary angiography. Circulation 68:321, 1983

108. Marshall RC, Tillisch JH, Phelps ME, et al: Identification and differentiation of resting myocardial ischemia and infarction in man with positron computed tomography 18-F-labeled fluorodeoxyglucose and N-13 ammonia. Circulation 64:766, 1981

109. Brunken R, Tillisch J, Schwaiger M, et al: Regional perfusion, glucose metabolism and wall motion in chronic electrocardiographic Q-wave infarctions. Circulation 13:951, 1986

110. Pohost GM, Ratner AV: Nuclear magnetic resonance: Potential applications in clinical cardiology. JAMA 251:1304, 1984

2
Radiopharmaceuticals for Cardiac Imaging

Ronald J. Callahan
Henry M. Chilton

CLASSES OF CARDIAC RADIOPHARMACEUTICALS

Evaluation of cardiac structure and function with radiopharmaceuticals continues to be a fast-growing segment of nuclear medicine. Cardiac nuclear medicine procedures are attractive because they are noninvasive and cost-effective and provide a wealth of diagnostic information in a variety of cardiac conditions, including coronary artery disease, as well as the delineation of myocardial infarction and the quantification of regional cardiac function. Currently, these studies are performed with a relatively small number of radiopharmaceuticals (listed in Table 2-1).

Considerable effort has been expended over the past several years on the development of new cardiac radiopharmaceuticals. This effort has been two fold: (1) the development of new drugs within existing classes of radiopharmaceuticals that represent improvements in either biodistribution and/or imaging properties (e.g., a myocardial perfusion agent labeled with ^{99m}Tc); and (2) the development of entirely new classes of radiolabeled drugs that permit the acquisition of information previously unattainable (e.g., cardiac metabolic agents). Some of the newer radiopharmaceuticals currently under evaluation are listed in Table 2-2. In addition, new information is becoming available on mechanisms of labeling and localization of all cardiac radiopharmaceuticals.

This chapter divides cardiac radiopharmaceuticals into four general categories: (1) myocardial infarction imaging agents, (2) myocardial perfusion agents, (3) metabolic agents, and (4) blood pool imaging agents. The general principles and properties of drugs in each class are reviewed. In addition, new drugs that show promise as clinically useful agents in these categories are introduced.

TABLE 2-1 Cardiac Radiopharmaceuticals Currently Available for General Use

Drug	Category	Indication
Technetium-99m pyrophosphate	Infarct-avid agent	Localization of damaged myocardium
Thallium-201 thallous chloride	Myocardial perfusion agent	Assessment of coronary artery disease
Technetium-99m autologous red blood cells	Blood pool imaging agent	Evaluation of dynamic cardiac function
Technetium-99m human serum albumin	Blood pool imaging agent	Evaluation of dynamic cardiac function

MYOCARDIAL INFARCTION IMAGING AGENTS

The ability to detect the presence, location, and size of necrotic myocardial tissue has long been a goal of nuclear medicine. Recently this goal has become increasingly important, since coronary artery bypass and the newer reperfusion therapies require the accurate assessment of patients who might benefit from these procedures.

Two radiopharmaceuticals are currently available for the detection of myocardial necrosis, each representing a different approach to assessing regional myocardial infarction: technetium-99m pyrophosphate and indium-111 antimyosin. Technetium-99m pyrophosphate is routinely available, whereas indium-111 antimyosin is currently undergoing clinical trials and appears promising for the diagnosis of myocardial infarction and myocarditis.

Technetium-99m Pyrophosphate

Direct imaging of damaged myocardium with technetium-99m pyrophosphate was introduced by Parkey et al.[1] In the visualization of acute experimental myocardial infarction. It was previously shown that calcium influx during irreversible myocardial damage results in the formation of a crystalline hydroxapatite-like substance that closely resembles the crystalline material of bone.[2] The use of a radiopharmaceutical that adsorbs onto hydroxyapatite of bone, such as technetium-99m pyrophosphate, for the detection of

TABLE 2-2 Cardiac Radiopharmaceuticals Currently Under Investigation and Potentially Useful as Diagnostic Agents

Drug	Category	Indication
Indium-111 Antimyosin	Infarct-avid agent	Diagnosis of myocardial infarction and myocarditis
Rubidium-82 C1	Myocardial perfusion agent	PET imaging of coronary artery disease
Technetium-99m isonitriles	Myocardial perfusion agent	Myocardial perfusion agent, possible substitute for ^{201}Tl
Fluorine-18 Fluorodeoxyglucose	Myocardial metabolic agent	Identification of viable myocardium
Iodine-123 modified fatty acid	Myocardial metabolic agent	Identification of viable myocardium
Technetium-99m BATO compounds	Myocardial perfusion agent	Assessment of coronary artery disease

PET, positron-emission tomography.

damaged myocardium logically follows from this observation.

Although several new technetium-99m phosphate and diphosphonate radiopharmaceuticals were developed as bone-seeking radiopharmaceuticals, clinical comparisons of these agents as myocardial infarct imaging agents failed to demonstrate their superiority over technetium-99m pyrophosphate. As a result, technetium-99m pyrophosphate remains the most widely used radiopharmaceutical for infarct-avid imaging.

Technetium-99m pyrophosphate clears rapidly from blood in a triphasic manner with the first component (74 percent of the injected dose) having a half-life $(t_{1/2})$ of 0.03 hour, the second component (18.3 percent) of 0.64 hour, and the third component (7.4 percent) of 53.7 hours. Less than 8 percent remains in the blood at 3 hours after intravenous (IV) injection. Of the total activity administered, 40 to 50 percent is deposited in bone. Cumulative urinary excretion up to 24 hours accounts for approximately 60 percent of the administered activity.[5]

It has been postulated that localization of technetium-99m pyrophosphate within acute myocardial infarction occurs in response to the calcium influx that accompanies cell death, although the precise uptake mechanism within the damaged myocardium is not completely understood. In addition to tissue calcification, uptake is dependent on local blood flow and the degree of tissue damage. Residual blood flow is required for the delivery of the radiopharmaceutical to the injury site. Following infarction, the highest concentration ratios of technetium-99m pyrophosphate between damaged and normal myocardium occurs when local blood flow is 20 to 40 percent of normal. With further reductions in blood flow, localization falls, and in regions of minimal blood flow (approximately 5 percent), uptake may appear normal.[6] Where there is no blood flow (such

as in the central infarct zone), no localization occurs. The area of radiopharmaceutical uptake corresponds to infarct size.[7]

The time-course relationship between the development of infarction and an abnormal technetium-99m pyrophosphate scintillation study has been studied in animal models. Technetium-99 pyrophosphate studies of experimental canine infarcts have shown that abnormal images are obtained within the 12 to 24 hours following a fixed coronary occlusion, becoming progressively more abnormal during the initial 24 to 72 hours.[8,9] Images remain positive up to 6 days after infarction and begin to fade thereafter, usually becoming normal by the fourteenth day after experimental canine coronary artery ligation. Willerson et al.[10] found that myocardial localization in humans begins approximately 10 to 12 hours after the onset of symptoms, with increasingly positive uptake demonstrated during the initial 24 to 72 hours after acute myocardial infarction.

Adult patients usually receive 15 to 20 mCi technetium-99m pyrophosphate via IV administration. No special patient preparation is necessary, except that the patients should be well hydrated, when possible, in order to facilitate the renal excretion of the radiopharmaceutical and reduce the blood background activity. Regions of acute myocardial infarction are reliably positive when performed as early as 12 to 18 hours following the acute episode or as late as 14 days after the event. Maximum localization in infarcts is limited, however, to a much shorter span, usually 2 to 3 days postinfarction.

Although the sensitivity of this procedure is quite high, the specificity is not especially high, since several conditions may lead to the accumulation of technetium-99m pyrophosphate by the myocardium, including unstable angina, ventricular aneurysm, pericarditis, cardiomyopathy, myocardial trauma, and radiation therapy.[11] Other limitations also apply, including the facts that the normal uptake of technetium-99m pyrophosphate by bone may limit its utility in the estimation of infarct size[10] and that the false-negative rate is relatively high during the initial 12 to 18 hours following infarction when the diagnosis is often critical.

Indium-111 Antimyosin

The first clinically significant diagnostic imaging application of radiolabeled antibodies in cardiac nuclear medicine was developed by Khaw et al.[12] using cardiac myosin as the target molecule. The cardiac myosin antibody system was chosen for in vivo visualization of myocardial infarction because cardiac myosin has certain immunologic properties that optimize its use in imaging (Table 2-3). Following myocyte necrosis from a myocardial infarct or any other cause, intracellular myosin is exposed to the extracellular space. A radiolabeled antibody could therefore penetrate disrupted cell membranes and bind to cardiac myosin, permitting its visualization by scintillation imaging.

Initially purified polyclonal antibodies labeled with radioisotopes of iodine were used to detect exposed cardiac myosin. With the advent of monoclonal antibody technology,[15] large quantities of purified murine antihuman cardiac myosin became available, and the antibody fragments—$(Fab')_2$ and Fab—were prepared. Studies have shown that the superior blood clearance of the Fab fragment renders it most suitable for imag-

TABLE 2-3 Properties of Cardiac Myosin Leading to Its Selection as an Antigen for Antibody Imaging of Necrotic Myocardium

Intracellular contractile protein
Exists in high concentrations
Readily isolated and purified
Immunogenic
Not exposed to extracellular environment in viable myocytes

ing. Because ^{131}I and ^{125}I possess undesirable physical properties and there is no ready supply of high-purity ^{123}I, other labeling strategies were investigated, including the use of ^{99m}Tc and [111]In.

Currently available preparations of antimyosin use the Fab fragment of antimyosin that is covalently linked to diethylenetriaminepentaacetic acid (DTPA) as described by Krejcarek and Tucker[16] and modified by Khaw et al.[17–19] Subsequently, DTPA-coupled antimyosin Fab has been labeled with ^{99m}Tc by the dithionite reduction system.[18,20] However, this method resulted in quite variable labeling efficiencies with the undesirable formation of the colloidal technetium impurity that localizes in the reticuloendothelial system. To eliminate the interference from liver activity and increase time available for imaging, a method was developed for labeling DTPA-antimyosin Fab with ^{111}In from the weak chelator sodium citrate (0.3 M) at pH 5.5. A commercially available kit for the labeling of DTPA-antimyosin Fab with ^{111}In with this method is currently undergoing clinical testing.

With ^{111}In-labeled antimyosin, experimental infarcts have been visualized at 5 hours after IV injection. However, because of the 2.8-day $t_{1/2}$ of ^{111}In, imaging studies can be carried out for up to 72 hours postadministration. In clinical studies with indium-111 DTPA antimyosin Fab, areas of infarcted myocardium are clearly visible at 20 to 24 hours postinjection.[20] The resulting images have been used to localize and quantify regions of myocardial necrosis in myocardial infarction.[20] Other myocardial imaging techniques, such as technetium-99m pyrophosphate and thallium-201 chloride, may not be sufficiently specific for assessment of irreversibly damaged myocardial tissue. For example, technetium-99m pyrophosphate may be sequestered by reversibly injured myocardium,[22] giving an overestimate of the extent of irreversibly damaged tissue.

Antimyosin antibody imaging is a reliable screening method for evaluating patients suspected of having myocarditis. In the diagnosis of acute myocarditis with indium-111 antimyosin, the optimal interval between injection and imaging is 48 hours.[21] A positive antimyosin scan indicates the need for ventricular biopsy to establish the histologic diagnosis. As with all antibodies of murine origin, the possibility of the production of human antimouse antibody (HAMA) must be considered when using indium-111 antimyosin in humans. Since multiple injections of the ^{111}In-labeled Fab antibody may be required for serial imaging in the evaluation of patients with myocarditis, the possible development of HAMA becomes even more important. In one study,[23] of 28 patients who received two to three injections of antibody, all sera tested showed absence of HAMA. Brown et al.[24] found no detectable HAMA in their large-scale study of sera from 1,832 patients.

MYOCARDIAL PERFUSION AGENTS

The use of radiopharmaceuticals to determine myocardial perfusion is based on a principle first described by Sapirstein and Moses.[25] This principle does not describe a specific class of radiopharmaceuticals, but rather specific kinetic parameters of tissue extraction and blood clearance. The Sapirstein principle states that the initial distribution of compounds which have a high extraction by the organ of interest (and rapid blood clearance) will be proportional to relative perfusion.

Thallium-201

Noninvasive nuclear medicine methods for the evaluation of myocardial perfusion have centered primarily on various radioisotopes of potassium and its analogues. Normally perfused myocardial cells have a high demand for intracellular potassium. While other muscles, tissues, and organs also use potassium, the myocardium has the highest concentration of this element per gram of tissue. The uptake of these substances by the myocardium occurs at a rate that is related to the coronary blood flow and the rate of exchange of the radioisotope between the circulating blood and viable myocardium. Localization of these monovalent substances ultimately depends on the intact cellular energy-transport mechanism involving the Na-K-ATPase pump. All monovalent alkaline metals behave similarly, although it has been demonstrated that the efficiency of the Na-K-ATPase mechanism for these ions appears to bear an inverse relationship to the size of the ion with evidence that larger ions are removed more slowly from blood.[26]

Thallium is in series IIIA of the periodic table and, therefore, is not a true potassium analogue. Nevertheless, thallium distributes in organs and tissues in a manner almost identical to that of potassium.[27] The reasons appear to involve physical and chemical similarities. Both potassium and thallium are monovalent cations, have hydrated ionic radii of similar size, and participate in the membrane Na-K-ATPase pump.[27,28]

The use of a radioisotope of thallium as a potassium analogue for imaging was initially made by Kawana et al.[29] In 1975, Lebowitz et al.[30] introduced ^{201}Tl ($t_{1/2}$ 73.1 hours) for medical use. The imaging properties of ^{201}Tl are not ideal; a lower energy spectrum with Hg x-ray emissions at 65 to 83 keV is not immediately attractive; however, it has become the radiopharmaceutical of choice for the evaluation of myocardial perfusion, since no other radiopharmaceutical currently available offers as desirable tissue distribution properties.

Thallium-201 is a cationic monovalent metal ion produced from the decay of ^{201}Pb, a radionuclide produced by the proton bombardment of stable ^{203}Tl. Thallium-201 is separated from ^{201}Pb by ion-exchange chromatography. The principal radionuclide impurities ^{200}Tl ($t_{1/2}$ phys 26.1 hours) and ^{202}Tl ($t_{1/2}$ phys 12.0 days) should be less than 2 percent and 2.7 percent of total radioactivity, respectively, at the time of calibration; ^{203}Pb should be less than 0.5 percent. The radionuclide purity of most commercially available formulations of ^{201}Tl thallous chloride at the time of calibration is typically 98 percent or greater. Significant amounts of these high-energy impurities may contribute substantially to image degradation.

Five minutes after IV administration, only 5 to 8 percent of the injected dose remains in blood.[31] Approximately 85 percent of ^{201}Tl that passes through the coronary circulation is extracted during each pass. Maximal concentration by the myocardium is reached at 10 minutes, with about 5 percent of the administered dose localizing within this organ. About 15 percent of ^{201}Tl is taken up by the liver and 3.5 percent by the kidneys. The biologic half-life for these organs is approximately 36 hours. About 4 to 8 percent of the injected dose is excreted in the urine during the first 24 hours. Fecal excretion is insignificant.

Approximately 0.15 percent of the injected dose is found in the testes of patients, while animal data have shown the total amount of ^{201}Tl in the ovaries and uterus to be 0.2 percent. Thallium-201 uptake occurs in the thyroid but appears to account for less than 0.2 percent.[32] Thallium-201 has been shown to be excreted in breast milk. It is therefore advised that patients who are breast feeding stop nursing for at least 3 weeks following the administration of thallium-201 thallous chloride.[35]

Thallium localization within the myocardium occurs intracellularly in proportion to regional blood flow. A close correlation exists between early ^{201}Tl distribution and microsphere-determined regional blood flow in canine coronary occlusion models.[31,33] In the normal and mildly reduced flow ranges, ^{201}Tl distribution closely approximates blood flow, while in the low-flow range (less than 10 percent of flow in the nonischemic zone), thallium concentration is usually found in excess of microsphere-determined regional blood flow.

Viable myocardium accumulates ^{201}Tl and appears as a region of relatively high activity, while ^{201}Tl uptake does not occur in infarcted tissues or in ischemic regions brought about by physical stress or pharmacologic intervention. After an interval of rest, however, ischemic regions will subsequently revert to areas of ^{201}Tl localization, whereas infarcted zones do not localize ^{201}Tl.

Approximately 8 to 10 percent of the administered dose is initially deposited in the lungs. This value will be greater in patients with increased left atrial pressure. Boucher et al.[34] reported that ^{201}Tl lung uptake correlates closely with the extent of coronary artery disease, the number of myocardial segmental thallium perfusion defects, and the prevalence of prior myocardial infarction.

Altered distribution patterns of ^{201}Tl have been shown to be caused by β-adrenergic blockers and nitrates, resulting in a loss of sensitivity of exercise ^{201}Tl imaging.[36–39] A decrease in both the number and size of exercise-induced perfusion defects results, creating the likelihood of false-negative exercise scans. These effects may stem from the drug-induced changes in the exercise performance of patients taking β-blockers by blunting the heart rate and systolic blood pressure elevations that occur in exercise. Nitrates may cause a beneficial redistribution of coronary blood flow, resulting in decreased myocardial ischemia.[40] If possible, β-blocker therapy should be discontinued 48 hours before performance of the study (by appropriate tapering of the dosage); nitrate therapy should also be discontinued before the ^{201}Tl study.[41,42]

Although the sensitivity and specificity of exercise ^{201}Tl imaging appear to be somewhat less dependent on the adequacy of exercise than does electrocardiography (ECG),[43] failure to exercise to the proper level of intensity can result in a significant decrease in the diagnostic sensitivity of this technique.[44] When exercise ^{201}Tl scintigraphy is not possible, the adjunctive use of dipyridamole, a potent coronary arteriolar vasodilator, can be employed to create a desirable stresslike condition for imaging. The validity of dipyridamole-assisted ^{201}Tl imaging as a highly sensitive and specific test for coronary artery disease has been determined in several reports.[45,46]

Positron-Emitting Myocardial Perfusion Agents

One of the major areas of expansion in nuclear medicine is positron emission tomography (PET). The use of PET in the evaluation of myocardial perfusion is possible, since a variety of positron-emitting radionuclides have been developed that demonstrate suitable myocardial uptake. These include the cyclotron-produced ^{13}N ($t_{1/2}$ phys 10 minutes) and ^{15}O ($t_{1/2}$ phys 2 minutes) and the generator-produced ^{82}Rb ($t_{1/2}$ phys 75 seconds).

The nonionic lipophilic properties of ^{13}N as ammonia (NH_3), has been used extensively for imaging myocardial blood flow at rest and during pharmacologic or physical stress imaging.[47–49] Nitrogen-13 as ammonia permits its rapid transit across the capillary and sarcolemmal membranes.[50] However, once intracellular, conversion back to the charged species occurs with subsequent utilization of ^{13}N by the glutamate-glutamine reaction. As a result, the exit of ^{13}N from the myocyte

is slowed and retention times of 60 to 120 minutes have been reported following IV administration.[56]

Regional ^{13}N concentrations relate to blood flow in a nonlinear fashion. With flow greater than 3 ml/min/g myocardium, only small increases in measured ^{13}N myocardial blood flow are observed. However, at 0.5 to 2.5 ml/min/g, an almost linear relationship exists with ^{13}N myocardial uptake.[52]

Oxygen-15 water has been used to make measurements of blood flow to the myocardium and brain.[53,54] Extraction of oxygen-15 water by the myocardium is essentially independent of metabolic variation due to the metabolically inert character of the radiopharmaceutical. As a result, its uptake is independent of metabolic variations that may affect other tracers. Since ^{15}O activity is relatively high in the vascular compartment and the lungs, subtraction techniques must be performed with a suitable blood pool marker, such as ^{15}O carbon monoxide, which binds to red blood cells (RBCs).

Whereas the short physical half-lives of ^{13}N and ^{15}O require on-site cyclotrons to produce adequate supplies of these positron-emitting radionuclides, some positron-emitting radionuclides, such as ^{82}Rb, are formed as generator products. Rubidium-82 is produced through the decay of ^{82}Sr ($t_{1/2}$ phys 23 days).[55,56] As an analogue of potassium, rubidium distributes according to Sapirstein's principle.[25] Because the generator supply mode obviates the need for a cyclotron and the generator may be eluted frequently (daughter build-up occurs rapidly), myocardial blood flow imaging with ^{82}Rb can be performed repeatedly over short time intervals. Blood flow as determined by radiolabeled microsphere technique, and ^{82}Rb myocardial uptake appear to be in close agreement. Single capillary transit extraction fractions average about 74 percent at control flows of 1 ml/min/g of myocardium but fall with higher flows.[57] As a result of the potential widespread availability due to its supply via a generator system, [82]Rb imaging is receiving considerable interest.

Technetium-99m Complexes for Myocardial Perfusion

A technetium-99m complex that distributes in myocardial tissues analogous to ^{201}Tl yet possesses the superior imaging properties of ^{99m}Tc has been attempted by several researchers. Recently, a number of compounds have been identified that are taken up by the myocardium in relationship to blood flow. Initially, Deutsch et al.[58] introduced 1,2-bis(dimethylphosphino)ethane (technetium-99m DMPE), which produced high-quality images of myocardial perfusion in a dog model.[59] Unfortunately, this compound demonstrated the effect of species variability with low myocardial and high lung uptake in humans when clinical studies were undertaken.[60] Jones et al.[61] introduced a new class of water-soluble technetium complexes, based on the isonitrile moiety, that are monovalent cations showing good myocardial localization. A variety of derivations of this class has emerged and are currently being tested in animal studies and/or clinical trials. Some of the promising compounds in this agent are shown in Table 2-4. Holman et al.[62] used technetium-99m TBI and performed imaging at 1 to 4 hours in humans to demonstrate high-quality myocardial images. The radiopharmaceutical showed high initial lung and liver uptake, which subsided at 40 to 60 minutes. A major distinction that has been noted between the ^{99m}Tc agents and ^{201}Tl is that no ^{99m}Tc agent yet developed undergoes myocardial redistribution. Although in delayed imaging with these agents, there has been a small degree of increased activity appearing in transiently ischemic areas, it is not sufficient for redistribution imaging. Such occurrence may be attributed to radiopharmaceutical efflux into blood from the activity that is initially deposited in the liver and lungs. The subsequent release of activity by these organs into blood permits uptake by the areas previously noted as ischemic during stress at the time of injection.[63] In the clinical setting, diagnostic evaluation of the myocardium immediately post-stress and subsequently at rest requires two separate injections of these ^{99m}Tc radiopharmaceuticals.

Comparison of thallium-201 and technetium-99m *t*-butyl isonitrile (TBI) in patients with suspected coronary artery disease found high liver uptake that obscured inferior segments of the left ventricle.[63] Liver-to-heart ratios with technetium-99m TBI were 3.4 at 60 minutes. Technetium-99m carboxymethoxyisopropyl isonitrile (CPI) has been found to produce high–quality images with

TABLE 2-4 Comparative List of Technetium-99m Labeled Myocardial Perfusion Agents

Common Name	Chemical Substitution	Characteristic Behavior
Technetium-99m TBI	*t*-Butyl isonitrile	Early lung and liver uptake, poor redistribution
Technetium-99m MIBI	Methoxyisobutyl isonitrile	Lowest lung and liver uptake
Technetium-99m CPI	Carboxymethoxyisopropyl isonitrile	Little liver and lung uptake
Technetium-99m MPIN	Methypropyl isonitrile	Lower heart to liver ratios, slightly faster washout
Technetium-99m BATO	Boron adducts of technetium oxime	Low lung and liver uptake, rapid myocardial clearance

less initial liver and lung uptake and relatively high myocardial-to-background ratios obtained at 10 minutes postinjection.[64] Still lower lung and liver levels have been noted with technetium-99m methoxyisobutyl isonitrile (MIBI). McKusick[65] compared technetium-99m TBI, CPI, and MIBI and found that MIBI yielded the least distracting lung and liver uptake. Myocardium-to-background ratios for TBI, CPI, and MIBI average 1.2, 1.9, and 2.5, respectively, at 30 minutes, and 1.3, 2.4, and 2.8, respectively, at 60 minutes. In a clinical comparison of MIBI and methoxypropyl isonitrile (MPIN) recently performed by Dudczak et al.[66] MIBI was found to be superior to MPIN with high heart-to-background ratios for MIBI. Respective ratios for MIBI and MPIN were 2.9 and 1.9 (at rest), and 3.1 and 2.3 (post-dipyridamole). Heart-to-liver ratios were approximately the same. MPIN demonstrated slightly faster myocardial washout than MIBI ($t_{1/2}$ 273 minutes versus 514 minutes).

Excretion of isonitrile agents appears to involve both renal and hepatobiliary mechanisms. Within 1 hour, renal excretion of the technetium-99m MIBI accounts for 16 percent of the administered dose, while excretion via the biliary pathway is about 8 percent at the same time.

BATO (Substituted Oxime) Complexes of Technetium-99m

Another new class of ^{99m}Tc agents are the boronic adducts of technetium oxime, called BATOs. These neutral, seven-coordinate technetium complexes have shown good myocardial uptake followed by rapid myocardial clearance and relatively low liver and lung uptake that clears rapidly. Good images of the myocardium have been obtained with SQ 30217 (chloro(methylboron(1-)-tris[1,2-cyclohexane-dionedioxime(1)]. Newer derivatives of this class, neutral trisoxime and chlorohydroxy-substituted oximes, have also shown excellent myocardial uptake with

slighly slower myocardial washout than that of the prototype agent (120 minutes versus 70 minutes).[67-70] Imaging with these types of agents may be initiated as soon as 2 to 3 minutes postinjection but must be completed within 15 to 20 minutes because of the rapid clearance.

The ultimate role of ^{99m}Tc myocardial perfusion agents relative to ^{201}Tl is yet to be determined, and the suitability of the different classes of agents and their application in myocardial perfusion imaging remains to be seen. The clinical information sought as well as cost and availability will all be significant factors in determining the role these agents will play.

METABOLIC HEART AGENTS

Several diverse agents have been studied in animals and human subjects in an attempt to identify severely ischemic but viable myocardium in patients with coronary artery disease. The promise of these agents is to provide definitive evidence that myocardial tissue, shown to be hypokinetic or akinetic by gated cardiac blood pool imaging, and/or hypoperfused by myocardial perfusion imaging, remains viable. This information is of increasing importance in light of newer reperfusion therapies for which a rapid technique for determining metabolic function on a regional basis becomes important.

Under aerobic conditions, the primary metabolic substrates of cardiac metabolism are fatty acids. The remainder of myocardial energy requirements are met by catabolism of lactate and glucose. Long-chain fatty acids of 14 to 18 carbons (C_{14} and C_{18}) account for 90 percent of myocardial energy requirements under aerobic conditions. However, when oxygen delivery is compromised,[71,72] the major substrate is glucose.[73] Metabolic cardiac agents have therefore been developed that are based on analogues of these varied metabolic substrates.

Glucose analogues have been developed that would be expected to show uptake in ischemic but viable tissue. Modified long-chain fatty acids would be expected to show a discordant distribution pattern with myocardial perfusion agents, thereby identifying areas of myocardium that are underperfused yet viable. Currently, the agents that show the most promise in these areas are the positron-emitting fluorodeoxyglucose and the branched-chain modified fatty acids labeled with [123]I.

Since metabolic substrates are in many cases rapidly catabolized with rapid tissue clearance of by-products, metabolic substrate radiopharmaceuticals are usually modified analogues that enter metabolic pathways and undergo at least one step in the metabolic pathway. These agents then become trapped intracellularly for a period sufficient to permit external imaging. Modified glucose and fatty acid analogues are available as metabolic cardiac agents.

Glucose Analogues

Regional myocardial uptake of glucose can be measured by the use of radiolabeled glucose analogues that trace the initial steps of glucose uptake and metabolism. The radiopharmaceutical of choice is 2-fluoro(^{18}F)-2-deoxyglucose (FDG). This glucose analogue can be suitably labeled with ^{18}F, a short-lived ($t_{1/2}$ phys 110 minutes) positron-emitting radionuclide.

FDG exchanges across capillary and cellular membranes in proportion to glucose metabolism and competes with glucose for phosphorylation by hexokinase to FDG-6 phosphate. At this step, however, this analogue of glucose is no longer competitive with glucose, since FGD-6 phosphate is not a substrate for glycolysis, nor can it be synthesized to glyco-

gen. Deoxyglucose-6 phosphate and 2-FDG-6 phosphate are then trapped in the tissue and released very slowly.[74,75] Kinetic models that substantiate the fact that PET images reflect glucose metabolism have been extensively studied.[74–79]

The synthesis of ^{18}F-labeled FDG was first developed by Ido et al.[80,81] at the Brookhaven National Laboratory. FDG for injection is readily prepared either by the electrophilic reaction of ^{18}F-enriched fluorine gas with 3,4,6-tri-O-acetyl-D-glucal or by the nucleophilic reaction of ^{18}F-labeled acetylhypofluorite with a suitably protected D-mannopyranose. The fluorinated product is hydrolyzed with acid to give a mixture of 2-fluoro-2-deoxy-D-glucose (FDG) and 2-fluoro-2-deoxy-D-mannose (FDM). It is purified by column chromatography and is dissolved in an appropriate solvent, most commonly 0.9 percent saline.

Increased demand for this product has resulted in modifications of the original method to include remote semiautomated procedures.[82,83] In fact, much of the promise of PET is based on automated synthesis modules using either the black box or robotics approach to the production of fluorine-18 FDG in a clinical setting. Many manufacturers of cyclotrons are including this type of technology in their PET facilities packages. It is not clear whether these automated synthesis modules are capable of producing products on a routine clinical basis and in a high-quality reproducible form for human use.

Modified Fatty Acids

Fatty acid radiopharmaceuticals that show promise for clinical use include the intrinsically labeled carbon-11 palmitate[84,85] and modified fatty acids labeled with either ^{123}I or [11]C.[86–88] Iodine-123-labeled modified fatty acids are particularly attractive for use with single photon emission computed tomography (SPECT), since they have greater availability than the positron-labeled (C-11) agents that require on-site cyclotrons.

In order to increase the residence time of fatty acids in the myocardium and allow sufficient time for imaging, the molecule can be chemically modified so that at least one step in the metabolic pathway is inhibited. This has been accomplished by the addition of a terminal phenyl group to inhibit terminal β-oxidation and by the synthesis of branched-chain fatty acids, primarily by methylation at the 3 position.[87] A molecule with a phenyl group in the Ω position has the added property of providing a moiety that can be iodinated easily and with good in vivo stability. The net result of these modifications has been an increase in residence time in the heart of up to 5 hours.[88,89] The extraction fraction for fatty acids is in the 50 to 60 percent range and serum $t_{1/2}$ is less than 2 minutes.[90]

The use of metabolic radiopharmaceuticals requires attention to the metabolic status of the patient. For example, the uptake of both fluorine-18 FDG and radiolabeled fatty acids is influenced by insulin and glucose, and free fatty acid (FFA) levels, respectively.[91–96] Therefore, dietary history becomes an important factor in evaluating images with metabolic agents.

The quantitative measurement of myocardial metabolism with these radiopharmaceuticals is very complex. Detailed mathematical models have been proposed for these agents, yet much work remains to be done. Currently, the comparison of the distribution patterns of these tracers with perfusion agents such as ^{201}Tl seems to be the preferred method of interpretation.

The ultimate role of cardiac metabolic radiopharmaceuticals in clinical cardiology remains to be determined. The availability of a commercially produced, ^{123}I-labeled modi-

fied fatty acid would accelerate the process of determining the role of this class of agents. For the increasing number of centers with PET capabilities, the availability of automated synthetic procedures for the preparation of fluorine-18 FDG will also increase the application of this compound in evaluating cardiac metabolism.

RADIOPHARMACEUTICALS FOR CARDIAC BLOOD POOL IMAGING

Measurements of ventricular function using radiopharmaceuticals can be made either during a single pass through the heart (first-pass study)[97] or after a blood pool tracer has equilibrated in the vasculature (gated blood pool study).[98,99] The physical and pharmacokinetic properties of radiopharmaceuticals for each of these indications are quite different.

In a first-pass study, the radiopharmaceutical only needs to reside within the intravascular space long enough to traverse the chamber(s) of interest. An additional requirement is the emission of suitable photons in sufficient abundance that adequate events can be acquired during very short imaging intervals. Also, the radiopharmaceutical should be obtainable in very small volumes (less than 3 ml), since bolus injection is desirable. If it is necessary to make repeated measurements, as during physiologic and/or pharmacologic interventions, the added property of rapid clearance from the blood pool either by radioactive decay or biologic clearance is required.

First-pass imaging requires no specific localization properties of the radiopharmaceutical, except that it present itself within the intravascular compartment sufficiently to permit observation of its passage through the heart and great vessels. With the exception of ^{99m}Tc-macroaggregated albumin (a radiopharmaceutical that localizes within the pulmonary capillary bed during its first pass through the lungs), most any other ^{99m}Tc radiopharmaceutical will suffice. Technetium-99m pertechnetate is usually the preferred radiopharmaceutical for first-pass imaging. Very short-lived radionuclides have also been used for first-pass imaging. These generator-produced radionuclides, ^{178}W-^{178}Ta, ^{191}Os-^{191m}Ir, and ^{195m}Hg-^{195m}Au, which have physical half-lives of several minutes or less, produce the very high flux of usable photons required for high-resolution first-pass imaging[100–102] and permit rapid sequential studies. Commercial availability of these short-lived generator radionuclides in the United States remains a problem.

In an equilibrium gated blood pool study, the radiopharmaceutical requirements are mainly related to the residence time in the intravascular compartment. This time should be such that there is a relatively constant volume of distribution of the radiopharmaceutical during the period of observation, that is, approximately 30 to 60 minutes.

Occasionally, first-pass imaging is performed in conjunction with equilibrium blood pool imaging by employing a first-pass radiopharmaceutical that will be suitably retained by the blood pool. Initial images of flow through the heart depict first-pass information, while later images demonstrate blood pool distribution. For this reason, the remainder of this section is devoted to presenting information on the agents used for equilibrium blood pool imaging.

Technetium-99m Human Serum Albumin

Technetium-99m will label human serum albumin (HSA) efficiently by a variety of methods, including electrolysis and stannous reduction. Commercially available formulations use stannous ions for the reduction of technetium-99m pertechnetate to permit complexation with albumin.[103] These kit preparations contain a lyophilized mixture of HSA, stannous ions (usually as stannous tartrate), and appropriate buffering substances. Following reconstitution of these kits with technetium-99m pertechnetate, labeling is relatively fast, with radiolabeling yields routinely in the 90 to 99 percent range.[103–105]

The initial distribution of technetium-99m HSA following IV injection is intravascular, followed by slow distribution to the extravascular fluid spaces.[104–106] The intravascular clearance half-time has been reported to be on the order of approximately 5 hours in humans.[106] In addition to the rate of clearance from the intravascular space, image quality is determined in part by the fraction of the administered dose remaining in the blood pool postinjection. For technetium-99m HSA, this value has been reported to be 82 percent, 60 percent, and 45 percent at 30 minutes, 2 hours, and 4 hours, respectively.[106]

Technetium-99m Red Blood Cells

The most commonly used radiopharmaceutical for equilibrium blood pool imaging is ^{99}Tc labeled autologous red blood cells. Red blood cells can be labeled with ^{99m}Tc by a variety of techniques, all of which use the stannous ion-assisted radiolabeling methodology.[107,109] With any of the commonly performed techniques, reasonably high labeling efficiencies can be achieved. However, because some of the variations employed for technetium-99m RBC labeling produce more effective labeling than others, it may be desirable to use one method over all others for certain clinical applications. For example, whenever technetium-99m RBC imaging is used for detection of gastrointestinal (GI) hemorrhage, the ^{99m}Tc-radiolabeled RBCs should have the highest tagging efficiency, since any amounts of unreacted technetium-99m pertechnetate would localize in gastric mucosa and potentially complicate an accurate diagnosis of active gastric bleeding.

In general, three parameters must be considered whenever stannous ions are used in the ^{99m}Tc radiolabeling of RBCs.

1. Treatment of RBCs with Stannous Ion

While it is technetium in the +7 (pertechnetate) oxidation state that crosses the intact RBC membrane,[110] only technetium that has been reduced to a lower oxidation state will bind hemoglobin (Hb) firmly[111,112] within the cell. Stannous ions (as stannous pyrophosphate) are most commonly employed for reduction of technetium. At physiologic pH, stannous ions are subject to hydrolysis and precipitation that causes their rapid clearance from blood by the reticuloendothelial system. When stannous ions are complexed with pyrophosphate or other soluble chelates, stannous ions are sufficiently soluble at physiologic pH to resist these effects, yet are not so strongly bound to pryophosphate to prevent transport by the RBC. In the in vivo[107] and modified in vivo methods,[109] treatment with stannous ion is accomplished by the direct IV administration of stannous pyrophosphate. Other chelates of stannous ions can also be used (e.g., pentetate, medronate) that will result in the radiolabeling of RBCs with varying degrees of efficiency.[113]

The quantity of stannous ion used in labeling RBCs with ^{99m}Tc is important. Insufficient amounts of stannous ion will not reduce ^{99m}Tc completely and thus decrease binding to Hb. Using the in vivo and modified in vivo methods, an excess of stannous ion will result in extracellular reduction of technetium, thereby preventing RBC membrane transport of technetium, resulting in decreased labeling efficiency.

This issue is further confused by the dose and dosage forms reported in the literature. For ease of comparison, all doses should be specified by the quantity of stannous ion (micrograms) per kg body weight. Pavel et al.[107] used a dose of 0.2 mg/kg stannous pyrophosphate equivalent to 30 μg stannous ion/kg. In animal studies, Jones et al.[113] observed changes in blood disappearance of technetium-99m pertechnetate at stannous ion doses of 1 μg/kg and a plateau of 10 μg Sn^{2+}/kg. Hamilton and Alderson[114] also found 10 μg Sn^{2+}/kg as the minimum dose to achieve satisfactory RBC labeling and noted no decrease in labeling efficiency at doses of up to 40 μg Sn^{2+}/kg. However, Khetigan et al.,[115] reported a threshold dose of 20 μg Sn^{2+}/kg before any alteration in pertechnetate biodistribution is noted. For technetium-99m RBC labeling, using either the in vivo or modified in vivo technique, most clinicians use 10 to 20 μg Sn^{2+}/kg. Depending on the commercial formulation chosen, it may be necessary to inject one-third to one-half the contents of a vial of stannous pyrophosphate or an entire vial to provide this amount of stannous ion. When the in vitro method of radiolabeling is employed, a much smaller amount of stannous ion is employed, usually 1 to 15 μg.[108,116]

2. Removal of Extracellular Stannous Ion

The presence of stannous ion in the serum can result in the undesirable reduction of technetium-99m pertechnetate prior to its entry into the RBC. Since only the oxidized form of ^{99m}Tc can be transported by the RBC membrane,[110] a decrease in labeling efficiency occurs.

In either the in vivo or the modified in vivo method, biologic clearance of excess stannous pyrophosphate is the method by which extracellular stannous ions are reduced. The optimal time between the injection of stannous pyrophosphate and the administration of technetium-99m pertechnetate (in vivo method) or the incubation of the stannous ion-pretreated cells (modified in vivo method) is 20 to 30 minutes.[107,109]

With the original in vitro labeling method,[108] extracellular stannous ion could be removed by centrifugation, a step that physically separates stannous-treated cells from the non–cell-bound stannous ions in serum. Recently, the in vitro labeling method has been modified to include the nonpenetrating oxidizing agent sodium hypochlorite to oxidize extracellular stannous ions, thus preventing reduction of technetium-99m pertechnetate.[116] With this technique, a small amount of sodium hypochlorite is added to whole blood that has been previously treated with stannous ion. Extracellular stannous ions are oxidized to the stannic form, thereby minimizing extracellular reduction of technetium. Intracellular stannous ions are not affected by the addition of sodium hypochlorite. Compared with the centrifugation method, the major advantage of this chemical method is that whole blood can be used for labeling, eliminating the need for centrifugation.

3. Addition of Technetium-99m Pertechnetate to Stannous-Pretreated Red Blood Cells

Actual RBC labeling with technetium-99m occurs whenever technetium-99m pertechnetate is brought into contact with RBCs that have been previously treated with stannous ion. Since the in vivo method requires only that technetium-99m pertechnetate be administered by the IV route, many clinicians find this the simplest method for RBC labeling. Unfortunately, poor-quality RBC labeling often results (compared with the in vitro incubation of technetium-99m pertechnetate), since IV administration of the pertechnetate ion is subject to some degree of partitioning between the intravascular and the extracellular spaces before RBC labeling can be achieved. It has been shown that the rate of technetium-99m RBC labeling is not instantaneous[117] and, therefore, ample time exists for pertechnetate to diffuse out of the intravascular compartment.

Care must be taken in interpreting reports on labeling efficiency with in vivo methods. While these figures may accurately represent the amount of radioactivity within the vascular space associated with RBCs, they do not distinguish the amount of pertechnetate that has distributed into the extracellular fluid space. Radioactivity within the extracellular spaces can significantly degrade image quality.

The Modified In Vivo Method

The modified in vivo method of RBC labeling[114] was developed primarily as a means to avoid the poor reproducibility and inferior quality images that often resulted with the traditional in vivo method. As in the in vivo method, the modified in vivo method also requires IV administration of stannous ions (as the stannous pyrophosphate complex). However, with the modified method, the stannous ion–treated RBCs are withdrawn directly into a syringe containing technetium-99m pertechnetate. A dilute solution of heparin (10 units/ml) is used as an anticoagulant within the indwelling line. The RBC/technetium-99m pertechnetate mixture is allowed to incubate at room temperature for 10 minutes after gentle mixing. Labeled cells are then reinjected. Since the entire labeling occurs within a closed system that is connected to an indwelling catheter, any likelihood that the cells will become contaminated or be misadministered to the wrong patient is minimized.

With this technique, the amount of ^{99m}Tc contained in the RBC fraction at the time of administration has been shown to be greater than 90 percent.[109] Some investigators have reported slighly higher labeling efficiencies using acid-citrate-dextrose (ACD) solution rather than heparin.[118] By labeling the stannous ion–treated RBCs within a syringe, extravascular distribution of ^{99m}Tc is prevented.

The labeling reaction taking place within the syringe has been well characterized. The rate of labeling is directly affected by hematocrit (Hct) and temperature.[117,119] In patients with low Hct values, such as in GI bleeding studies, incubation time should be increased to 20 minutes. The temperature of the labeling mixture can be kept close to body temperature by using lead shields that have been stored in a warmer. The lead acts as a source of heat, lessening the rate of blood cooling after it is withdrawn from the patient.

The in vivo behavior of technetium-99m RBCs has been studied in patients and normal volunteers.[120,121] After IV injection of pertechnetate during in vivo labeling, maximum whole blood activity is not reached until at least 30 minutes postinjection. However, maximum activity is present at 5 minutes when the in vitro method is used. The maximum blood levels are 18 percent higher for the in vitro method as compared with the in vivo. For up to 8 hours following injection, the in vitro method results in higher blood levels, whereas 24–hour retention is slightly higher for the in vivo method. Whole-body clearance has been found to be biexponential for both methods. Clearance data from Atkins et al.[121] are presented in Table 2-5. Several studies have compared the use of technetium-99m HSA and technetium-99m RBCs prepared by either the in vitro or in vivo method of radiolabeling.[104,106,114,121,122]

On the basis of these studies, the following conclusions can be made.

1. Whenever technetium-99m HSA is compared with ^{99m}Tc-labeled RBCs prepared by any method, labeled RBCs are determined to be superior.
2. When in vivo and modified in vivo methods of labeling RBCs are compared, the modified in vivo method is judged superior.
3. When in vitro labeled RBCs are compared with in vivo and/or modified in vivo methods and judged on labeling efficiency and image quality, in vitro labeled cells are judged superior.
4. When availability and ease of labeling are considered in comparisons among all RBC labeling methods, the in vitro kit is found inferior because of the increased manipulation required and the potential for misadministration of cells to the wrong patient.
5. Comparison of all methods of RBC labeling demonstrates that the modified in vivo method provides image quality approaching that of in vitro methods but is far more easily performed with readily available components.

For any given clinical situation, therefore, the actual selection of a blood pool agent will depend on the level of acceptable image quality, the number of studies performed daily, and the level of expertise of the techni-

TABLE 2-5 Whole-body Clearance Rates for Technetium-99m Red Blood Cells Labeled In Vivo and In Vitro

| | Fast Component $(t_{1/2})$ | | Slow Component $(t_{1/2})$ | |
Method	hr	%	hr	%
In vivo	2.5 ± 0.7	10.9 ± 6	176.6 ± 163.6	90.5 ± 5
In vitro	2.7 ± 1.5	25.4 ± 10.4	75.6 ± 25.3	82.2 ± 7.7

Data from Atkins et al.[121]

TABLE 2-6 Drugs Reported to Interfere with the Labeling of Red Blood Cells with ^{99m}Tc

Drug	Possible Mechanism
Heparin	Formation of Tc-99m labeled heparin
Methyldopa, hydralazine	Oxidation of stannous ion
Methyldopa, quinide	Formation of RBC antibodies
Digoxin	Mechanism unknown
Prazocin, propranolol	Mechanism unknown
Iodinated contrast media	Iodide competes with transport of pertechnetate by RBC membrane

Data from Ponto et al.[41]

cal staff. Several drug interactions have been reported with technetium-99m RBCs for equilibrium blood pool imaging. Poor radiolabeling of RBCs with ^{99m}Tc or early dissociation of ^{99m}Tc from the labeled RBC brought about by concomitant drug therapy can adversely affect image quality. Table 2-6 lists several of the drugs known to interfere with technetium-99m RBC labeling or that may be responsible for deterioration of the labeled cell.

REFERENCES

1. Parkey RW, Bonte FJ, Meyer SL, et al: A new method for radionuclide imaging of acute myocardial infarctions in humans. Circulation, 50:540, 1974
2. D'Agostino AN, Chiga M: Mitochondrial mineralization in human myocardium. Am J Clin Pathol 53:820, 1970
3. Kelly RJ, Chilton HM, Hackshaw BT, et al: Comparison of TC-99m pyrophosphate and Tc-99m methylene diphosphonate in acute myocardial infarction: Concise communication, J Nucl Med 20:402, 1979
4. Wakat MA, Chilton HM, Hackshaw BT, et al: Comparison of Tc-99m pyrophosphate and Tc-99m hydroxymethylene diphosphonate in acute myocardial infarction. J Nucl Med 21:203, 1980
5. Subramanian G, McAfee JG, Blair RJ, et al: Technetium-99m-methylene diphosphate—a superior agent for skeletal imaging: Comparison with other technetium complexes. J Nucl Med 16:744, 1975
6. Zaret BL, DiCola VC, Donabedian RK, et al: Dual radionuclide study of myocardial infarction. Relationships between myocardial uptake of potassium-43, technetium-99m stannous pyrophosphate, regional myocardial blood flow and creatine phosphokinase depletion. Circulation, 53:422, 1976
7. Wahner HK, Dewanjee MK. Drug-induced modulation of Tc-99m pyrophosphate tissue distribution: What is involved? J Nucl Med 22:555, 1981
8. Buja LM, Parkey RW, Stokely EM, et al: Morphologic correlates of technetium-99m stannous pyrophosphate imaging of acute myocardial infarcts in dogs. Circulation 52:596, 1975
9. Buja LM, Parkey RW, Stokely EM, et al: Pathophysiology of technetium-99m stannous pyrophosphate and thallium-201 scintigraphy of acute anterior myocardial infarcts in dogs. J Clin Invest 57:1508, 1976
10. Willerson JT, Parkey RN, Bonte FJ, et al: Pathophysiologic consideration and clinicopathological correlates of technetium-99m stannous pyrophosphate myocardial scintigraphy. Semin Nucl Med 10:54, 1980
11. Lyons KP, Olson HG, Aronow WS: Pyrophosphate myocardial imaging. Semin Nucl Med 10:168, 1980
12. Khaw BA, Beller GA, Haber E, Smith TW: Localization of cardiac myosin-specific antibody in myocardial infarction. J Clin Invest 58:439, 1976
13. Khaw BA, Beller GA, Haber E: Experimental myocardial infarct imaging following intravenous administration of iodine-131 labeled antibody (Fab)$_2$ fragments specific for cardiac myosin. Circulation 57:743, 1978
14. Khaw, BA, Gold HK, Leinbach RC, et al: Early imaging of experimental myocardial infarction by intracoronary administration of ^{131}I-labeled anticardiac myosin (Fab′)$_2$ fragments. Circulation 58:1137, 1978
15. Kohler G, Milstein C: Continuous cultures of fused cells secreting antibody of prede-

fined specificity. Nature (Lond) 256:495, 1975

16. Krejcarek GE, Tucker KL: Covalent attachments of chelating groups of macromolecules. Biochem Biophys Res Commun 77:581, 1977

17. Khaw BA, Fallon JT, Strauss HW, Haber E: Myocardial infarct imaging with Indium-111-diethylene triamine pentaacetic acid-anticanine cardiac myosin antibodies. Science 209:295, 1980

18. Khaw BA, Strauss HW, Carvalho A, et al: Technetium-99m labeling of antibodies to cardiac myosin Fab and to human fibrinogen. J Nucl Med 23:1011, 1982

19. Khaw BA, Mattis JA, Melincoff G, et al: Monoclonal antibody to cardiac myosin: Imaging of experimental myocardial infarction. Hybridoma 3:11, 1984

20. Khaw BA, Gold HK, Yasuda T, et al: Scintigraphic quantification of myocardial necrosis in patients after intravenous injection of myosin specific antibody. Circulation 74:501, 1986

21. Yasuda T, Palacios I, Dec W, et al: Indium-111 monoclonal antimyosin antibody in the diagnosis of acute myocarditis. Circulation 76:306, 1987

22. Gerber KH, Higgins CB: Quantitation of size of myocardial infarcts by computerized transmission tomography. Comparison with hot-spot and cold-spot radionuclide scans. Invest Radiol 18:238, 1983

23. Nichol P, Yasuda T, Locke E: Multiple intravenous administration of In-111 antimyosin Fab: Determination of antimurine Fab response in patients with myocarditis. J Nucl Med 29:939, 1988

24. Brown JM, Dean RT, Kaplan P, et al: Absence of Human Antimouse (HAMA) response in patients given antimyosin Fab-DTPA monoclonal antibody. J Nucl Med 29:851, 1988

25. Sapirstein LA, Moses JE: Cerebral and cephalic blood flow in man: Basic consideration of the indicator fraction technique. Dynam Clin Stud Radioisotopes 3:135, 1964

26. Love WD, Ishihara Y, Lyon LD, et al: Differences in the relationships between coronary blood flow and myocardial clearance of isotopes of potassium, rubidium, and cesium. Am Heart J 76:353, 1968

27. Gehring PJ, Hammond PB: The uptake of thallium by rabbit erythrocytes. J Pharmacol Exp Ther 145:215, 1964

28. Britten J, Blank M: Thallium activation of Na-K-ATPase of rabbit kidney. Biochim Biophys Acta 159:169, 1968

29. Kawana M, Krizek H, Porter J, et al: Use of T1-199 as a potassium analog in scanning. J Nucl Med 11:333, 1970 (abst)

30. Lebowitz E, Greene MW, Fairchild R, et al: Thallium for medical use. J Nucl Med 16:151, 1975

31. Atkins HL, Budinger TF, Lebowitz E, et al: Thallium-201 for medical use. Part 1. Human distribution and physical imaging properties. J Nucl Med 18:133, 1977

32. Mueller TM, Marcus ML, Ehrhardt JC, et al: Limitations of thallium-201 myocardial perfusion scintigrams. Circulation 54:640, 1976

33. Pohost GM, O'Keefe DD, Gewirtz H, et al: Thallium redistribution in the presence of severe fixed coronary stenosis. Clin Res 26:260A, 1978 (abst)

34. Boucher CA, Zir LM, Beller GA, et al: Increased lung uptake during exercise myocardial imaging: Clinical, hemodynamic and angiographic implications in patients with coronary artery disease. Am J Cardiol 46:189, 1980

35. ICRP Publication 52. Protection of the Nuclear Medicine Patient. Pergamon, Oxford, 1988

36. Hockings G, Saltissi S, Croft DN, et al: Effect of beta adrenergic blockade on thallium-201 myocardial perfusion imaging. Br Heart J 49:83, 1983

37. Henkin RE, Chang W, and Provus R: The effect of beta blockers on thallium scans. J Nucl Med 23:63, 1982 (abst)

38. Pohost GM, Alpert NM, Ingwall JS, et al: Thallium redistribution: mechanisms and clinical utility. Semin Nucl Med 10:70, 1980

39. Osbakken MD, Okada RD, Boucher CA, et al: The effect of inderal, exercise level, and subcritical disease on the specificity of exercise thallium-201 imaging. J Nucl Med 22:41, 1981 (abst)

40. Wolf R, Pretschner P, Engel HJ, et al: Effect of isosorbide dinitrate on thalium-201 myocardial imaging in coronary heart disease. Am J Cardiol 43:432, 1979 (abst)

41. Hladik WB, Ponto JA, Lentle BC, et al: Iatrogenic alterations in the biodistribution of radiotracers as a result of a drug therapy: Reported instances. p. 189. In Hladik WB III, Sada G, Study KT (eds): Essentials of Nuclear Medicine Science. Williams & Wilkins, Baltimore, 1987

42. Hamilton GW, Narahara KA, Yee H, et al: Myocardial imaging with thallium-201: Effect of cardiac drugs on myocardial images J Nucl Med 19:10–16, 1978

43. Berman DS, Garcia EV, Maddahi J, et al: Thallium-201 myocardial perfusion scintigraphy. p. 479. In Freeman LM (ed): Freeman and Johnson's Clinical Radionuclide Imaging. 3rd Ed. Grune & Stratton, Orlando, FL, 1984.

44. McLaughlin PR, Martin RP, Doherty P, et al: Reproducibility of thallium-201 myocardial imaging. Circulation 55:497, 1979

45. Leppo J, Boucher CA, Okada RD, et al: Serial thallium-201 myocardial imaging after dipyridamole infusion: Diagnostic utility in detecting coronary stenoses and relationship to reginal wall motion. Circulation 66:649, 1982

46. Francisco DA, Collins SM, Go RT, et al: Tomographic T1–201 myocardial perfusion scintigrams after maximal coronary artery vasodilation with intravenous dipyridamole. Circulation 66:370, 1982

47. Gould KL, Schelbert HR, Phelps ME, et al: Non-invasive assessment of coronary stenoses with myocardial perfusion imaging during pharmacologic coronary vasodilation. V. Detection of 47% diameter coronary stenoses with intravenous nitrogen-13 ammonia and emission-computer transaxial tomography in intact dogs. Am J Cardiol 43:200, 1979

48. Schelbert HR, Wisenberg G, Phelps ME, et al: Non-invasive assessment of coronary stenoses by myocardial imaging during pharmacologic coronary vasodilation. VI. Detection of coronary artery disease in man with intravenous N-13 ammonia and positron computed tomography. Am J Cardiol 49:1197, 1982

49. Tamaki N, Yonekura Y, Senda M, et al: Myocardial positron computed tomography with ^{13}N-ammonia at rest and during exercise. Eur J Nucl Med 11:246, 1985

50. Schelbert HR, Phelps ME, Huang SC, et al: N-13 ammonia as an indicator of myocardial blood flow. Circulation 63:1259, 1981

51. Bergman ST, Hack S, Tewson T, et al: The dependence of accumulation of ^{13}NH$_3$ by myocardium on metabolic factors and its implication for the quantitative assessment of perfusion. Circulation 61:34, 1980

52. Shah A, Schelbert HR, Schwaiger M, et al: Measurement of regional myocardial blood flow with N-13 ammonia and positron emission tomography in intact dogs. J Am Coll Cardiol 5:92, 1985

53. Mazziotta JC, Phelps M: Positron emission tomography studies of the brain. p. 493. In Phelps M, Mazziotta J, Schelbert H (eds): Positron Emission Tomography and Autoradiography: Principles and Application for the Brain and Heart. Raven Press, New York, 1986.

54. Bergmann SR, Fox KAA, Rand AL, et al: Quantification of regional myocardial blood flow in vivo with H$_2$^{15}O. Circulation 70:724, 1984

55. Horlock P, Clark J, O'Brien HA, et al: The preparation of rubidium-82 radionuclide generator. J Radioanal Chem 64:257, 1981

56. Neirinckx RD, Kronauge JF, Gennaro GP, et al: Evaluation of inorganic absorbance for the rubidium-82 generators: I. Hydrous SnO$_2$. J Nucl Med 23:245, 1982

57. Grover M, Schwaiger M, Hansen H, et al: Coronary artery occlusion and reperfusion alters rubidium-82 extraction fraction. Circulation 70:II–124, 1984 (abst)

58. Deutsch E, Glavan KA, Sodd VJ, et al: Cationic Tc-99m complexes as potential myocardial imaging agents. J Nucl Med 22:897, 1981

59. Nishiyama H, Deutsch E, Adolph RJ, et al: Basal kinetic studies of Tc-99m DMPE as a myocardial imaging agent in the dog. J Nucl Med 23:1093, 1982

60. Dudczak R, Angelberger P, Homan R, et al: Evaluation of ^{99m}Tc-dichlorobis (1,2-dimethylphosphino)ethane (^{99m}Tc-DMPE) for myocardial scintigraphy in man. Eur J Nucl Med 8:513, 1983

61. Jones AG, Abrams MJ, Davison A: A new class of water soluble low valent technetium unipositive cations: Hexakisisonitrile tech-

netium (I) salts. J Nucl Med All Sci 26:149, 1982

62. Holman BL, Jone AG, Lister-James J, et al: A new Tc-99m-labeled-myocardial imaging agent, hexakis (t-butylisonitrile) technetium (I) [Tc-99m TBI]: Initial experience in the human. J Nucl Med 25:1350, 1984

63. McKusick KA, Holman BL, Rigo P, et al: Human myocardial imaging with Tc-99m isonitriles. Circulation 74:II–296, 1986B

64. Sporn V, Perez-Balino N, Holman BL, et al: Myocardial imaging with Tc-99m CPI: Initial experience in the human. J Nucl Med 27:878, 1986 (abst)

65. McKusick KA, Holman BL, Jones AG, et al: Comparison of 3 Tc-99m isonitriles for detection of ischemic heart disease in humans. J Nucl Med 27:878, 1986 (abst)

66. Dudczak C, Leitha T, Kletter K, et al: Comparison of Tc-99m-methoxypropyl-isonitrile (MPIN) and Tc-99m-methoxyisobutyl-isonitrile (MIBI) for myocardial imaging in man. J Nucl Med 29:794, 1988

67. Nunn AD, Treher EN, Feld T: Boronic acid adducts of technetium oxime complexes (BATO's): A new class of neutral complexes with myocardial imaging capabilities. J Nucl Med 27:893, 1986 (abst)

68. Narra RK, Kuczunski BL, Feld T, et al: A comparison of the pharmacokinetics of a new Tc-99m-labeled myocardial imaging agent, SQ 32, 014 with SQ 30,217. J Nucl Med 28:674, 1987 (abst)

69. Hirth W, Jurisson S, Linder K, et al: Chlorohydroxy substitution on technetium dioxime complexes: Chemical and biological comparison of TcCl(dioxime)$_3$Br and TcOH(dioxime)$_3$Br. J Nucl Med 29:800, 1988 (abst)

70. Linder KE, Treher EN, Juri PN, et al: Neutral tris oxime complexes of technetium-(III): Chemistry and biodistribution of TcX(oxime)$_3$. J Nucl Med 29:800, 1988 (abst)

71. Opie L: Carbohydrates and lipids. Heart 10:118, 1984

72. Marshall RC, Huang SC, Nash WW, et al: Assessment of the [18F]fluorodeoxyglucose kinetic model in calculations of myocardial glucose metabolism during ischemia. J Nucl Med 24:1060, 1983

73. Liedtke JA: Alterations in carbohydrate and lipid metabolism in the acutely ischemic heart. Prog Cardiovasc Dis 23:321, 1981

74. Phelps ME, Huang SC, Hoffman EJ, et al: Tomographic measurement of local cerebral glucose metabolic rate in humans with (f-18)1-fluoro-2-deoxy-D-glucose: Validation of method. Ann Neurol 6:371, 1979

75. Huang SC, Phelps ME, Hoffman EJ, et al: Noninvasive determination of local cerebral metabolic rate of glucose in man. Am J Physiol 238:E69, 1980

76. Phelps ME: Emission computed tomography. Semin Nucl Med 7:337, 1977

77. Phelps ME, Hoffman EJ, Huang SC, et al: ECAT: A new computerized tomographic imaging system of positron-emitting radiopharmaceuticals. J Nucl Med 19:635, 1978

78. Kuhl DE, Edwards RQ, Ricci AR, et al: The MARK IV system for radionuclide computed tomography of the brain. Radiology 121:405, 1976

79. Budinger TF, Derenzo SE, Gullbear GT, et al: Emission computer assisted tomography with single-photon and positron annihilation photon emitters. J Comp Assist Tomog 1:131, 1977

80. Ido T, Cuan CN, Fowler JS, et al: Fluorination with F$_2$-A convenient synthesis of 2 deoxy-2 fluroro-D-glucose. J Org Chem 42:2341, 1977

81. Ido T, Wan CN, Casella V, et al: Labeled 2-deoxy-D-glucose analogs. [18F]-labeled 2 deoxy-2 fluoro-D-glucose, 2-deoxy-2-fluoro-D-mannose and [14C]-2-deoxy-2-fluoro-D-glucose. J Label Comp Radiopharm 14:174, 1978.

82. Barreo JR, McDonald NS, Robinson GD, et al: Remote, semiautomated production of F-18 labeled 2-deoxy-2-fluoro-D-glucose. J Nucl Med 22:372, 1981

83. Fowler JS, MacGregor RR, Wolf AP, et al: A shielded synthesis system for production of 2-deoxy-2-[18F]fluoro-D-glucose. J Nucl Med 22:376, 1981

84. Schon H, Schelbert HR, Henze E, et al: Quantification of regional C-11 palmitate kinetics by positron tomography (PET). Circulation 70:11, 1984 (abst)

85. Geltman EM, Biello D, Welch MJ, et al: Characterization of non-transmural myocardial infarction by positron emission tomography. Circulation 65:747, 1982

86. Freundlieb C, Hock A, Vyska K, et al: Myocardial imaging and metabolic studies with 17-(I-123)-iodoheptadecanoic acid. J Nucl Med 21:1044, 1980

87. Livini E, Elmalch DR, Levy S, et al: Beta-methayl (1-C-11) heptadecanoic acid: A new myocardial metabolic tracer for positron emission tomography. J Nucl Med 23:169, 1982

88. Livini E, Elmalch DR, Barlai-Kovach M, et al: Radioiodinated beta-methyl phenyl fatty acids as potential tracers for myocardial imaging and metabolism. Eur Heart J 6:85, 1985

89. Miller DD, Gill JB, Barlai-Kovach M, et al: Modified fatty acid analog imaging: Correlation of SPECT and clearance kinetics in ischemic reperfused myocardium. J Nucl Med 23:84, 1985

90. Miller DD, Strauss HW: Radionuclides for Cardiac Imaging. p. 18. In Miller DD, Burns RJ, Gill JB, Ruddy TD (eds): Clinical Cardiac Imaging. McGraw-Hill, New York, 1988

91. Neely JR, Morgan HE: Relationship between carbohydrate and lipid metabolism and the energy balance of heart muscle. Annu Rev Physiol 36:413, 1974

92. Opie LH, Owen P, Riemersma RA: Relative rates of oxidation of glucose and free fatty acids by ischemic myocardium after coronary artery ligation in the dog. Eur J Clin Invest 3:419, 1973

93. Rovetto MJ, Lamberton WF, Neely JR: Mechanisms of glycolytic inhibition of ischemic rat heart. Circ Res 37:742, 1975

94. Hillis LD, Braunwald E: Myocardial ischemia. N Engl J Med 296:971, 1977

95. Wildenthal K, Morgan HR, Opie LH, et al: Regulation of Cardiac Metabolism. p. 49. In American Heart Association Monograph, American Heart Association, Dallas, 1976

96. Braunwald E: Protection of the ischemic myocardium. p. 48. In American Heart Association Monograph. American Heart Association, Dallas 1976

97. Schelbert HR, Verba JW, Johnson AD, et al: Non-traumatic determination of left ventricular ejection fraction by radionuclide angiocardiography. Circulation 51:902, 1975

98. Strauss HW, Zaret BL, Hurley PJ, et al: A scintiphotographic method for measuring left ventricular ejection fraction in man without cardiac catheterization. Am J Cardiol 28:575, 1971

99. Zaret BL, Strauss HW, Hurley PJ, et al: A non-invasive scintiphotographic method for detection of regional ventricular dysfunction in man. N Engl J Med 284:1165, 1971

100. Cheng C, Treves S, Samuel A, et al: A new osmium-191/iridium-191m generator. J Nucl Med 21:1169, 1980

101. Brihaye C, Butler TA, Knapap FF, Jr, et al: A new osmium-191/iridium-191m radionuclide generator system using activated charcoal. J Nucl Med 27:380, 1986

102. Dymond DS, Elliot AT, Flatman W, et al: Clinical validation of gold-195m: A new short half-life radiopharmaceutical for rapid sequential first-pass angiography in man. J Am Coll Cardiol 2:85, 1983

103. Nusynowitz ML, Straw JD, Benedetto AR, et al: Blood clearance rates of technetium-99m albumin preparations. (Concise communication. J Nucl Med 19:1142, 1978

104. Thrall JH, Freitas JE, Swanson D, et al: Clinical comparison of cardiac blood pool visualization with technetium-99m red blood cells labeled in vivo with the technetium-99m human serum albumin. J Nucl Med 19:796, 1978

105. Yang SSL, Nickolff EL, McIntyre PA, et al: Tc-99m human serum albumin: A suitable agent for plasma volume measurements in man. J Nucl Med 19:804, 1978

106. Atkins HL, Klopper JF, Ansari AN, et al: A comparison of Tc-99m-labeled human serum albumin and in vitro labeled red blood cells for blood pool studies. Clin Nucl Med 5:166, 1980

107. Pavel D, Zimmer ZM, Patterson VN: In vivo labeling of red blood cells with [99m]Tc: A new approach to blood pool visualization. J Nucl Med 18:305, 1977

108. Smith TD, Richards P: A simple kit for the preparation of ^{99m}Tc labeled red blood cells. J Nucl Med 17:126, 1976

109. Callahan RJ, Froelich JW, McKusick KA, et al: A modified method for the in vivo labeling of RBC with [99m]Tc. J Nucl Med 23:315, 1982

110. Rabito CA, Callahan RJ, McKusick KA, et al: Transport of pertechnetate by human

erythrocyte membrane. J Nucl Med 27:946, 1986

111. Dewanjee M: Binding of [99mTc] ion to hemoglobin. J Nucl Med 15:703, 1974

112. Rehani MN, Sharma SK: Site of [99mTc] binding to the red blood cell: Concise communication. J Nucl Med 21:676, 1980

113. Jones AG, Davis MA, Uren RF, et al: In vivo red cell labeling with [99mTc]. J Nucl Med 18:637, 1977

114. Hamilton RG, Alderson PO: A comparative evaluation of technique for rapid and efficient in vivo labeling of red blood cells with [99mTc] pertechnetate. J Nucl Med 18:1010, 1977

115. Khentigan A, Garret M, Lum D, Winchell HS: Effects of prior administration of SN(11) complexed on in vivo distribution of [99mTc] pertechnetate. J Nucl Med 17:380, 1976

116. Srivastava SC, Babich JB, Richards P: A new kit method for the selective labeling of erythrocytes in whole blood with technetium-99m. J Nucl Med 24:128, 1983

117. Callahan RJ, Froelich JW, McKusick KA, and Strauss HW: Factors affecting the rate and extent of incorporation of Tc-99m into pre-tinned red blood cells (RBC). J Nucl Med 23:109, 1982b.

118. Porter WC, Dees SM, Freitas JE, Dworking HJ: Acid-Citrate-Dextrose compared with heparin in the preparation of in vivo-in vitro technetium-99m RBC. J Nucl Med 24:282, 1983

119. Callahan RJ: Radiolabeled red blood cells as diagnostic radiopharmaceuticals. p. 50. In Fritzberg AR (ed): Radiopharmaceuticals: Progress and Clinical Perspectives. Vol. II. CRC Press, Boca Raton, FL, 1986

120. Hegge FN, Hamilton GW, Larson SM: Cardiac chamber imaging: A comparison of red blood cells labeled with [99mTc], in vitro and in vivo. J Nucl Med 19:129, 1978

121. Atkins HL, Srivfistava SC, Meinken GE et al: Biological behavior of erythrocytes labeled in vivo and in vitro with 99m-Tc. J Nucl Med Technol 13:136, 1985

122. Graham MM, Nelp WB: Cardiac blood pool activity after in vivo and in vitro red blood cell (RBC) labeling. J Nucl Med 21:7, 1980

3

Assessment of Myocardial Injury with Labeled Antimyosin Antibodies

Peter P. Liu
Tsunehiro Yasuda
Ban-an Khaw

Labeled antimyosin antibody imaging is maturing into an important clinical tool to assess irreversible myocardial injury and cellular viability. This technique originated in the basic science laboratory, where careful research was initially carried out, and was followed meticulously by improvements in antibody labeling and imaging. Currently, it is undergoing phase III clinical trials in North America and Europe. Once they are clinically available, labeled antimyosin antibodies will represent a significant step forward in the diagnosis and management of cardiac patients with a suspected myocardial injury. This chapter addresses the principles of antimyosin antibody imaging and the relevant basic and clinical applications of this new and exciting imaging modality.

IMPORTANCE OF ASSESSING MYOCARDIAL VIABILITY

During a severe insult or injury to the heart, the amount of myocardium that is irreversibly damaged will have a direct bearing on the subsequent myocardial function and in turn will determine the patient's ultimate prognosis.[1,2] Because the human myocyte loses its ability to replicate soon after birth, myocytes damaged during an insult can never be replaced. Normal myocardial function is maintained by each viable myocyte acting in concert. However, with significant myocyte injury, initially regional, and ultimately global, myocardial dysfunction is found. Excessive myocyte death, such as occurs in a large myocardial infarction or severe myocarditis, will lead to acute left ventricular failure and cardiogenic shock, rapidly followed by the death of the patient. Therefore, interventions designed to preserve myocyte viability in the face of a serious damaging process, such as thrombolytic therapy during acute myocardial infarction, or immunosuppressive treatment in myocarditis, are aimed to preserve the myocyte viability and ventricular function and ultimately to improve the patient's prognosis.

In order to assess the extent of irreversible injury and the effectiveness of intervention, a marker to detect the presence of irreversible myocardial cell death is crucial. Clinically, a hot spot imaging agent that will permit accurate and early localization of the cells destined for irreversible injury would supply such a marker. Previously, technetium-99m pyrophosphate scanning has been the gold standard in labeling myocardial injury, based on the presence of calcium deposition in irreversibly injured cells.[3,4] However, the various practical limitations have prompted the search for a better agent for this purpose. By combining the understanding of mechanisms of cellular injury and modern molecular immunology, labeled antimyosin antibodies now challenge the previous gold standard as the best technique to define myocardial injury.

TECHNIQUES OF ASSESSING MYOCARDIAL VIABILITY IN VIVO

Identifying irreversible myocardial injury is a challenging process in the best of situations. This becomes especially difficult when one attempts to identify precisely the point at which irreversible cell death occurs. The commonly associated pathologic ultrastructural markers for irreversibly injured myocytes are the presence of amorphous matrix densities in mitochondria and breaks in the plasma membrane of the sarcolemma.[5,6] The latter leads to unrestricted entry of extracellular constituents into the damaged myocytes, as well as to loss of critical low-molecular-weight enzymes to the extracellular space. The sudden increase in osmotic load causes cell swelling and rupture. The loss of magnesium and potassium ions as well as the entry of calcium ions result in extensive disruption of the metabolic machinery of the myocytes, finally bringing on the termination of cellular function and cell death.

Morphologic techniques are therefore the most accurate for determining cellular necrosis, but their use is neither feasible nor practical for the in vivo situation, except for direct pathologic examination of myocardial samples obtained from a myocardial biopsy. Other methods of detecting myocardial necrosis rely on the presence of leaked cellular contents in the serum, such as myocardial creatine kinase (CK-MB), and metabolic enzymes, such as SGOT and LDH.[7] However, they are limited in their ability to localize and rapidly quantitate the extent of necrosis.

Because excessive calcium deposition does take place in the necrotic myocardial cell, coprecipitation of the calcium in the mitochondria with radiolabeled pyrophosphate has become a commonly used method to localize and judge the size of the area of necrosis.[3,8] Unfortunately, this technique is useful only after an obligatory delay of a few hours to, more commonly, a few days after the initial injury event and is often only clinically useful for retrospective diagnosis.

To obviate some of the limitations of pyrophosphate scanning, Khaw et al.[9,10] developed radiolabeled antimyosin antibodies that are capable of in vivo binding of cardiac myosin in the presence of myocyte membrane damage, which is the most reliable indicator of irreversible cell injury. Recent studies have shown this technique to be highly specific in delineating irreversible myocardial necrosis.[11–13]

posed myosin molecule can be delivered to the extracellular space. One such successful technique is the administration of labeled antibodies specific for the myosin heavy-chain molecule into the extracellular space.

THE MYOSIN MOLECULE AND ITS PROPERTIES DURING NECROSIS

Myosin is a large contractile protein (470,000 M_r) that represents the thick filaments on ultrastructural analysis of cardiac myocytes. It is found in large quantities in the myocyte and is responsible for cardiac contraction in conjunction with the protein actin. The myosin molecule consists of two heavy chains, made up of two globular heads joined to two 150-nm-long tails. Two light-chain fractions (18,000 and 26,000 M_r) are also associated with each globular head. The light-chain fraction is soluble, whereas the heavy-chain fraction is highly insoluble in physiologic fluids.

During myocyte necrosis, the cell membrane is disrupted, and the myosin molecule becomes exposed to the extracellular space. The soluble light chains will be released into the bloodstream and can be detected in the serum by sensitive radioimmunoassay (RIA) techniques.[14] Recent studies have demonstrated the feasibility of this approach in detecting the presence of myocardial infarction, as well as quantitating myocardial infarct size.[15,16]

In order to localize and size the infarcted myocardium itself, the tracer used must attach specifically to the necrotic myocardial cells, to the exclusion of viable cells. Because of the relatively insoluble properties of the myosin heavy-chain fraction, even in the presence of myocyte necrosis and membrane dissolution, the heavy chain will remain in place for a considerable time after cell death. This lends itself to an excellent opportunity for infarct localization, if a radiolabeled radiotracer that can specifically attach to the ex-

LABELED ANTIMYOSIN ANTIBODIES

The progressive interest in labeling antibodies dates back to the early days, when Pressman and Keighley[17] in 1948 used labeled immunoglobulins against rat kidney to demonstrate in vivo localization. This evolved over the next 40 years from isolation of the immunoglobulin fraction, to the characterization of individual whole antibodies, to the development of monoclonal antibodies and purification of its Fab fragments. Advances in labeling technology also developed in parallel and expanded from the original techniques of radioiodination to the development of multivalent cationic isotopes, including ^{111}In and ^{99m}Tc. Currently there is tremendous interest in the use of labeled antibodies in many areas of medicine, including tumor detection and treatment, labeling of inflammation and thrombosis, and the use of antimyosin antibodies for the localization of myocardial necrosis.

The myosin molecule is, in fact, an ideal antigen for labeled antibody techniques, because (1) it is an intracellular protein, which only becomes exposed to the extracellular space during the process of necrosis; (2) it is present in large concentrations; (3) due to the insolubility of the myosin, it is not washed out of the cells after membrane disruption; (4) it can be readily purified to act as an antigen; and (5) it is very immunogenic and results in large quantities of antibody production using both polyclonal and monoclonal techniques.

The development of antimyosin antibody labeling began with polyclonal antimyosin antibodies derived from rabbits immunized with purified cardiac myosin (human and canine) delivered in Freund's adjuvant. The polyclonal antibody isolated by affinity chromatography was labeled with radioiodine and was used to provide the first in vivo evidence that it can localize in necrotic myocardium.[9] The labeling chemistry was further refined and modified for complex cationic isotopes, such as ^{99m}Tc and ^{111}In.[18,19]

To increase specificity, monoclonal techniques were employed that fuse immunized murine spleen cells with myeloma cells to form a hybridoma capable of producing monoclonal antimyosin.[20] Finally, to improve the kinetics of antibody clearance from nonspecific organs, and to improve the target to background ratio, the antibodies were cleaved by papain digestion, and the resultant Fab fragment purified by molecular sieve and affinity chromatography.[10,20] This is the agent that is currently of greatest clinical interest.

ANTIMYOSIN ANTIBODY-LABELING TECHNIQUES

Iodination

The earliest and most reliable, as well as the easiest, technique for antibody labeling is the substitution of one of the —OH groups of the tyrosine residues of the antibody with radioactive iodine, similar to preparing antibodies for RIA. This technique has been favored for its ease of labeling, but it has major deficiencies when used for imaging due to both in vivo dehalogenation and the poor imaging properties of the commonly used ^{131}I or ^{125}I. The best iodine isotope for imaging is ^{123}I; however, a pure source of high-quality ^{123}I supply is not always readily available. Therefore, imaging using ^{125}I or ^{131}I was performed during the developmental stages of this antibody. Several techniques can be used to iodinate an antibody; a few examples are discussed briefly in this chapter.

The first and simplest technique is iodination using iodine monochloride, which has an efficiency similar to labeling using iodine alone.[21] In this case, radioactive iodine is added to the monochloride before mixing with the protein antibody. The specific activity, however, is low compared with other techniques.

A second method of iodination is using chloramine-T to achieve high specific activity, which has been successfully used for human growth hormone.[22] Either ^{125}I or ^{131}I is mixed with the antibody in the presence of chloramine-T, and the entire reaction can be terminated by the addition of sodium metabisulfite. A variation of this basic technique that has proved extremely successful is the use of immobilized chloramine-T on plastic beads. Radioiodination is accomplished by the addition of radioactive iodine and the antibodies to the beads. The reaction can be terminated by removing the chloramine-T beads from the reaction mixture. Unfortunately, this labeling technique can be harsh on the protein structure and denaturation of the antibody sometimes results.

To avoid excessive denaturation of immunoglobulins, an extremely gentle method of radioiodination was developed by Marchalonis that uses lactoperoxidase derived from fresh skimmed milk and causes very little alteration of antibody affinity. This technique has been used by Khaw et al.[9,11,23] in earlier studies to maintain a high level of antibody reactivity.

Bifunctional Chelation with Multivalent Cationic Isotopes

To potentially simplify the labeling procedure and permit labeling of antibodies with isotopes other than iodine, alternative techniques incorporating multivalent cationic isotopes have been sought. This generally involves the covalent coupling of bifunctional chelating agents such as EDTA or

DTPA. For example, the DTPA molecule can be most readily and reliably attached to the antibody by mixed anhydride or bicyclic anhydride reactions. The chelate-bound antibody can then be labeled with a multivalent cationic-isotope such as ^{111}In or reduced [99m]Tc. To permit radiolabeling with ^{99m}Tc, a dithionite reduction technique has been found to be most feasible.

These techniques, when applied to the antimyosin molecule, can be used either to label whole antibodies or the papain digested Fab fragments.[18–20] The simple and easy binding of ^{111}In chloride to the previously linked Fab-DTPA complex is now available in kit form (Centocor, Malvern, PA) that is currently undergoing clinical trials.

BASIC SCIENCE STUDIES WITH LABELED ANTIMYOSIN

Cell Culture Studies

To use antimyosin antibodies effectively, it must be shown that the uptake of this tracer is related to irreversible myocardial injury. To prove that antimyosin binds to myocytes with disrupted membrane (irreversibly injured cells) but not to cells with intact cell membranes, an experiment using neonatal myocyte cultures was carried out.[24] The antimyosin was linked to tiny fluorescent polystyrene beads and was introduced into the cell culture medium, in which irreversible injury was applied to some of the cells. Scanning electron microscopy (SEM) demonstrated that the antimyosin did not bind to any normal myocytes but bound extensively to the intracellular myocyte contents through regions of membrane disruption. In fact, in those cells that showed antimyosin uptake, myofilaments containing myosin were seen to wrap around the antimyosin beads.

Antimyosin can also be localized in myocardial infarction in vivo. Transmission electron microscopy (TEM) with immunoperoxidase staining showed localization of dark stains of antimyosin antibodies in myocytes with disrupted cell membranes, whereas there was no localization in the myocytes with intact membranes (Fig. 3-1). Immunofluorescent staining of ischemic rat ventricular myocardium using monoclonal antimyosin antibody also showed visualization of damaged myocardial cells using this technique and confirmed the localization of the border zone.[25]

Therefore, it appears that the localization of antimyosin antibodies is very specific for myocytes with significant membrane disruption (generally gaps greater than 50 μm in diameter), a feature indicative of irreversible cellular death.

Imaging Studies in Models of Myocardial Infarction

After successful demonstration of the specific localization properties of labeled antimyosin antibody, the question arises as to whether this antibody could be labeled with a gamma imaging isotope and still permit actual visualization of the location and extent of the infarction process.

The first set of experiments used canine models of myocardial infarction and imaged with F(ab')$_2$ fragments of antimyosin antibody labeled with [131]I.[9] Left anterior descending (LAD) coronary artery occlusion to create experimental infarction was first performed. After ^{131}I antimyosin antibody injection, there was discrete localization of the antibody in the infarct zone, which closely corresponded to the pathologically identified area of infarction using tetrazolium stain (Fig. 3-2).

Because of the poor imaging properties of ^{131}I, the next step was to improve the radiolabel attached to the antimyosin antibody. Since ^{99m}Tc has many desirable characteristics in terms of gamma camera imaging and

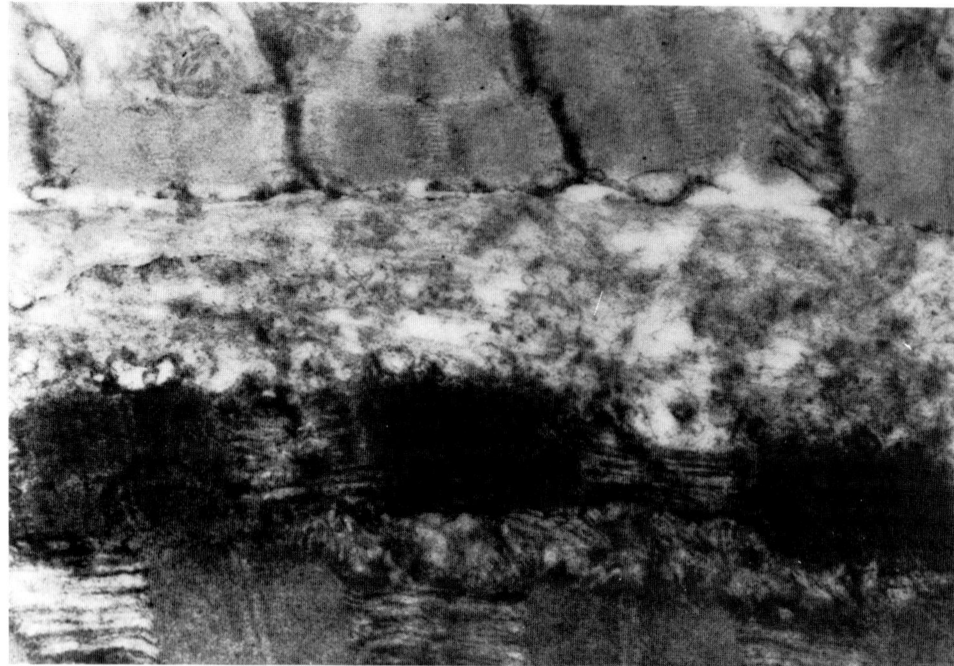

Fig.3-1 Transmission electron micrograph using immunoperoxidase stain showing localization of monoclonal antimyosin Fab (dark stains) in the necrotic myocyte (bottom). No staining is observed in the intact myocyte (top).

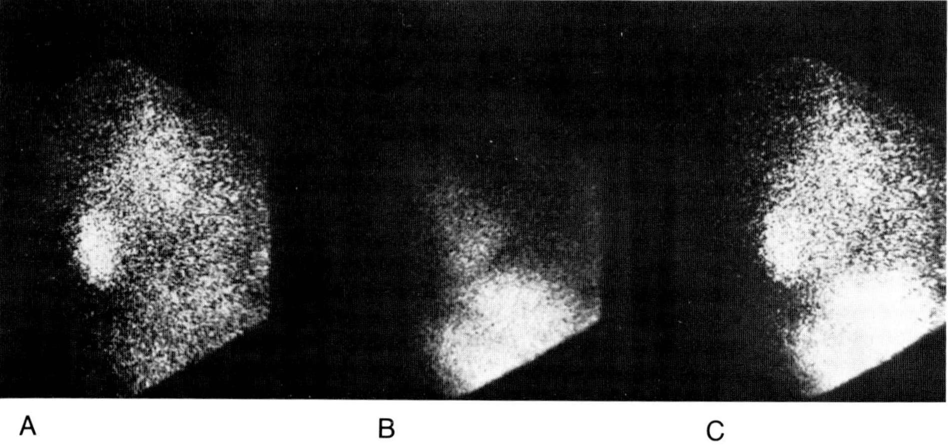

Fig. 3-2 In vivo gamma camera images in a canine model of infarction. **(A)** Iodine-131 antimyosin F(ab′)$_2$ localization in an infarct. **(B)** Thallium-201 distribution in the same animal. **(C)** Composite of both.

is much more readily available, attempts were made to label the antibody fragments with [99m]Tc. After the monoclonal antimyosin antibody Fab fragment was labeled with ^{99m}Tc using the dithionite method described earlier, it was injected into dogs undergoing 3 hours of coronary occlusion followed by reperfusion.[20] There was excellent visualization of the area of the infarction, which became even more intense by 18 hours. However, the presence of ^{99m}Tc colloids during this labeling process led to excessive liver activity, making visualization of the adjacent myocardium difficult. In addition, the labeling process was rather tedious, prompting further search into alternative labeling techniques with different isotopes.

The next step in the development of labeled antibody was the successful labeling of the antimyosin Fab fragments with indium-111 chloride, using DTPA-linked antibodies.[12,19] A transchelation process was carried out using citrate as a weak chelator. The resulting simple addition of indium-111 citrate with DTPA-antibody led to transchelation in about 15 minutes, yielding ^{111}In labeled Fab antibodies.

The use of [111]In Fab antibodies in myocardial necrosis resulted in excellent images with less liver activity and higher specific infarct site localization (Fig. 3-3A,B). The ^{111}In-labeling process seems to be a simple and straightforward procedure that results in excellent image quality. Therefore, this procedure has been adapted for commercial production of the indium-antimyosin antibody-labeling kit.

Comparison with Other Infarct-Imaging Agents

Other agents frequently used in patients with acute myocardial infarction include technetium-99m pyrophosphate and thallium-201. Thallium-201 indicates myocardial perfusion; therefore, areas of myocardial in-farction generally show up as regions of no thallium uptake (cold spots), making quantitation more difficult. By contrast, like antimyosin antibody, technctium-99m pyrophosphate labels the infarcted region, which shows up on the gamma camera image as a hot spot. Technetium-99m pyrophosphate has traditionally been used as the imaging agent to localize the process of myocardial infarction.[3,4] However, recent evidence suggests that localization of pyrophosphate might not be as specific as previously thought, and it may in fact be taken up by reversibly damaged, but ultimately viable, myocardial cells.[26,27] This is especially apparent in the early reperfused myocardium, in which calcium may enter myocardial cells that will ultimately recover but that may transiently take up technetium-99m pyrophosphate nevertheless.[28]

Therefore, a comparison of technetium-99m pyrophosphate and indium-111 antimyosin in infarct localization and infarct sizing was performed in canine models of myocardial infarction using LAD coronary artery occlusion and reperfusion.[29] Initial in vitro studies were carried out to compare blood flow, technetium-99m pyrophosphate, and antimyosin uptake. It was found that in the border zone of the infarct region, where blood flow was intermediate in value between the normal and infarcted area, the pyrophosphate uptake was paradoxically high at 40:1, whereas the antimyosin uptake in the same region was 2:1. This added further evidence to the hypothesis that pyrophosphate may be taken up by noninfarcted myocardium in the margins of infarction receiving borderline blood flow.

Further studies using in vivo imaging confirmed the above findings.[12] When compared with pathologically stained infarct size, the pyrophosphate-delineated area was consistently larger than that from concurrently administered antimyosin (Fig. 3-4). From actual measurements taken, the pyrophosphate

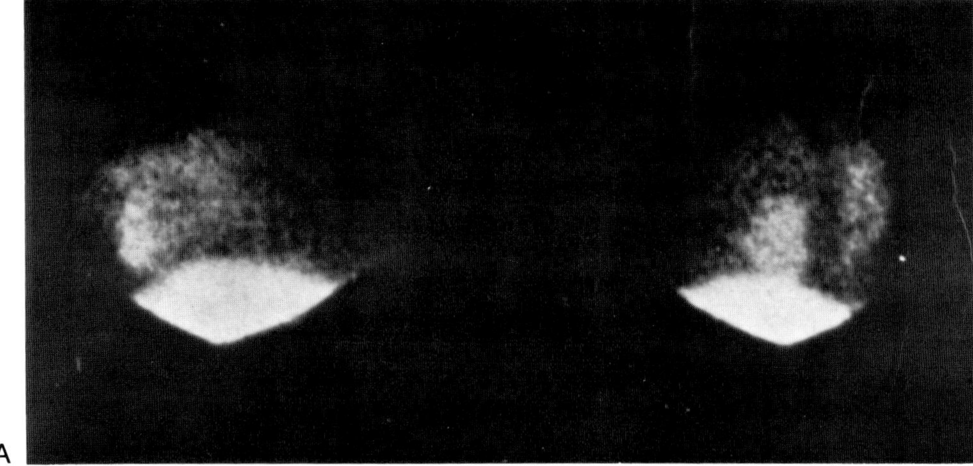

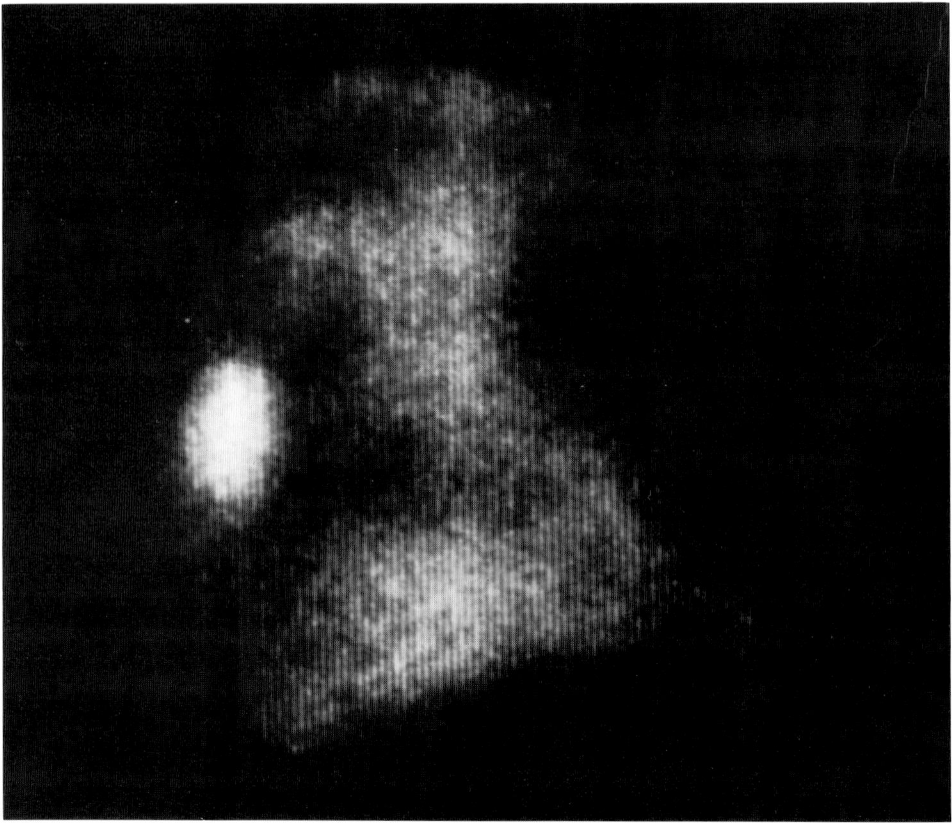

Fig. 3-3 Indium-111 monoclonal antimyosin antibody images in a canine model of infarction. **(A)** Lateral (*left*) and anteroposterior (*right*). There was good myocardial localization of labeled antibody. **(B)** Five hours after IV injection. Note high specific localization in the myocardial infarct region, with low blood pool and liver activity.

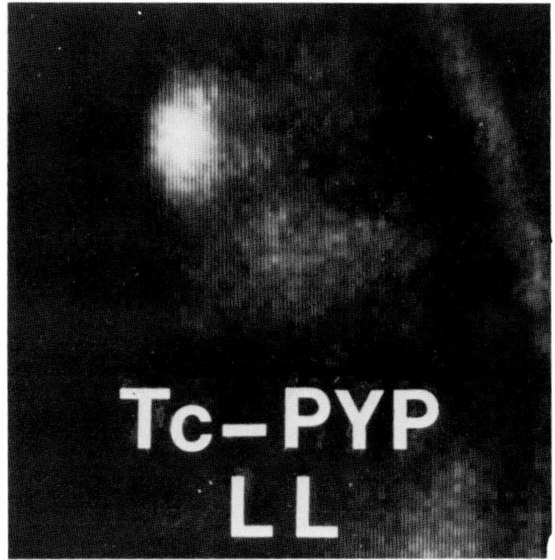

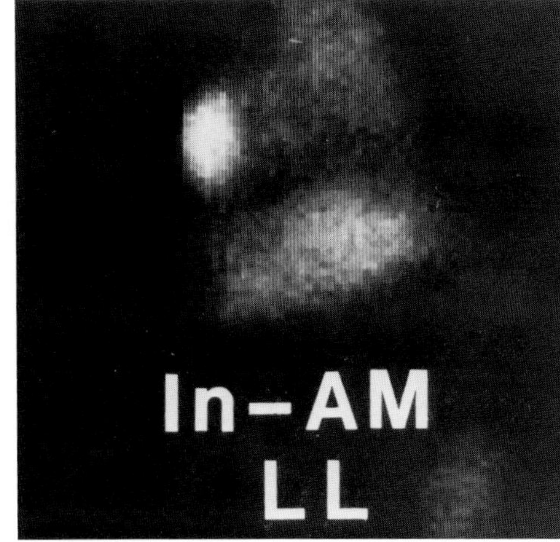

Fig. 3-4 Images of simultaneously administered technetium-99m pyrophosphate **(A)** and indium-111 antimyosin Fab **(B)** obtained in a canine 3-hour occlusion-reperfusion model of infarction. As can be seen, the pyrophosphate infarct uptake is larger than the corresponding antimyosin uptake.

infarct size is approximately 1.4 times that of the antimyosin infarct size. This does not mean that technetium-99m pyrophosphate is not clinically useful, but it may overestimate the area of irreversible injury, especially in the setting of early reperfusion, by including areas of ischemic but not irreversibly injured cells.

Acute Myocarditis

Beyond ischemic myocardial injury, other disease processes that result in myocardial necrosis may also be diagnosed by labeled antimyosin antibody imaging. Ohkusa et al.[30] produced a model of murine myocarditis using encephalomyocarditis virus inoculation. Labeled antimyosin uptake into the myocardium was found to be related to the degree of cellular necrosis and injury. Since myocarditis tends to be a patchy process, and its diagnosis may be missed by myocardial biopsy, labeled antimyosin may evolve to be an extremely important diagnostic tool.

Acute Cardiac Allograft Rejection

Another clinical situation involving generalized necrosis of myocardial cells is that of cardiac transplant rejection. Addonizio et al.[31] studied the efficacy of ^{111}In-labeled antimyosin Fab to quantify canine cardiac allograft rejection with both planar and tomographic scans.[31] Indium-111 antimyosin uptake was not seen in native untransplanted healthy hearts, but the faint diffuse uptake in the nonrejecting transplanted hearts that were undergoing long-term immunosuppression suggested mild chronic myocyte loss. However, there was dramatic and intense uptake of labeled antimyosin antibody in allograft hearts showing electrocardiographic (ECG) evidence of transplant rejection. The uptake of antimyosin correlated closely with the histopathologic score of rejection. These encouraging results suggest that ^{111}In antibody can detect the presence, location, and severity of cardiac transplant rejection.

TECHNIQUES OF IMAGING PATIENTS WITH ANTIMYOSIN ANTIBODIES

The successful completion of the above experimental studies led to the clinical trial of the labeled antibodies in patients with acute myocardial infarction, as seen in the typical acute care setting, and with other disease processes involving myocardial necrosis.

Imaging Protocol with Antimyosin Antibodies

The first clinical experience with antimyosin antibodies was with the [99mTc]-labeled Fab fragments in patients with acute myocardial infarction. The patients were studied soon after their presentation to the hospital with acute myocardial infarction, and 30 mCi of [99mTc]-labeled antimyosin Fab antibody was injected intravenously to permit localization and quantitation of their myocardial infarction.

Because of relatively prolonged blood pool residence of the antibody prior to specific infarct localization, a gated radionuclide angiogram in multiple views can be carried out in the standard views soon after injection, either in the intensive care unit or in the nuclear medicine laboratory. Using this strategy, information on wall-motion abnormalities can also be obtained in conjunction with the infarct estimation, without exposing the patient to any additional radiation.

The initial blood pool activity disappears with time, and the image for infarct localization and sizing can be obtained as early as 9 to 12 hours after injection. Avoidance of colloidal contamination by using fresh dithionite reducing agents can further enhance the target-to-background ratio. An example

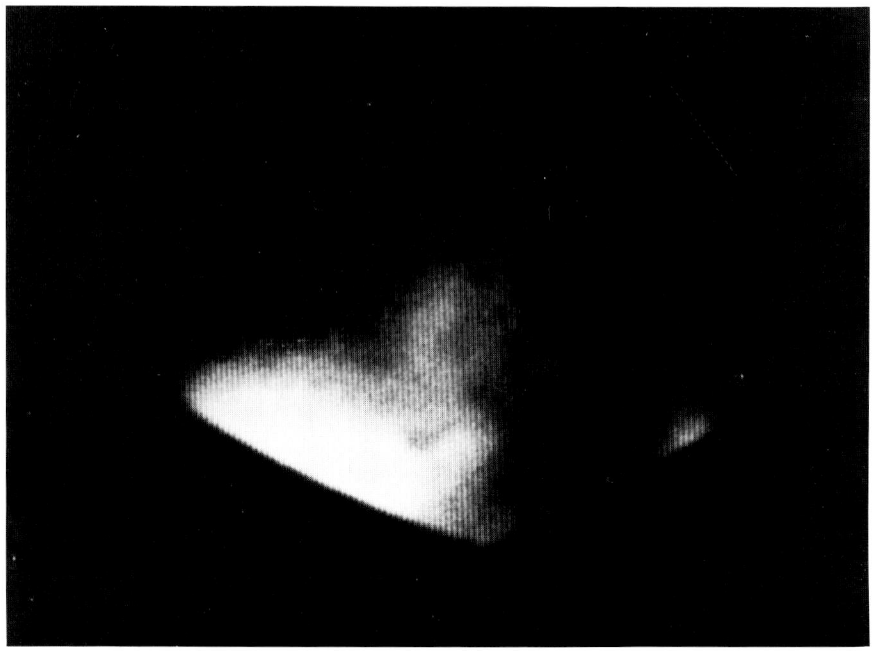

Fig. 3-5 Example of a left lateral [99mTc]-labeled antimyosin Fab image in a patient with acute myocardial infarction. Note the liver uptake due to colloidal contamination.

of a ^{99m}Tc-labeled antimyosin antibody image is shown in Figure 3-5.

In an acute care setting, ungated images in the anterior and LAO 45-degree views are the most useful and practical. The images can be taken with either a general-purpose or a high-resolution parallel hole collimator, with the image accumulated for 1 million counts. For improved infarct localization, emission tomographic images can also be obtained by imaging the patient continuously in a circular orbit at 3-degree increments for a total of either 180 or 360 degrees. The images can then be reconstructed in transverse or short axis views for visualization and quantitation of infarct size.

Indium-111-labeled monoclonal antimyosin can be employed in a manner similar to the ^{99m}Tc-labeled antibody. Because the DTPA, a bifunctional chelate, is already covalently linked to the antibody, preparation of the imaging agent is extremely easy. The only step required is the actual mixing of indium-111 chloride with the prechelated antibody in citrate. Because of the much longer half-life of ^{111}In (67 hours as compared with 6 hours for ^{99m}Tc), imaging can be performed 16 to 48 hours after injection, adding to the flexibility of timing in imaging using this agent. The image is usually taken with a medium-energy collimator and accumulated for 1 million counts. An example is shown in Figure 3-6. Similar to ^{99m}Tc-labeled antimyosin antibodies, tomographic images can also be readily obtained with ^{111}In-labeled antimyosin antibody. An example is illustrated in Figure 3-7.

CLINICAL STUDIES WITH LABELED ANTIMYOSIN ANTIBODIES

Acute Myocardial Infarction

Clinical studies using ^{99m}Tc-labeled antimyosin antibodies are being evaluated in patients with acute myocardial infarction. Khaw et

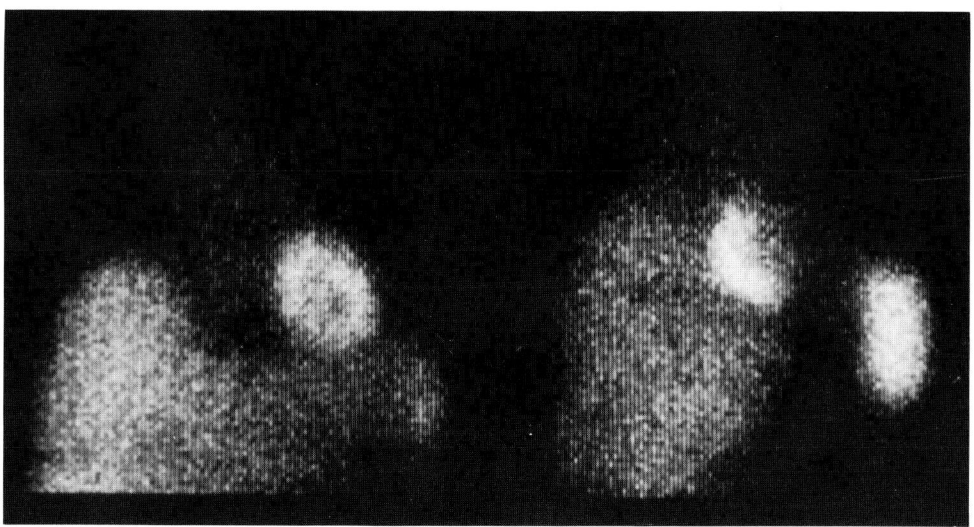

Fig. 3-6 Example of indium-111 antimyosin Fab images in the anterior (*left*) and LAO (*right*) views from a patient with acute anterior wall myocardial infarction. Note the excellent target-to-background ratio.

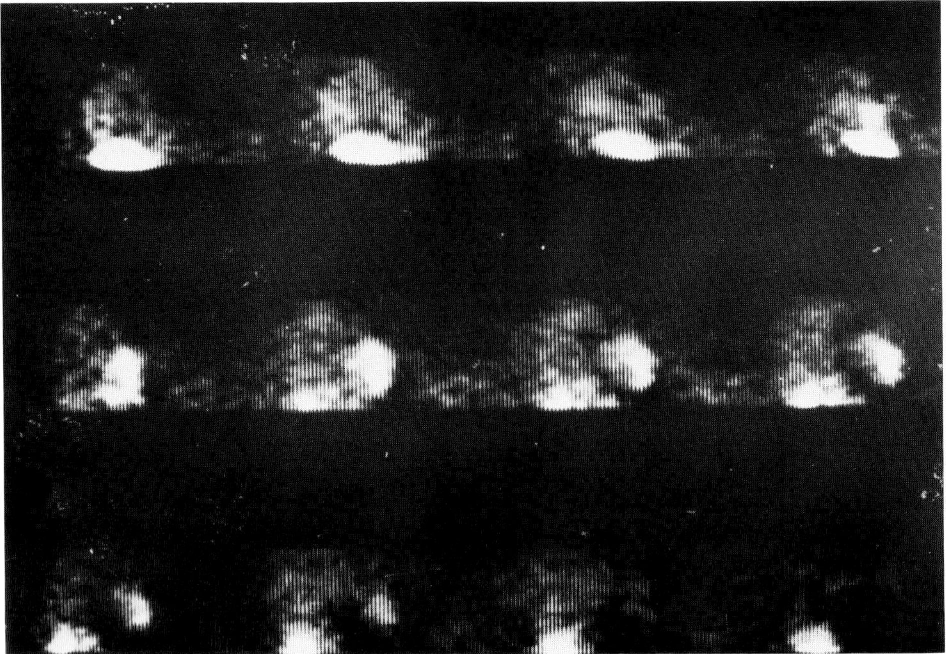

Fig. 3-7 Single photon sagittal tomograms in a patient with acute myocardial infarction given IV indium-111 antimyosin Fab. The sagittal images were reconstructed from the patient's right to left side and show good infarct localization.

al.[32] studied 30 patients who presented to the emergency department of the Massachusetts General Hospital with acute myocardial infarction, characterized by typical chest pain, ST-segment elevation with evolution to infarct pattern, and CK elevation above twice normal. Technetium-99m-labeled antimyosin Fab fragment was given within 24 hours of admission to the hospital, imaged using the above protocol between 6 to 24 hours after injection. Compared with quantitative regional wall-motion analysis using contrast angiography at 10 to 14 days and peak CK release, there was a good correlation between the size of myocardial necrosis indicated by labeled antibody and the extent of hypokinetic segments on angiography ($r=0.79$, $P=0.002$), and peak creatine kinase ($r=0.90$, $P=<0.01$).

Therefore, it is very clear that antimyosin antibody can detect the extent of myocardial necrosis in patients, and correlates closely with the degree of myocardial dysfunction. It is interesting that when compared with the technetium-99m pyrophosphate scan done in the same patients 3 days later, the infarct localization is similar using the two agents, but again the infarct size is distinctly bigger in the pyrophosphate scan (average 1.7 times). Therefore, labeled antimyosin antibody may be a more accurate technique with which to estimate the myocardial infarct size, especially during acute myocardial infarction with or without coronary reperfusion.

To quantitate myocardial infarct size more precisely, Yasuda et al.[33] used tomography and ^{99m}Tc-labeled monoclonal antimyosin antibody in patients with myocardial infarction. The results showed a good correlation with CK release and corresponding angiographic abnormalities.

The important clinical question that arises in this setting is whether antimyosin antibody has any prognostic value, bearing in mind the original relationship between infarct size and prognosis. Liu et al.[34] studied a similar group of patients with acute myocardial infarction and quantitated their infarct size with ^{99m}Tc-labeled antimyosin antibody. Subsequent follow-up at an average of 15 months indicated that when compared with other acute peri-infarction prognostic indicators, such as peak CK, ejection fraction, ST-segment changes, or Killip's hemodynamic classification using logistic regression analysis, the best indicator of future complication and mortality is, in fact, infarct size by antimyosin antibody scanning. Thus, antimyosin antibody has now been shown to have clinical value not only in the detection of myocardial infarction, but also in the localization and sizing of infarcts to provide prognostic information regarding mortality and morbidity.

In the current setting of interventional treatment during acute myocardial infarction, patients often receive reperfusion therapy using either intravenous thrombolytic agents or percutaneous transluminal angioplasty alone or in combination. Therefore, the ability to assess the extent of myocardial necrosis accurately will be extremely important in both determining the success of therapy and deciding on follow-up treatment. For example, in a patient showing excellent successful reperfusion with little necrosis, but evidence of ongoing ischemia, further revascularization procedures such as angioplasty or bypass surgery are indicated. By contrast, if extensive necrosis has already occurred, further reperfusion or revascularization is unlikely to be of immediate benefit and, in fact, may be detrimental.

Clinical Myocarditis

In parallel with the studies done in animal models of myocarditis, clinical myocarditis has now been studied with indium-111 antimyosin antibody and compared with pathologic evidence of myocarditis on myocardial biopsy. An example of a patient with myo-carditis and a positive antimyosin scan is shown in Figure 3-6. Yasuda et al.[35,36] performed both right ventricular biopsy and antimyosin antibody imaging in 24 patients with suspected clinical myocarditis. The antimyosin antibody scan was shown to be extremely sensitive. Of seven patients showing myocarditis on biopsy, all had positive antimyosin scans. None of the negative scans had a positive biopsy. But an additional seven patients with no evidence of myocarditis on biopsy also had positive antimyosin scans. All these patients had distinct clinical symptoms of myocarditis, while 5 had rapid improvement in ejection fraction with time, compatible with the course of myocarditis. This supports the contention that the antimyosin scan is probably more sensitive in detecting myocarditis than myocardial biopsy, perhaps because of the patchy nature of the myocarditic process itself, which can easily be missed on a selective myocardial biopsy.

A follow-up study in patients with dilated cardiomyopathy imaged with indium-111 antimyosin antibody was recently reported by Palacios et al.[37] Of 30 patients with dilated cardiomyopathy who underwent antimyosin antibody scans, 17 patients demonstrated initial antibody uptake. Subsequently, improvement in ejection fraction at 6 months follow-up was seen in a significant number of patients, but it most frequently occurred in patients with initial positive antimyosin antibody scans. In addition, those who did show improvement with initially positive scans had negative antibody scans on subsequent follow-up. These studies indicate again that the antimyosin antibody scan is not only useful in the diagnosis of myocarditis with high sensitivity but also has a significant prognostic role in these patients.

Other Clinical Uses of Antimyosin Antibodies

Preliminary work is also now under way in patients with cardiac transplants, to detect potential sensitivity and timing of transplant rejection using labeled antibodies.[38] Other studies have also shown preliminary encouraging results in patients with right ventricular infarction, in delineating the extent of right ventricular infarct, and in quantitating its size.[39]

Safety of Use of Antimyosin Antibodies

The use of antibodies in clinical situations always engenders the potential possibility of eliciting an acute allergic reaction or late serum sickness because of the presence of foreign protein derived from the antibody source. However, the amount of Fab fragments of the antibody used (100 to 600 μg) is unlikely to elicit any antibody or recall response in patients. The amount of antibody is much less than that used in current tumor-detection or -treatment protocols. Khaw et al.[40] performed intradermal tests on all patients before administering antimyosin antibody, and did not have any positive skin-test reaction to either the rabbit polyclonal antibody or the murine monoclonal antibody. More recently, in patients with cardiac transplantation imaged repeatedly with antimyosin antibody, there also has not been any adverse reaction on rechallenge with the same labeled agent. Therefore, antimyosin antibody appears to be an effective imaging agent that is safe for human use.

FUTURE TRENDS

Further improvement on the labeled antimyosin antibody is currently under way. One of the present limitations of antibody imaging is the prolonged half-life of Fab fragments in the plasma, precluding earlier imaging. To accelerate blood clearance and permit earlier imaging, monoclonal antimyosin antibody has been linked to DTPA-succinylpolylysine.[40] There is no loss of antigen affinity using this labeling technique, but there is a dramatic change in the in vivo biodistribution properties favoring greater target-to-background activities.[41] In canine models of myocardial infarction, the first images can be obtained within ½ hour of injection, showing great promise of this approach to permit earlier imaging.[40]

Other possible modifications include the use of other isotopes and labeling techniques, such as ^{123}I, with its excellent gamma camera imaging characteristics. Khaw et al.[42] showed that infarction can be visualized within 1 hour of administration with excellent 5-hour images showing little blood pool activity by using ^{123}I-labeled antimyosin antibody.[42] In addition, there was no hepatic uptake at all. This finding suggests that iodinated antibody may indeed be better than chelated antibody for myocardial infarct imaging purposes. Other alternative techniques of labeling antibody with ^{99m}Tc are also being explored by several groups and may still ultimately turn out to be the best label for these agents. However, significant research would be necessary before this improvement could be realized in a clinical application.

SUMMARY

Labeled antimyosin antibodies represent a significant step forward in the diagnosis and quantitation of myocardial necrosis. The labeling process has also improved from initial iodination of antibodies to current complexing with multivalent cationic isotopes using chelating agents. Basic science studies have demonstrated the extreme specificity of these agents in delineating myocardial necrosis, which appear to be more accurate than technetium-99m pyrophosphate. Preliminary clinical studies have shown exciting results in the detection, quantitation, and prognostication of acute myocardial infarction, myocarditis, and cardiac transplantation. Further improvements in techniques of antibody labeling and increasing clinical experience will establish the place of these agents in diagnostic nuclear medicine.

REFERENCES

1. Rude RE, Muller JE, Braunwald E: Efforts to limit the size of myocardial infarcts. Ann Intern Med 95:736, 1981
2. Sobel BE, Bresnahan GF, Shell WE, Yoder RD: Estimation of infarct size in man and its relation to prognosis. Circulation 46:640, 1972
3. Buja LM, Parkey RW, Dees JH, et al: Morphologic correlates of technetium-99m stannous pyrophosphate imaging of acute myocardial infarction in dogs. Circulation 52:596, 1975
4. Falkoff M, Parkey RW, Bonte FJ, et al: Technetium-99m stannous pyrophosphate myocardial scitigraphy: Serial imaging to detect myocardial infarcts in patients. Clin Cardiol 1:163, 1978
5. Jennings RB, Reimer KA: Lethal myocardial ischemic injury. Am J Pathol 102:241, 1981
6. Reimer KA, Jennings RB, Tatum AH: Pathobiology of acute myocardial ischemia: Metabolic, functional and ultrastructural studies. Am J Cardiol 52:72A, 1983
7. Roberts R, Sobel BE. Creatine kinase isoenzymes in the assessment of heart disease. Am Heart J 95:521, 1978
8. Reimer KA, Martonffy K, Schumacher BL, et al: Localization of 99m-Tc-labeled pyrophosphate and calcium in myocardial infarcts after temporary coronary occlusion in dogs. Proc Soc Exp Biol Med 156:272, 1977
9. Khaw BA, Beller GA, Haber E: Experimental myocardial infarct imaging following intravenous administration of iodine-131 labeled antibody F(ab')$_2$ fragments specific for cardiac myosin. Circulation 57:743, 1978
10. Khaw BA, Fallon JT, Beller GA, Haber E: Specificity of localization of myosin specific antibody fragments in experimental myocardial infarction: Histologic, histochemical, autoradiographic and scintigraphic studies. Circulation 60:1527, 1979
11. Khaw BA, Gold HK, Leinbach RC, et al: Early weighing of experimental myocardial infarction by intracoronary administration of ^{131}P-labeled anti–cardiac myosin (Fab')$_2$ fragments. Circulation 58:1137, 1978
12. Khaw BA, Beller GA, Haber E, Smith TW: Localization of cardiac myosin-specific antibody in myocardial infarction. J Clin Invest 58:439, 1976
13. Khaw BA, Strauss HW, Moore R, et al: Myocardial damage delineated by Indium-111 antimyosin Fab and Technetium-99m pyrophosphate. J Nucl Med 28:76, 1987
14. Khaw BA, Gold HK, Fallon JT, Haber E: Detection of serum cardiac myosin light chains in acute experimental myocardial infarction: Radioimmunoassay of cardiac myosin light chains. Circulation 58:1130, 1978
15. Katus HA, Yasuda T, Gold HK, et al: Diagnosis of acute myocardial infarction by detection of circulating cardiac myosin light chains. Am J Cardiol 54:964, 1984
16. Liu P, Yasuda T, Strauss HW, et al: Infarct sizing using serial radioimmunoassay of serum myosin light chains. J Am Coll Cardiol 7(suppl):115A, 1986
17. Pressman D, Keighley G: The zone of activity of antibodies as determined by the use of radioactive tracers: The zone of activity of nephritoxic antikidney serum. J Immunol 59:141, 1948
18. Khaw BA, Strauss HW, Carvalho A, et al: Technetium-99m labeling of antibodies to cardiac myosin Fab and to human fibrinogen. J Nucl Med 23:1011, 1982
19. Khaw BA, Mattis JA, Melincoff G, et al: Monoclonal antibody to cardiac myosin: Imaging of experimental myocardial infarction. Hybridoma 3:11, 1984
20. Eckelman WC, Paik CH, Reba RC: Radiolabeling of antibodies. Cancer Res 40:3036, 1980
21. Hunter WM, Greenwood FC: Preparation of iodine-131 labeled human growth hormones of high specific activity. Nature (Lond) 194:495, 1962
22. Khaw BA, Gold HK, Leinbach RC, et al: Early imaging of experimental myocardial infarction by intracoronary administration of I-131-labeled anticardiac myosin (Fab')$_2$ fragments. Circulation 58:1137, 1978
23. Khaw BA, Fallon JT, Strauss HW, Haber E: Myocardial infarct imaging with indium-111-diethylene triamine pentaacetic acid-anticanine cardiac myosin antibodies. Science 209:295, 1980

24. Khaw BA, Scott J, Fallon JT, et al: Myocardial injury: Quantitation by cell sorting initiated with antimyosin fluorescent spheres. Science 217:1050, 1982

25. Nolan AC, Clark WA, Karwoski T, Zak R: Patterns of cellular injury in myocardial ischemia determined by monoclonal antimyosin. Proc Natl Acad Sci USA 80:6046, 1983

26. Bianco JA, Kemper AJ, Taylor A, et al: Technetium-99m pyrophosphate in ischemic and infarcted dog myocardium in the early stages of acute coronary occlusion: Histochemical and tissue-counting comparisons. J Nucl Med 24:485, 1983

27. Gerber KH, Higgins, CB: Quantitation of size of myocardial infarctions by computerized transmission tomography. Comparison with hot-spot and cold-spot radionuclide scans. Invest Radiol 18:238, 1983

28. Jansen ED, Corbett JR, Buja LM, et al: Quantification of myocardial injury produced by temporary coronary artery occlusion and reflow with technetium-99m-pyrophosphate. Circulation 75:611, 1986

29. Beller GA, Khaw BA, Haber E, Smith TW: Localization of radiolabeled cardiac myosin-specific antibody in myocardial infarcts: Comparison with technetium-99m stannous pyrophosphate. Circulation 55:74, 1977

30. Ohkusa T, Matsumori A, Matoba Y, et al: Antimyosin monoclonal antibody Fab imaging of experimental viral myocarditis. Circulation 78(II):492, 1988

31. Addonizio LJ, Michler RE, Marboe C, et al: Imaging of cardiac allograft rejection in dogs using indium-111 monoclonal antimyosin Fab. J Am Coll Cardiol 9:555, 1987

32. Khaw BA, Gold HK, Yasuda T, et al: Scintigraphic quantification of myocardial necrosis in patients after intravenous injection of myosin-specific antibody. Circulation 74:501, 1986

33. Yasuda T, Khaw BA, Gold HK, et al: Quantitation of myocardial necrosis with Tc-99m-monoclonal antimyosin Fab and single photon emission tomography. J Nucl Med 24:P37, 1984 (abst)

34. Liu P, Yasuda T, Newell J, et al: Infarct sizing by Tc-99m labeled antimyosin antibody: A powerful predictor of complications of myocardial infarction. Circulation 70(II):123, 1984

35. Yasuda T, Palacios IF, Dec W, et al: In-111 monoclonal antimyosin antibody imaging in the diagnosis of acute myocarditis. Circulation 76:306, 1987

36. Yasuda T, Palacios IF, Khaw BA, et al: Monoclonal indium-111 antimyosin antibody imaging versus right ventricular biopsy in the diagnosis of acute myocarditis. J Nucl Med 28:910, 1987

37. Palacios I, Yasuda T, Khaw BA, et al: Indium-111 antimyosin antibody imaging in the follow-up of patients with acute dilated cardiomyopathy. Circulation 74(II):142, 1986

38. Ueda K, Takeda K, LaFrance ND, Solez K, et al: Is In-111 antimyosin antibody a useful diagnostic marker for evaluation of early cardiac allograft rejection? Transplant Proc 20:778, 1988

39. Yamaoki K, Isobe M, Tsuchimochi H, et al: Imaging for right ventricular infarction by single photon emission tomography with labeled anticardiac monoclonal antibody in dog. Circulation 74(II):297, 1986

40. Khaw BA, Torchilin VP, Struass HW, et al: DTPA-polylysine linked monoclonal antimyosin localization in acute experimental myocardial infarction. J Nucl Med 27:909, 1986

41. Torchilin VP, Klibanov AL, Nossiff ND, et al: Monoclonal antibody modification with chelate-linked high-molecular-weight polymers: Major increase in polyvalent cation binding without loss of antigen binding. Hybridoma 6:229, 1987

42. Khaw BA, Kanke M, Powers J, et al: Improved selective localization of experimental myocardial infarcts utilizing new I-123 labeled monoclonal antimyosin Fab. Circulation 74(II):296, 1986

4

Radionuclide Imaging of Resting Cardiac Function

Mark R. Starling
Ralph Blumhardt

The application of radionuclide imaging to assessing left ventricular ejection fraction is well accepted. There are, however, two major developments in radionuclide imaging of the heart, which have expanded the indications for this technique: (1) the development of radionuclide methods for assessing both right and left ventricular volumes and performance, and (2) the use of radionuclide imaging for assessing prognosis in patients with cardiopulmonary pathology. The emphasis in this chapter is, therefore, on the application of radionuclide imaging to these important areas of recent development.

ASSESSING THE LEFT VENTRICLE

Left Ventricular Volumes

Several techniques employing first-transit or equilibrium radionuclide imaging have been developed for assessing left ventricular volumes.[1-9] There are two general approaches to calculating left ventricular volumes: (1) geometric, and (2) count-based approaches. Massie et al.[1] compared radionuclide geometric and count-based methods for calculating left ventricular volumes; these investigators reported that the equilibrium radionuclide count-based (i.e., nongeometric) approach provided the highest correlation and lowest standard error compared with multiple first-transit and/or equilibrium radionuclide geometric approaches for estimating left ventricular volumes. Thus, this count-based approach proved the most accurate radionuclide technique and permitted multiple determinations of left ventricular volumes to be accomplished from a single dose of radioisotope.

Several equilibrium radionuclide count-based methods of calculating left ventricular volumes have been evaluated.[2-8] These methods have all used background-corrected left ventricular end-diastolic and end-systolic counts obtained from semiautomated or hand-drawn regions of interest that have also been normalized for frame duration, cardiac cycles acquired, and plasma count activity. Dehmer et al.[2] compared count-based equilibrium radionuclide left ventricular volume indices with left ventricular volumes obtained using cineangiography and reported correlations (r = 0.98–0.99). These investigators further validated this approach by comparing radionuclide stroke volume indices to stroke volumes obtained using the thermodi-

lution technique.[3] Calculating radionuclide left ventricular volume indices,[2,6,7] however, requires regression equation correction of these indices to absolute left ventricular volumes. This regression equation correction represents an average attenuation correction. This kind of correction may not be appropriate for all patients, since each patient attenuates differently.

There are theoretical advantages to individualizing the correction for attenuation in each patient to obtain absolute left ventricular volumes. Starling et al.,[6] in fact, demonstrated

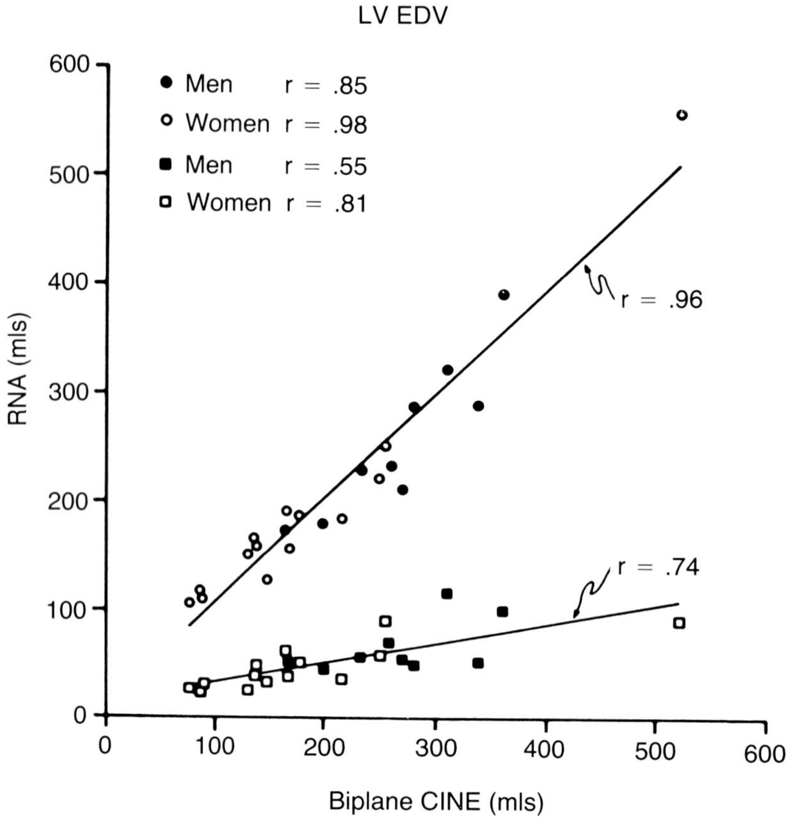

Fig. 4-1 Relationship between uncorrected (□, ■) and attenuation-corrected (○, ●) gated equilibrium radionuclide angiographic (RNA) left ventricular (LV) end-diastolic volumes (EDV), on the ordinate, is compared with the corresponding biplane contrast cineangiographic (CINE) LV EDV measures, on the abscissa. Individual regression lines and correlation coefficients are shown. (From Starling et al.,[6] with permission.)

that the correlation coefficients and range of left ventricular volume estimates obtained using an individualized attenuation-correction technique are superior to those obtained from regression equation–corrected left ventricular volume indices (Fig. 4-1). This has also been demonstrated by Burow et al.[7] for radionuclide stroke volumes. Thus, individualizing the attenuation correction for calculating left ventricular volumes is important for improving the precision of the radionuclide volume estimates.

The methods of obtaining individualized attenuation correction factors in patients have varied.[5–8] One simple geometric approach, described by Starling et al.,[5,6] uses anatomic landmarks identified on the equilibrium radionuclide angiogram in the left anterior oblique (LAO) and anterior view to obtain a distance measurement (Fig. 4-2). Using this distance and the camera obliquity, the distance from the left ventricular geometric center of mass to the gamma camera in the LAO view is calculated. This distance, combined with an approximate linear attenuation coefficient for ^{99m}Tc in water of 0.15 cm^{-1}, yields an individualized attenuation correction factor. Other investigators have obtained this distance by computer algorithm,[4] while still others have calculated individual buildup factors assuming a constant distance to obtain these correction factors.[8] Irrespective of the technique employed, one or another assumption is made that establish these methods as approximations. In contrast, Corbett et al.[9] demonstrated that tomographic equilibrium radionuclide left ventricular end–diastolic and end–systolic volumes correlated with the corresponding cineangiographic left ventricular volume measurements ($r = 0.82$ and 0.93, respectively). The tomographic approach also provided a better detection of left ventricular wall-motion abnormalities in patients with coronary artery disease, as compared with the standard radionuclide technique.

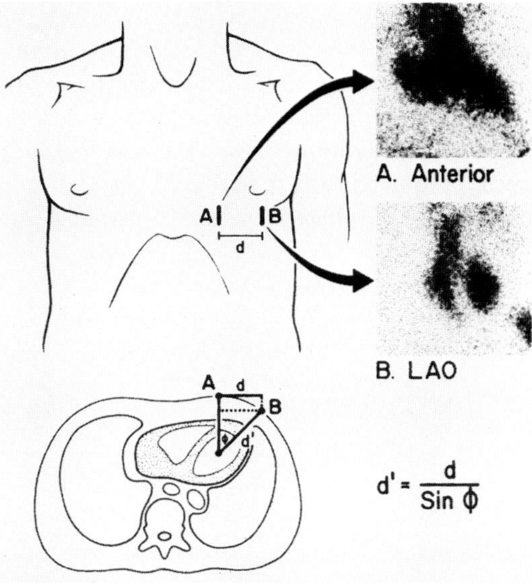

Fig. 4-2 Method of obtaining the horizontal distance d for calculating the distance from the left ventricular (LV) center of mass to the camera in the 45-degree left anterior oblique (LAO) projection for attenuation correction. With the camera in the anterior **(A)** and LAO **(B)** projections, the ^{99m}Tc point source is placed over the LV and marks are placed on the anterior chest wall (left). The horizontal distance between the two marks is measured and the distance d' from the LV center of mass to the camera in the LAO projection is calculated (lower right). (From Starling et al.[5] with permission.)

Similar findings have been reported by Bunker et al.[10] Thus, this tomographic approach to calculating left ventricular volumes may alleviate the necessity for attenuation correction and provide additional information concerning regional wall-motion abnormalities.

Left Ventricular Contractility

One of the most interesting applications of these radionuclide left ventricular volume techniques is calculating contractile function based on the pressure-volume analysis described by Sagawa.[11] This concept of left ventricular contractility suggests that when end-systolic pressure-volume points obtained from multiple pressure-volume loops in the same heart are linearly regressed, the maximum slope value E_{max} reflects contractile function as long as heart rate and basal contractile state remain unaffected by changes in loading condition (Fig. 4-3). Kronenberg et al.[12] evaluated this pressure-volume relationship using radionuclide and contrast cineangiographic left ventricular volumes and high-fidelity pressure recordings in animals. Although the mean slope of the radionuclide end-systolic pressure-volume relations underestimated that calculated by cineangiography, the slope values correlated ($r = 0.81$). Similar comparisons have been made in patients, by Starling et al.[13] These investigators demonstrated that the radionuclide and biplane cineangiographic end-systolic pressure-volume relations also correlated ($r = 0.98$). Thus, these data in animals and in human subjects suggest that equilibrium radionuclide left ventricular volumes may be combined with high-fidelity left ventricular

pressure measurements to obtain indices of left ventricular contractility, which may be very important in understanding the effects of pathologic processes on the left venticular myocardium.

Left Ventricular Ejection Fraction

GLOBAL EJECTION FRACTION

Both the first-transit and equilibrium radionuclide approach to obtaining measures of left ventricular systolic function, (i.e., ejection fraction) have correlated with the corresponding cineangiographic measurements. Folland et al.[14] demonstrated that first-transit left ventricular ejection fractions correlated with those by cineangiography ($r = 0.86$), the equilibrium radionuclide ejection fraction determinations also correlated with those by cineangiography ($r = 0.84$), and the two radionuclide techniques correlated with each

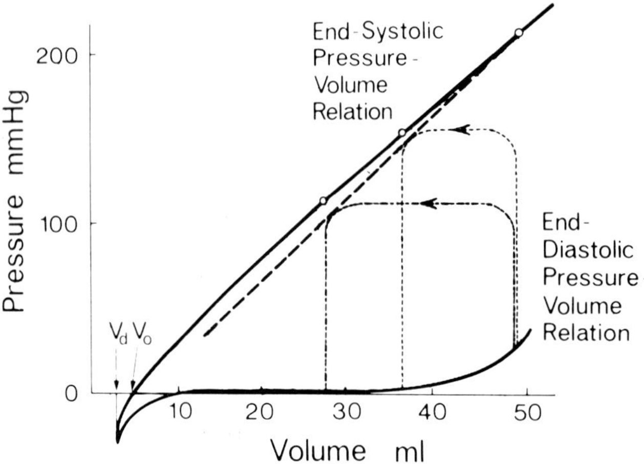

Fig. 4-3 Schematic diagram showing the end-systolic pressure-volume relationships and its extrapolated volume-axis intercept V_0 are shown (O—O—O). Three isovolumic pressures with the slope of the line representing the isovolumic length-tension relations. (---) End-systolic pressure-volume relationship obtained from two ejecting contraction loops from the same heart, Note the similarity to the isovolumic, length-tension relations. (From Sagawa,[11] with permission.)

other ($r = 0.87$). These correlations for both the first-transit and equilibrium radionuclide left ventricular ejection fraction calculations in comparison with the cineangiographic left ventricular ejection fractions have been confirmed by several investigators. The technique used to process the equilibrium radionuclide images for left ventricular ejection fraction may be very important. Generally, a semiautomated edge detection algorithm is used to produce a variable region of interest from end-diastole throughout the cardiac cycle to obtain end-diastolic and end-systolic counts for calculation of the ejection fraction. This assumes that (1) left ventricular counts are proportionate to volumes, (2) the change in counts is proportionate to the change in volume, (3) the change in counts divided by end-diastolic counts yields an accurate ejection fraction, and (4) the radioisotope is evenly distributed within the left ventricular blood pool and also that the contribution of count activity within the regions of interest due to overlying and underlying structures can be excluded by background subtraction. The accuracy of the left ventricular ejection fraction calculation is therefore dependent on the accuracy of the left ventricular regions of interest determined by the edge detection algorithm and the background region of interest. Background can significantly influence the left ventricular ejection fraction in that overestimation of background will artificially increase ejection fraction, while underestimation of background can artificially reduce ejection fraction. The radionuclide methodology used in determining left ventricular ejection fraction must therefore be well validated in each laboratory to establish the accuracy of the left ventricular performance estimates.

REGIONAL EJECTION FRACTION

Several methods have been developed for assessing regional left ventricular ejection frac-

tions from radionuclide images.[15,16] Maddox et al.[15] demonstrated that a single modified LAO projection yielded regional changes in background-corrected counts in each of three anatomic regions (i.e., septal, inferoapical, and posterolateral) that separated normal from hypokinetic and akinetic segments. The individual regions used in the analysis of regional left ventricular function can be correlated with individual coronary perfusion beds.

Functional images have also been developed to assist with the visual analysis of left ventricular wall motion. Stroke volume images can be obtained by subtracting the end-systolic from the end-diastolic image, and an ejection fraction image can be constructed by dividing the stroke volume image by the end-diastolic image.[17] In addition, a paradox image can be derived by subtracting an end-diastolic from an end-systolic image so that dyskinetic regions can be identified by positive counts, indicating relatively greater volume during systole than during diastole.[18] These observations have been shown to be reasonably accurate determinations of regional dyskinesia in comparison with that noted on contrast cineangiography. Thus, in clinical circumstances in which regional function is important, these parametric radionuclide images may enhance our subjective interpretation of left ventricular wall motion.

Prognostic Importance of Left Ventricular Ejection Fraction

One of the areas in which the radionuclide determination of left ventricular ejection fraction has been of particular value is in defining prognosis in patients with various cardiovascular disease processes. Patients can be stratified on the basis of the prediction of in-hospital mortality and complications following an acute myocardial infarction, the long-term prognosis for patients surviving an acute myocardial infarction, long-term survival in patients with valvular heart disease, and the prediction of the effects of certain antineoplastic medications on myocardial performance.

ACUTE MYOCARDIAL INFARCTION

The initial studies employing radionuclide imaging in acute myocardial infarction attempted to establish the effects of acute myocardial infarction on left ventricular performance and to prognosticate in-hospital cardiac events. Schelbert et al.[19] reported that the radionuclide left ventricular ejection fraction averaged 52 ± 5 percent in 27 patients with an uncomplicated myocardial infarction, 40 ± 5 percent in patients with mild to moderate left ventricular failure (P<0.001), and 33 ± 7 percent in patients with pulmonary edema (P<0.001). Importantly, during the early postinfarction period, the radionuclide left ventricular ejection fraction demonstrated improvement in 55 percent of patients and remained unchanged or decreased in the remaining 45 percent. Patients with an initial low or decreasing radionuclide left ventricular ejection fraction had a significantly greater incidence of early mortality or left ventricular dysfunction compared with those in whom ejection fraction was normal or improved early after infarction (P<0.02).

These observations on early morbidity and mortality have been confirmed by others. Shah et al.[20] reported that in patients experiencing their first acute transmural myocardial infarction, subsequent complications, including congestive heart failure, hypotension, shock, postinfarction angina, or death, developed in patients with a lower mean radionuclide left ventricular ejection fraction (34 ± 10 percent) than in patients whose hospital course was uncomplicated (52 ± 13 percent, P<0.001). In their population of 56 patients,

7 patients died acutely within 14 days of their infarction, and their radionuclide left ventricular ejection fraction was only 27 ± 11 percent compared with survivors in whom it was 46 ± 13 percent (P<0.001). Similarly, Abrams et al.[21] evaluated the importance of the radionuclide left ventricular ejection fraction in patients with an acute myocardial infarction and mild left ventricular failure (class II). They also reported that, in addition to a history of prior myocardial infarction, the left ventricular regional wall motion index or ejection fraction determined by radionuclide angiography or two-dimensional echocardiography improved the prediction of in-hospital complications. These data indicate that radionuclide angiography performed early in the setting of acute myocardial infarction may be able to identify subgroups of patients in whom early cardiac events might be more frequent. Consequently, a radionuclide determination of left ventricular ejection fraction may be of value in some patients with acute myocardial infarction to identify high-risk subgroups for more aggressive medical and/or interventional therapy to reduce their short-term morbidity and mortality.

Left ventricular ejection fraction determined by radionuclide angiography has also been shown to be very useful in predicting long-term survival in patients who are discharged from the hospital following acute myocardial infarction. Schulze et al.[22] reported that long-term survivors of acute myocardial infarction had higher left ventricular ejection fractions than did patients who died of sudden death (P<0.02). More importantly, patients who had a left ventricular ejection fraction of less than 40 percent had a worse 1-year survival than did patients in whom the left ventricular ejection fraction was 40 percent or more. Notably, the mortality was particularly high (20 percent) during the first 6 months. These data have been further expanded by the Multicenter Postinfarction Research Group, which demonstrated that four risk factors were independent predictors of mortality in patients following acute myocardial infarction.[23] These included a radionuclide left ventricular ejection fraction of less than 40 percent, ventricular ectopy of 10 or more depolarizations per hour, advanced New York Heart Association functional class prior to infarction, and rales heard in the upper two-thirds of the lung fields in the coronary care unit. The importance of the radionuclide left ventricular ejection fraction determination can be appreciated in Figure 4-4. Note that the 1-year mortality was less than 5 percent in patients with a left ventricular ejection fraction of more than 40 percent. However, there was an exponential increase in mortality as the radionuclide left ventricular ejection fraction decreased from 40 to 20 percent, with a mortality at 1 year of 10 to 15 percent; EF decreased to less than 20 percent, when mortality exceeded 45 percent during the first year postinfarction.

It must be appreciated that several methods of risk stratifying patients following an acute myocardial infarction have been previously investigated. These include holter monitoring, electrocardiographic (ECG) treadmill exercise testing, and determinations of left ventricular ejection fraction. In a recently published investigation by Starling et al.,[24] 72 patients with an uncomplicated acute myocardial infarction were evaluated clinically by ECG treadmill exercise testing and by radionuclide angiography. The radionuclide left ventricular ejection fraction was identified as the optimal predictor of cardiac mortality during the 1-year follow-up by multiple logistic regression analysis, while ECG treadmill exercise testing was predictive of subsequent ischemic cardiac events. Thus, it would appear that the major use of radionuclide left ventricular ejection fraction prior to hospital discharge would be to determine a relative risk of cardiac death in the

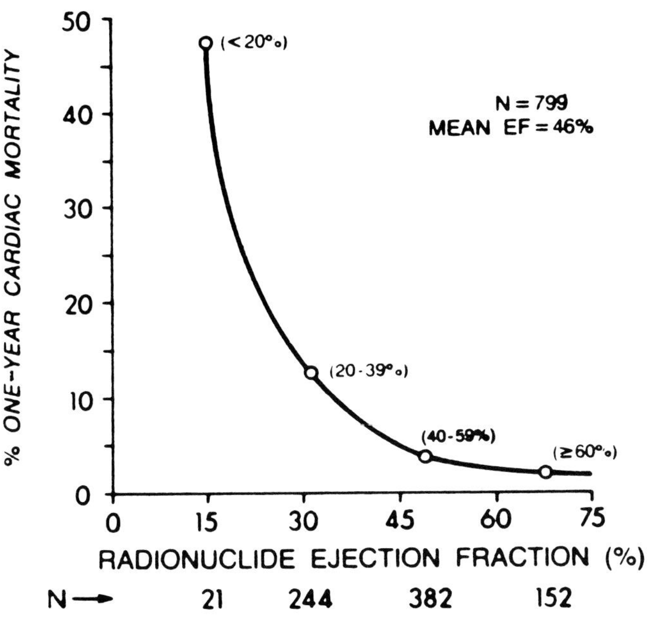

Fig. 4-4 Cardiac mortality in four categories of radionuclide left ventricular ejection fraction (EF) determined prior to hospital discharge is illustrated. Note the logarithmic increase in 1-year cardiac mortality as left ventricular ejection fraction falls below 50 percent. (From the Multicenter Post-Infarction Research Group,[23] with permission.)

year following infarction, while other forms of risk stratification (i.e., ECG treadmill exercise testing) may be useful in identifying patients in whom ischemic events will occur more frequently in the ensuing year.

VALVULAR HEART DISEASE

An additional important application of the radionuclide left ventricular ejection fraction determination has been the prediction of outcome following valve replacement, particularly in patients with mitral regurgitation. Hochreiter et al.[25] reported that patients in whom the preoperative radionuclide left ventricular ejection fraction was less than 45 percent had a high mortality rate prior to valve replacement, compared with patients with

mitral regurgitation in whom the ejection fraction was 45 percent or more ($P<0.02$) (Fig. 4-5). In addition, it was noted that the radionuclide right ventricular ejection fraction was also predictive of outcome prior to valve replacement in these patients with mitral regurgitation. Patients who had a radionuclide right ventricular ejection fraction of less than 30 percent also had a high mortality rate prior to valve replacement, in contrast to patients with a right ventricular ejection fraction of 30 percent or more ($P<0.01$) (Fig. 4-5). Finally, the combined radionuclide assessment of left and right ventricular ejection fraction further enhanced the predictive power for outcome prior to mitral valve replacement. Thus, radionuclide angiography has been established as an exceedingly important tool in determining prognosis in patients

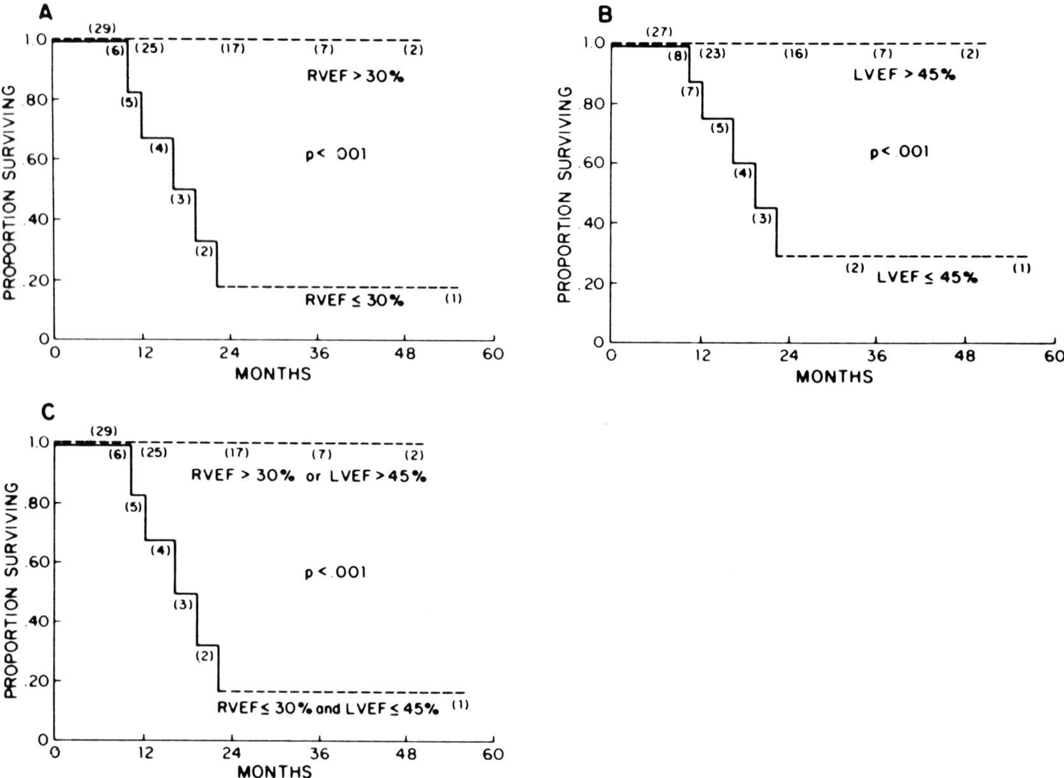

Fig. 4-5 Survival in medically treated patients as a function of **(A)** right ventricular ejection fraction (RVEF), **(B)** left ventricular ejection fraction (LVEF), and **(C)** both RVEF and LVEF, illustrated for patients with chronic severe mitral regurgitation. (From Hochreiter et al.,[25] with permission.)

with mitral regurgitation prior to valve replacement.

CARDIOMYOPATHY

The sequential assessment of left ventricular ejection fraction by radionuclide angiography for predicting the dose-response effects of the anthracycline antibiotic, doxorubicin, given for cancer therapy has been well established. As reported by Alexander et al.,[26] sequential radionuclide left ventricular ejection fraction determinations in patients given doxorubicin in excess of 350 mg/m^2 demonstrated that the left ventricular ejection fraction fell in these patients. In five patients, severe cardiotoxicity with congestive heart failure and an ejection fraction of less than 30 percent was noted. All patients demonstrated some cardiotoxicity with a drop in the radionuclide left ventricular ejection fraction. Moderate cardiac toxicity with a reduction in left ventricular ejection fraction upon completion of the accumulated doxorubicin dose was not ameliorated with discontinuation of the drug (Fig. 4-6). In fact, long-term left ventricular dysfunction was documented. Similar observations were reported by Gottdiener et al.[27] Thus, the sequential assessment of radionuclide left ventricular ejection fraction during doxorubicin therapy should be performed routinely. If the left ventricular ejection fraction falls by 15 percent or below a value to 45 percent, the primary physician should be alerted to the possibility of permanent left ventricular dysfunction due to doxorubicin.

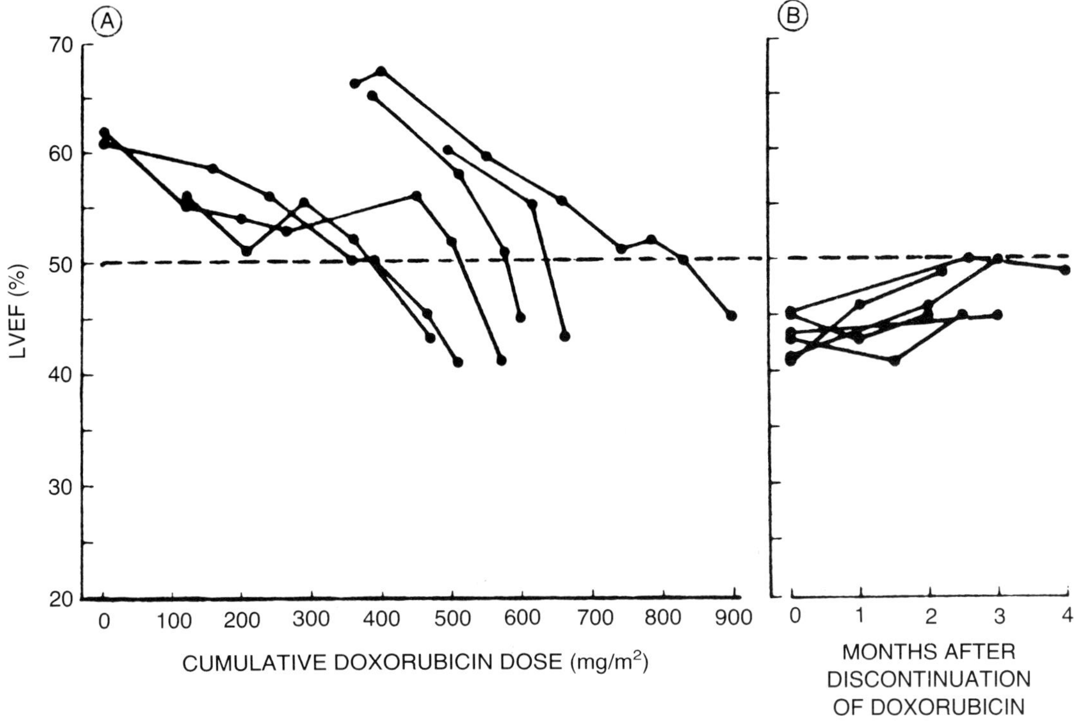

Fig. 4-6 Sequential measurements of left ventricular ejection fraction (LVEF) in six patients in whom doxorubicin was discontinued after the demonstration of moderate cardiotoxicity. **(A)** The relationship between LVEF, on the ordinate, and cumulative doxorubicin dose on the abscissa and **(B)** the relationship between LVEF, on the ordinate, and time in months, on the abscissa, in the same patients. (—) Lower limit of normal for LVEF (50 percent). Note that the LVEF increased in all six patients but remained below the lower limit of normal after discontinuation of doxorubicin. (From Alexander et al.,[26] with permission.)

These data indicate that in various pathologic processes, a radionuclide left ventricular ejection fraction obtained at rest is exceedingly valuable for predicting the development of left ventricular dysfunction, symptoms of left heart failure, and survival. Consequently, it is recommended that patients who have sustained an acute myocardial infarction have a radionuclide left ventricular ejection fraction obtained at least prior to hospital discharge for predicting long-term mortality. It should also be obtained routinely in patients with mitral regurgitation, and it should be used serially in these patients to assess left ventricular ejection fraction changes over time. Once a progressive reduction in ejection fraction occurs, but not below 45 percent, more aggressive invasive evaluation should be undertaken prior to valve replacement. Similarly, sequential radionuclide left ventricular ejection fractions are imperative during anthracycline antibiotic therapy to establish when this therapy has induced cardiotoxicity.

Left Ventricular Diastolic Function

Analysis of the left ventricular semiautomated time–activity curve for determining the maximal rate of rapid filling (i.e., peak filling rate) has been performed using a derivative function or third order polynomial approximation of the left ventricular volume curve. Bacharach et al.[28] explored the temporal resolution necessary for analyzing the peak filling rate using a differential approximation of time–activity curves; these workers reported that the peak filling rate can be measured with a 40-msec frame duration on either first-transit or equilibrium radionuclide studies. The radionuclide peak filling rate was applied by Bonow et al. in patients with hypertrophic obstructive cardiomyopathy[29] and coronary artery disease.[30,31] Bonow et al.[30] reported that the radionuclide peak filling rate was abnormal in patients with coronary artery disease, irrespective of whether they had normal or abnormal resting left ven-

tricular ejection fractions (Fig. 4-7). An abnormal radionuclide peak filling rate also was evident in patients with coronary artery disease and normal resting left ventricular ejection fractions, irrespective of the extent of coronary artery disease.

The value of the radionuclide peak filling rate in assessing changes in diastolic function in patients with coronary artery disease who have undergone percutaneous transluminal coronary angioplasty has also been evaluated.[31] In 25 patients with single-vessel coronary artery disease, Bonow et al.[31] reported that despite normal radionuclide global and regional left ventricular ejection fractions at rest, left ventricular diastolic filling was abnormal in 17 patients. After percutaneous transluminal angioplasty, the left ventricular peak filling rate improved from 2.3 ± 0.6 to 2.8 ± 0.5 end-diastolic volumes/sec ($P<0.001$). These data indicate that in patients with coronary artery disease and normal resting ejection fractions, abnormal diastolic function can be detected by peak filling rate in a high percentage of patients and that it is a reversible manifestation of impaired coronary blood flow. This was further confirmed by Yamagishi et al.,[32] who demonstrated that abnormalities in radionuclide peak filling rate in patients with left anterior descending coronary artery disease and no previous infarction were due to asynchronous diastolic filling in the affected region, which may then impair global left ventricular filling.

Several studies have been performed to establish the hemodynamic correlates of the radionuclide peak filling rate. Magorien et al.[33] demonstrated that the radionuclide peak filling rate was inversely correlated with maximum negative dP/dt ($r = -0.85$), the rate of isovolumic left ventricular pressure decline ($r = -0.49$), and left ventricular end-diastolic pressure ($r = 0.62$). Further investigation in animals has been performed by Ishida et al.,[34] who demonstrated that the peak filling rate

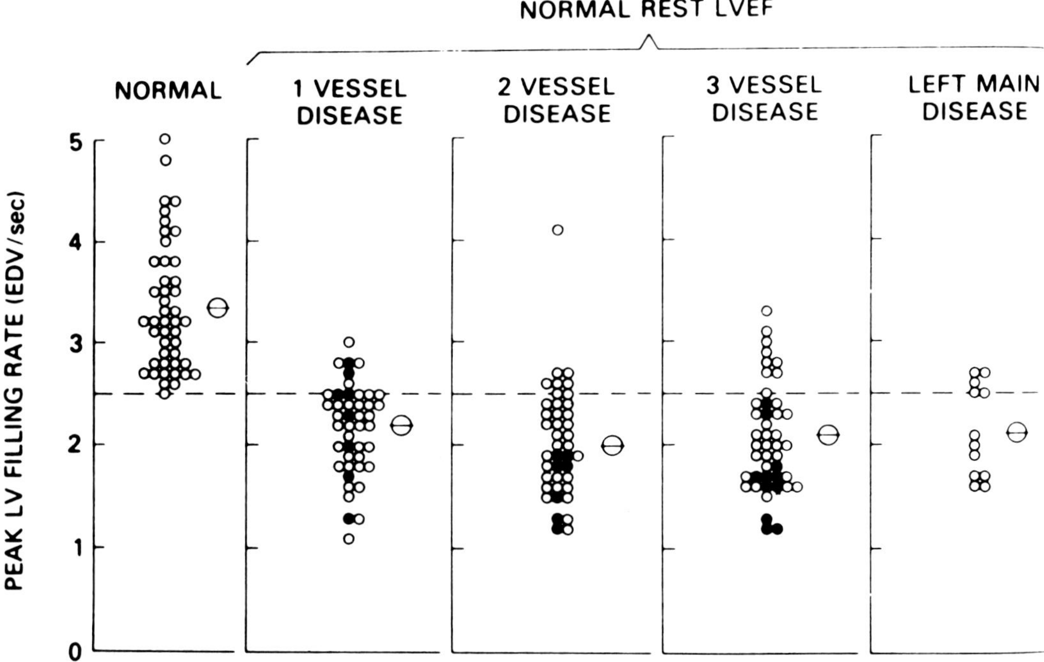

Fig. 4-7 Left ventricular (LV) peak filling rates in patients with coronary artery disease and normal LV ejection fractions (LVEF) are divided into patients with stenosis of one, two, or three coronary arteries or patients with stenosis of the left main coronary artery. Note that despite normal resting LVEF, all the mean peak filling rates in end-diastolic volumes/sec in these patients were depressed in comparison with normal subjects irrespective of the extent of coronary artery stenosis. (From Bonow et al.,[30] with permission.)

was related to the diastolic atrioventricular pressure difference ($r = 0.90$). Moreover, there were also correlations with the rate of isovolumic left ventricular pressure decline ($r = 0.37$) and left atrial pressure at the antrioventricular pressure crossover ($r = 0.60$). Thus, these investigators concluded that the radionuclide peak filling rate was determined both by left atrial pressure and the left ventricular relaxation rate and should be used with some caution as an index of left ventricular diastolic function. Iskandrian and Hakki[35] showed that there is also an age-related decline in the radionuclide peak filling rate ($r = -0.47$, $P<0.001$). The peak filling rate is therefore determined by several hemodynamic variables and may be influenced significantly by age, so that differences between patient groups and the effects of cardiovascular pathology on peak filling rate must be interpreted with these potential limitations in mind. Nevertheless, this may be a useful indicator of alterations in filling dynamics produced by such interventions as medical or interventional therapy in patients used as their own control.

Left Ventricular Phase Analysis

Fourier analysis is a mathematical technique by which any periodic function (i.e., equilibrium radionuclide left ventricular time-activity curves) can be represented by the sine and cosine functions of different frequencies, each characterized by a specific amplitude and phase.[36] In a gated equilibrium radionuclide angiogram, most of the change in count activity within the heart occurs at the fundamental frequency, the heart rate. By convention, the pixel whose fundamental frequency is maximally positive in the first frame of a gated radionuclide study has a phase of 0. Thus, those pixels representing the ventricles are clustered around 0 degrees, while those representing the atria, which beat out of phase with the ventricles, have a phase of around 180 degrees.

Using this mathematical approximation, several investigators have identified characteristic abnormalities in the phase histogram associated with right and left bundle branch block (RBBB and LBBB),[37,38] Wolff-Parkinson-White syndrome,[38,39] ventricular tachycardia,[40] and left ventricular regional wall-motion abnormalities.[41,42] It is this latter application that is most interesting. Botvinick et al.[42] showed that the phase delay is generally related to the degree of contraction abnormality; that is, the mean phase in hypokinetic segments differs from that in normal kinetic segments in the same patient ($P<0.025$). The phase delay of akinetic and dyskinetic segments differs from the normal kinetic segments ($P<0.001$), and the phase delay in dyskinetic segments differs from that in akinetic segments ($P<0.005$). Nevertheless, these investigators cautioned that there was significant overlap in the phase delay in the normal and hypokinetic segments. Starling et al.[43] reported in animals that various phase and amplitude parameters are correlated with changes in regional segment crystal fractional shortening during graded alterations in regional function produced by transient ischemia. Once again, there was substantial overlap in the phase parameter changes as alteration in regional crystal fractional shortening progressively worsened. These data do suggest, however, that phase shifts may be proportionate to the extent of regional contraction abnormality induced by transient ischemia.

ASSESSING THE RIGHT VENTRICLE

Right Ventricular Volumes

The application of equilibrium radionuclide techniques to the calculation of right ventricular volumes has demonstrated encouraging results. The advantage of this approach is the relative geometric independence of the count-based equilibrium radionuclide technique for assessing the complex shaped right ventricle. The ability of equilibrium radionuclide techniques to obtain absolute right ventricular volumes has been evaluated both in children[44] and in adults.[45] Using the attenuation-correction radionuclide technique described by Starling et al.,[5,6] Dell'Italia et al.[45] applied this approach to the right ventricle. They compared radionuclide right ventricular volume indices and attenuation-corrected right ventricular volumes to biplane contrast cineangiographic volumes calculated using a cast-validated Simpson's rule algorithm. The correlation coefficients between the radionuclide right ventricular end-diastolic and end-systolic volume indices and the biplane contrast cineangiographic right ventricular volumes were significantly lower than those obtained with attenuation correction. Also, substantially narrower 95 percent confidence intervals for the predicted cineangiographic volumes were reported for the attenuation-corrected radionuclide right ventricular volume determinations. These data indicate that a count-based method, which is relatively independent of geometric considerations, can be used to calculate accurate right ventricular volumes.

An alternative approach to calculating right ventricular volumes is the analysis of radio-isotope dilution curves obtained from first-transit radionuclide angiograms. Nusynowitz et al.[46] used this technique to obtain right ventricular stroke volumes from regions of interest over the right ventricle or lung and demonstrated correlations with both Fick and green dye stroke volumes ($r = 0.76$ to 0.88). By employing the right ventricular ejection fractions obtained from the radionuclide first-transit technique and the right ventricular stroke volumes, right ventricular volumes could be calculated. Although these radionuclide right ventricular volume estimates have not been compared with those obtained by biplane contrast cineangiography, this is a promising alternative approach employing a first-transit technique rather than an equilibrium technique that may yield accurate right ventricular volumetric data.

Right Ventricular Ejection Fraction

Both the first-transit and equilibrium radionuclide approaches have demonstrated their ability to obtain accurate right ventricular ejection fractions. Initially, Steele et al.[47] compared first-transit radionuclide and biplane contrast cineangiographic estimates of right ventricular ejection fraction and reported a correlation ($r = 0.80$) (Fig. 4-8). Subsequently, Maddahi et al.[48] developed a multiple region-of-interest method of estimated right ventricular ejection fraction from gated equilibrium radionuclide images. As shown in Figure 4-9, when a single region

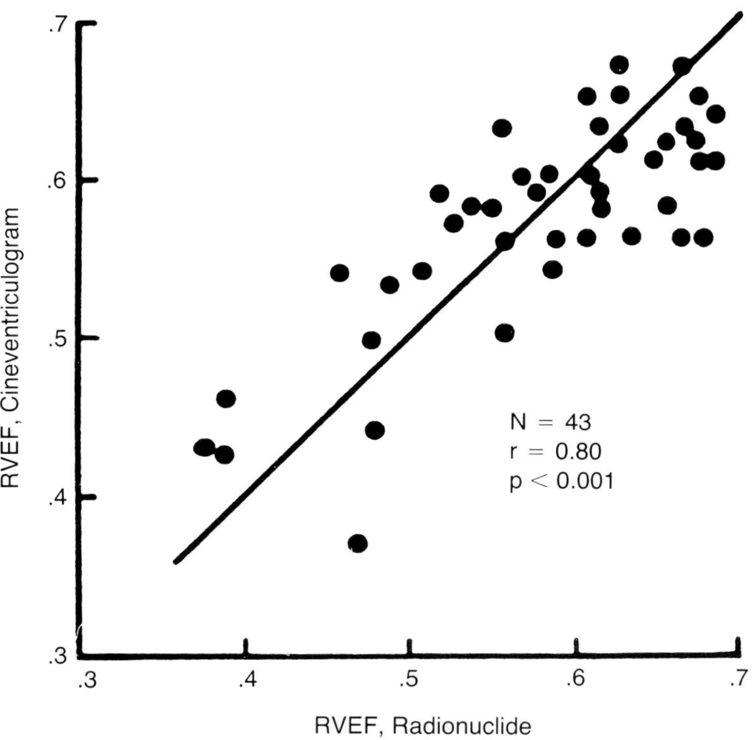

Fig. 4-8 Right ventricular ejection fraction (RVEF) values from biplane contrast cineventriculograms, on the ordinate, are compared with the RVEF values obtained from first-transit radionuclide angiograms, on the abscissa. Note the correlation over the range of RVEF values studied. (From Steele et al.,[47] with permission.)

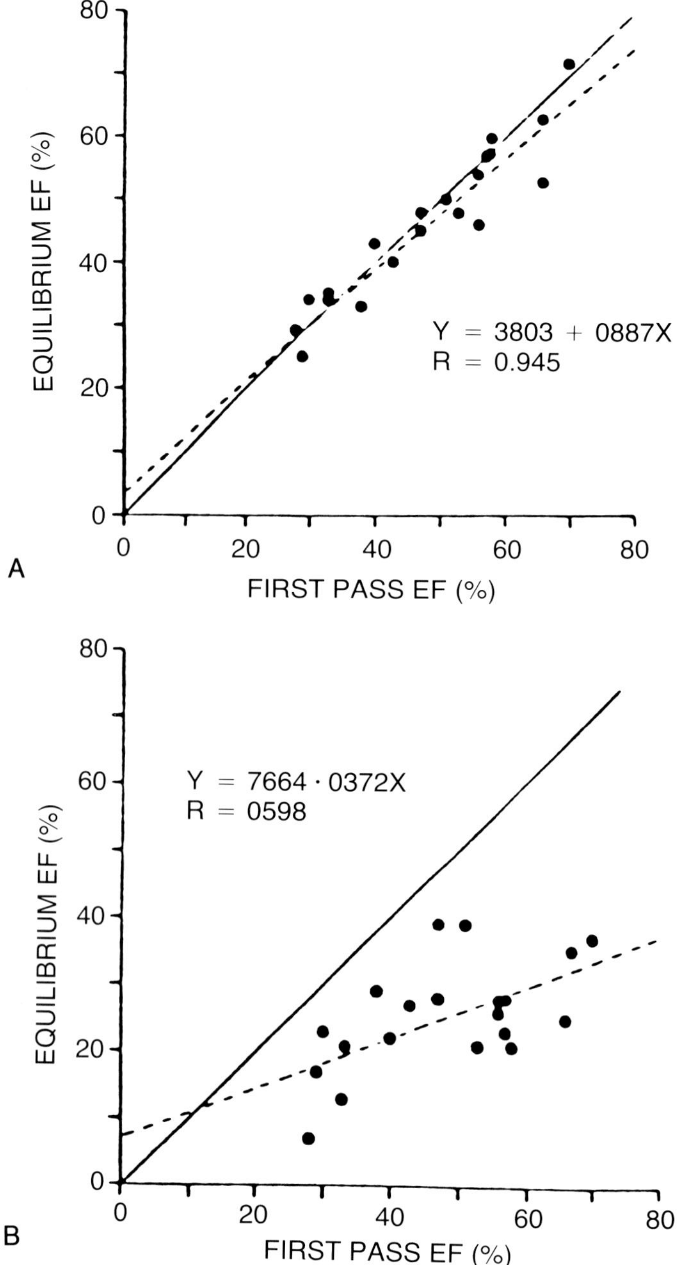

Fig. 4-9 (A) Correlation between multiple-gated equilibrium and first-transit radionuclide techniques for measuring right ventricular ejection fraction (EF) when a single end-diastolic region of interest was used to evaluate the equilibrium radionuclide images is shown. A poor correlation was noted. The equilibrium radionuclide technique using this single region-of-interest selection technique substantially underestimated the first-transit RVEF. **(B)** By contrast, the RVEF measurements obtained using a dual region-of-interest selection technique at end-diastole and end-systole on the equilibrium radionuclide images correlated well with the first-transit radionuclide technique, and there was no underestimation of the RVEF. (From Maddahi et al.,[48] with permission.)

of interest was used, significant underestimates of the first-transit right ventricular ejection fraction measures were noted, but when dual regions of interest were used, which permitted exclusion of the right atrium at end-systole, the right ventricular ejection fraction measures correlated and were not different.

Similar to the first-transit technique, further validation of this equilibrium radionuclide approach to calculating right ventricular ejection fraction has been performed in comparison with biplane contrast cineangiography. Parrish et al.[44] reported that right ventricular ejection fraction determinations by equilibrium radionuclide angiography and biplane contrast cineangiography correlated, and the slope of the regression line was close to identity. Moreover, they reported, as had Maddahi et al.,[48] that the reproducibility of the radionuclide technique was high for these right ventricular ejection fraction determinations. The correlation noted between the equilibrium radionuclide and cineangiographic right ventricular ejection fraction measures was less strong when atrial separation was not optimal compared with when it was excellent ($r = 0.78$ versus 0.91, respectively). Thus, it is clear from these data that both first-transit and equilibrium radionuclide techniques are accurate and reproducible noninvasive approaches to the assessment of right ventricular ejection fraction.

Since both the first-transit and equilibrium radionuclide techniques provide accurate estimates of right ventricular ejection fraction, a clear understanding of their potential limitations is important. The potential errors in the ejection fraction measurements using these techniques can be characterized as either statistical or systematic. Statistical uncertainty is apparent in the first-transit radionuclide ejection fraction determinations, since it is dependent on the number of scintigraphic events detected. By contrast, systematic errors are evident in the equilibrium technique,

since they are related to incorrect definitions of regions of interest. One potential method for overcoming the statistical uncertainty in the first-transit radionuclide acquisition has been suggested by Harolds et al.[49] Their technique demonstrated that gating the first-transit radionuclide acquisition could enhance statistical reliability of the right ventricular ejection fraction technique compared with the standard first-transit technique. By contrast, the equilibrium radionuclide technique, which has much higher count rates and therefore less statistical uncertainty, has the problem of overlap of the right atrium and ventricle. Holman et al.[50] approached this problem using a 30-degree slant-hole collimator, which provides a left anterior oblique projection with a 30-degree caudal tilt and delineates right atrial and ventricular borders more clearly. This approach, coupled with parametric images for region-of-interest selection, demonstrated an excellent correlation with first-transit right ventricular ejection fractions ($r = 0.76$ to 0.95). The lower correlations noted occurred when background was chosen around the right ventricle rather than around the left ventricle. Thus, gating the first transit or using caudal tilt for the radionuclide equilibrium technique may minimize the statistical and systematic errors inherent in these two radionuclide approaches to calculating right ventricular ejection fraction.

The absence of systematic errors in the first-transit radionuclide right ventricular ejection fraction determination make it a particularly appealing approach for assessing this functional parameter in normal subjects and patients with cardiopulmonary pathology. When performed with ^{99m}Tc, the number of serial studies that can be performed is limited. Several newer short-lived radionuclides or inert gases have been evaluated for assessing right ventricular ejection fraction in comparison with the standard ^{99m}Tc approach. These short-lived radionuclides include ^{81m}Kr,[51–53] ^{195m}Au,[54] and ^{191}Ir,[55] and the inert gas ^{133}Xe.[56,57] All these radionuclides have been compared with first-transit and/or equilibrium radionuclide right ventricular ejection fraction determinations and have demonstrated correlations. Thus, these radionuclides provide accurate determinations of right ventricular ejection fraction that can be repeated frequently; in addition, the radiation dose to the body and specific organs is markedly reduced. Therefore, the use of these radionuclides may increase in the future due to these beneficial characteristics.

To interpret the right ventricular ejection fraction calculation appropriately, an understanding of the hemodynamic correlates that determine the right ventricular ejection fraction in normal subjects and patients with cardiopulmonary pathology is necessary. Korr et al.[58] demonstrated the inverse linear relationship between equilibrium radionuclide right ventricular ejection fractions and mean pulmonary artery pressure and right ventricular end-diastolic pressure (Fig. 4-10). The investigation by Brent et al.[59] also showed a comparable relationship between the first-transit radionuclide right ventricular ejection fraction measurements and peak pulmonary artery pressure and pulmonary vascular resistance ($r = -0.81$ and -0.73, respectively) and right ventricular end-diastolic volume index and right atrial pressure ($r = -0.56$ and -0.51, respectively). These data suggest that right ventricular ejection fraction obtained using these radionuclide techniques is strongly affected by the loading conditions on the right ventricle.

Prognostic Implications of Right Ventricular Ejection Fraction

The ability of the radionuclide right ventricular ejection fraction to identify specific cardiovascular disease processes and its prognostic importance have been areas of intensive research in recent years. In several pathophysiologic processes, the radionuclide right ventricular ejection fraction can determine not only diagnosis and function but prognosis as well.

RIGHT VENTRICULAR INFARCTION

The hallmark of right ventricular infarction has been the disproportionate elevation of right atrial pressure in comparison to pulmonary artery wedge pressure in patients with an acute inferior transmural myocardial infarction. Initially, Tobinick et al.[60] and Reduto et al.[61] employed first-transit radionuclide techniques to assess both right and left ventricular function in patients with acute myocardial infarction, and they reported a greater reduction in right ventricular ejection fraction in patients with inferior compared to anterior transmural myocardial infarctions. In addition, Tobinick et al.[60] demonstrated that this reduction in right ventricular ejection fraction was associated with a positive myocardial scintigraphic examination for both inferior and right ventricular infarction. Recently, using both first-transit and equilibrium radionuclide angiographic techniques, Starling et al.[62] defined criteria for identifying hemodynamically significant right ventricular infarction. For both radionuclide imaging techniques, a right ventricular regional wall-motion abnormality, with or without an associated right ventricular ejection fraction of 40 percent or less, was reported to be a valuable criterion for detecting hemodynamically significant right ventricular ischemic dysfunction. Subsequently, Dell'Italia et al.[63] evaluated patients prospectively with acute inferior transmural myocardial infarction to define the relative value of various imaging modalities for identifying this entity. Radionuclide angiography demonstrated the highest sensitivity and specificity in comparison with two-dimensional echocardiography and technetium-99m pyrophosphate imaging. Moreover, both first-transit and equilibrium radionuclide techniques have been used to assess the long-term hemodynamic effects of right ventricular ischemic dysfunction. The acute radionuclide

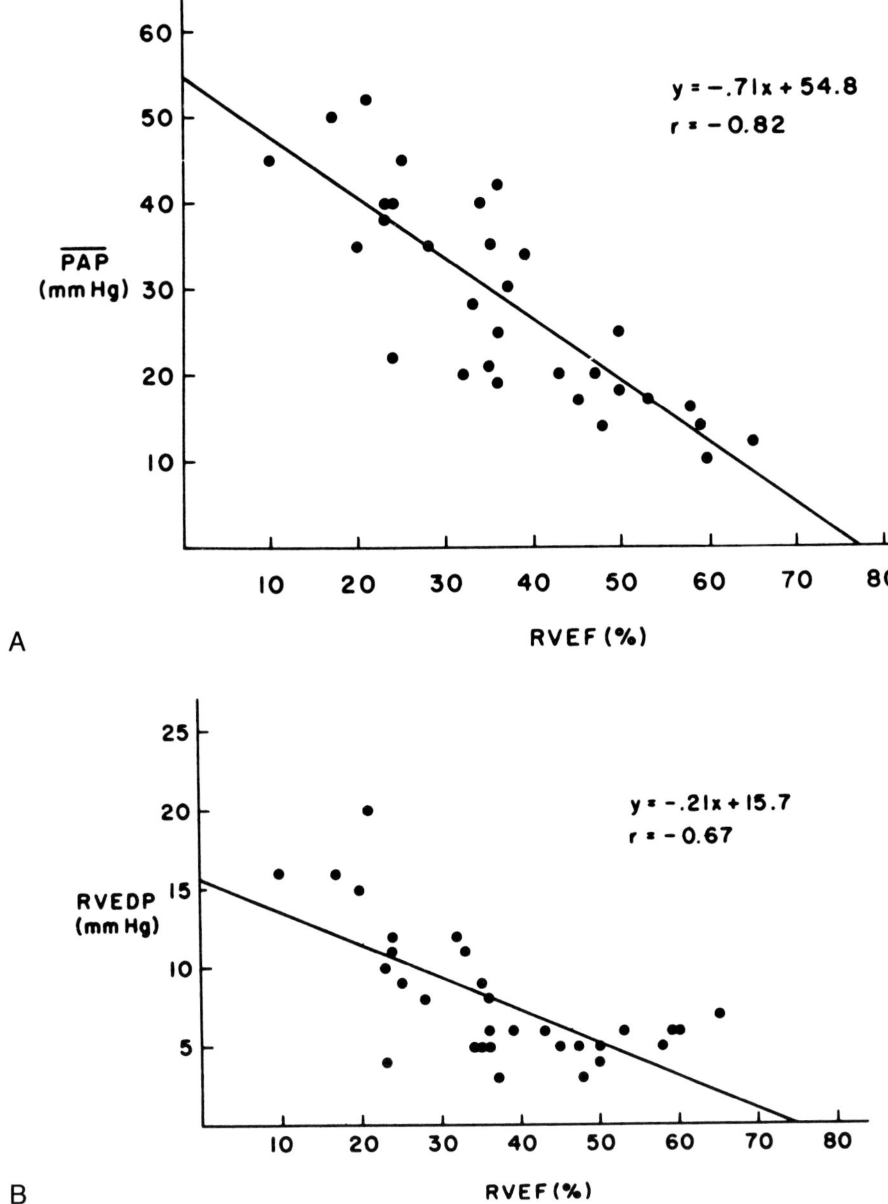

Fig. 4-10 (A) Relationship between mean pulmonary artery pressure (PAP) and the radionuclide right ventricular ejection fraction (RVEF). **(B)** Relationship between right ventricular end-diastolic pressure (RVEDP) and the radionuclide right ventricular ejection fraction (RVEF). Note the strong inverse linear correlations between mean pulmonary artery pressure and RVEDP and the radionuclide RVEF determinations. (From Korr et al.,[58] with permission.)

abnormalities consistent with right ventricular infarction improved over a 6- to 12-month period as manifest by an increase in right ventricular ejection fraction.[64] In addition, Dell'Italia et al.[63] showed that radionuclide angiography can be used to evaluate right ventricular volume and ejection fraction changes during therapeutic interventions, which further our understanding of the pathophysiologic mechanisms of hemodynamic impairment in patients with acute right ventricular infarction. Thus, these data suggest that either first-transit or equilibrium radionuclide angiography should be used as the noninvasive test of choice in patients with suspected right ventricular infarction to confirm the diagnosis, to follow right ventricular size and performance during recovery, and to assess treatment interventions given acutely to improve right ventricular performance.

Valvular Heart Disease

The prognostic importance of right ventricular ejection fraction has been recently emphasized by Hochreiter et al.[25] in patients with chronic severe mitral regurgitation. Using radionuclide angiography to assess both right and left ventricular ejection fractions, these investigators reported that the right ventricular ejection fraction at rest was the only independent predictor of symptoms and exercise performance. Cardiac deaths during medical therapy were clustered among a group of patients with a depressed right ventricular ejection fraction (30 percent or less) and left ventricular ejection fraction (45 percent or less), but this was not the case for patients who were treated surgically. The survival analysis demonstrated the independent predictive power of right and left ventricular ejection fractions. Thus, these data demonstrate the importance of assessing right ventricular ejection fraction in patients with chronic severe mitral regurgitation for deter-

mining long-term prognosis and the timing of operative correction.

Congestive Cardiomyopathy

The clinical value of right ventricular ejection fraction for determining prognosis, the response to exercise, and efficacy of therapy in patients with chronic congestive cardiomyopathy has been evaluated extensively using radionuclide angiography. Polak et al.[65] demonstrated that, in patients with chronic congestive heart failure with left ventricular ejection fractions of less than 40 percent by radionuclide angiography, survival was lower in patients with a reduced right ventricular ejection fraction (Fig. 4-11). This reduction in right ventricular ejection fraction was also associated with worse functional class, higher pulmonary artery wedge pressure, and higher mean pulmonary artery pressure and resistance. Baker et al.[66] subsequently reported that right ventricular ejection fraction at rest correlated with maximal oxygen consumption during upright bicycle exercise ($r = 0.70$), but left ventricular ejection fraction did not. This correlation appeared to be stronger among patients with ischemic heart disease than among patients with idiopathic dilated cardiomyopathy. It would appear from the work of Franciosa et al.[67] that pulmonary hemodynamics determine the right ventricular ejection fraction at rest and both determine functional capacity in patients with left ventricular failure. These data suggest that monitoring right ventricular performance in these patients may be very useful in assessing therapeutic responses in patients with left ventricular failure.

In light of these observations, therapeutic interventions with vasodilators and inotropic agents have been performed and their effects evaluated with radionuclide right ventricular ejection fraction determinations. Colucci et al.[68] demonstrated an increase in right ventricular ejection fraction from 29 ± 5 to 38

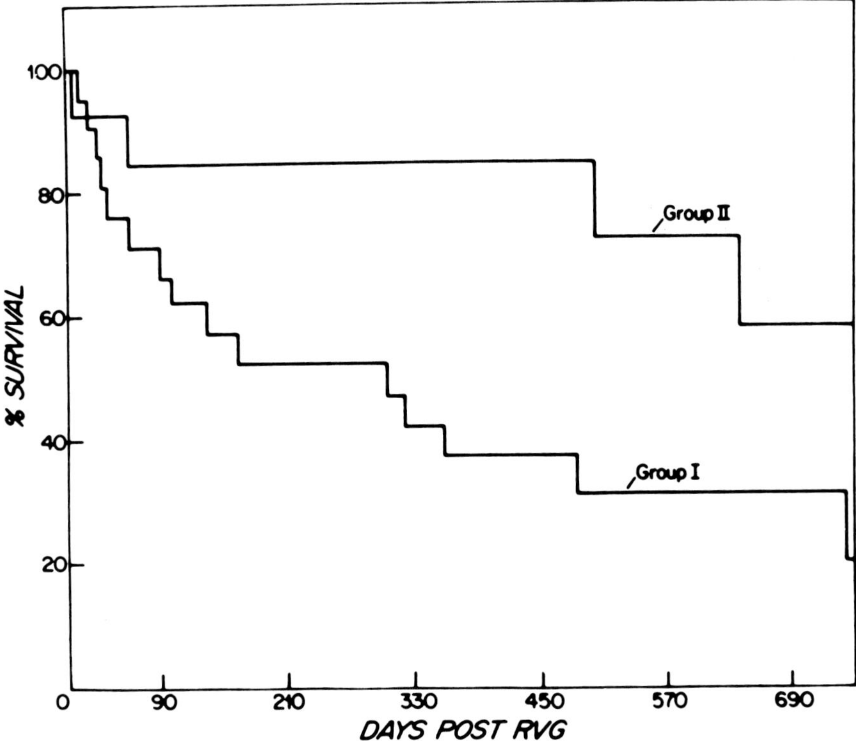

Fig. 4-11 Cumulative probability of survival for patients with a right ventricular ejection fraction (RVEF), either 35 percent or more (group II) or less than 35 percent (group I). Significantly different probabilities ($P<0.05$) are evident at 6, 12, and 24 months after radionuclide ventriculography (RVG). (From Polak et al.,[65] with permission.)

± 6 percent ($P<0.02$) following a single oral dose of prazosin. This improvement in right ventricular ejection fraction was associated with other hemodynamic improvements. Also, Konstam et al.[69] demonstrated the relative effects of the bipyridine, amrinone, and nitroprusside on right ventricular size and performance. Amrinone produced a greater reduction in right ventricular end-systolic volume than did nitroprusside for comparable reductions in end-systolic pressure demonstrating the marked positive inotropic effect of this agent. Thus, radionuclide techniques are useful tools for determining prognosis and exercise performance, for assessing the effects of therapeutic intervention on right ventricular ejection fraction, and for

determining the mechanism of action of various drugs in patients with congestive heart failure.

Chronic Obstructive Pulmonary Disease

The use of radionuclide imaging techniques to obtain right ventricular ejection fraction measures in patients with chronic obstructive pulmonary disease has produced important diagnostic, therapeutic, and prognostic information.[70–75] Berger et al.[70] evaluated right ventricular ejection fraction at rest using the first-transit radionuclide technique and demonstrated a wide range of ejection fraction values (19 to 71 percent) in these patients.

In patients with chronic obstructive pulmonary disease and cor pulmonale, an abnormally depressed right ventricular ejection fraction was seen. Among the additional patients with a reduced right ventricular ejection fraction, nearly 50 percent subsequently developed acute respiratory decompensation and/or cor pulmonale, while no patient with a normal right ventricular ejection fraction did so, during the ensuing year. Furthermore, patients with a reduced right ventricular ejection fraction had a lower arterial oxygen tension and forced respiratory volume in 1 second, but no difference in left ventricular ejection fraction. Consequently, radionuclide assessment of right ventricular ejection fraction at rest may be very useful for predicting subsequent respiratory and/or hemodynamic deterioration in patients with chronic obstructive pulmonary disease.

Radionuclide techniques have also been used to evaluate the response of right and left ventricular performance in patients with chronic obstructive pulmonary disease to therapeutic interventions. The response of resting right ventricular ejection fraction in these patients to oxygen,[71] digoxin,[72] aminophylline,[73] terbutaline,[74] and vasodilator therapy[75] has been evaluated. Oxygen[71] produced no significant effect on resting right ventricular ejection fraction. By contrast, digoxin improved the right ventricular ejection fraction only when left ventricular ejection fraction was depressed at rest.[72] Both aminophylline and terbutaline have significantly improved right ventricular ejection fraction at rest,[73,74] while the response of right ventricular ejection fraction to vasodilator therapy has been variable.[75] The variability in the right ventricular ejection fraction response to vasodilators is probably related to their differing effects on pulmonary artery pressure and resistance and right ventricular preload. Thus, the first-transit and equilibrium radionuclide assessment of right ventricular ejection fraction is valuable for assessing the effects of therapeutic interventions in patients with chronic obstructive pulmonary disease.

ASSESSING CARDIAC OUTPUT, SHUNTS, AND VALVULAR REGURGITANT FRACTIONS

Shunt Analysis

The most commonly used method for assessing intracardiac left-to-right shunts has been the first-transit radionuclide technique. Askenazi et al.[76] evaluated 105 patients with left-to-right shunts using list mode radionuclide acquisitions and a gamma variate model for fitting both the initial and recirculation curves. Analysis of the radionuclide initial and recirculation lung activity curves allowed quantitation of pulmonary-to-systemic flow ratios for comparison to those obtained at cardiac catheterization (Fig. 4-12). The correlation between this radioisotope technique and the oximetry pulmonary to systemic flow ratios was $r = 0.94$. This approach is now a well-accepted radionuclide method for quantitating shunts in children and adults. An alternative approach has been used to quantitate left-to-right shunts in adults with atrial septal defects. Sorenson et al.[77] demonstrated that the equilibrium radionuclide approach could quantitate left-to-right shunts at the atrial level. They could also be serially followed to assess the adequacy of the surgical repair. This approach, however, necessitates the assumption that the stroke counts from the right and left ventricles are proportionate to pulmonary and systemic flow and that there is no intraventricular or arterial mixing. Thus, this technique can be used only for atrial septal defects and not for detecting ventricular septal or patent ductus arteriosis defects, which can be detected with the first-transit approach. Thus, the equilibrium technique has limited applicability.

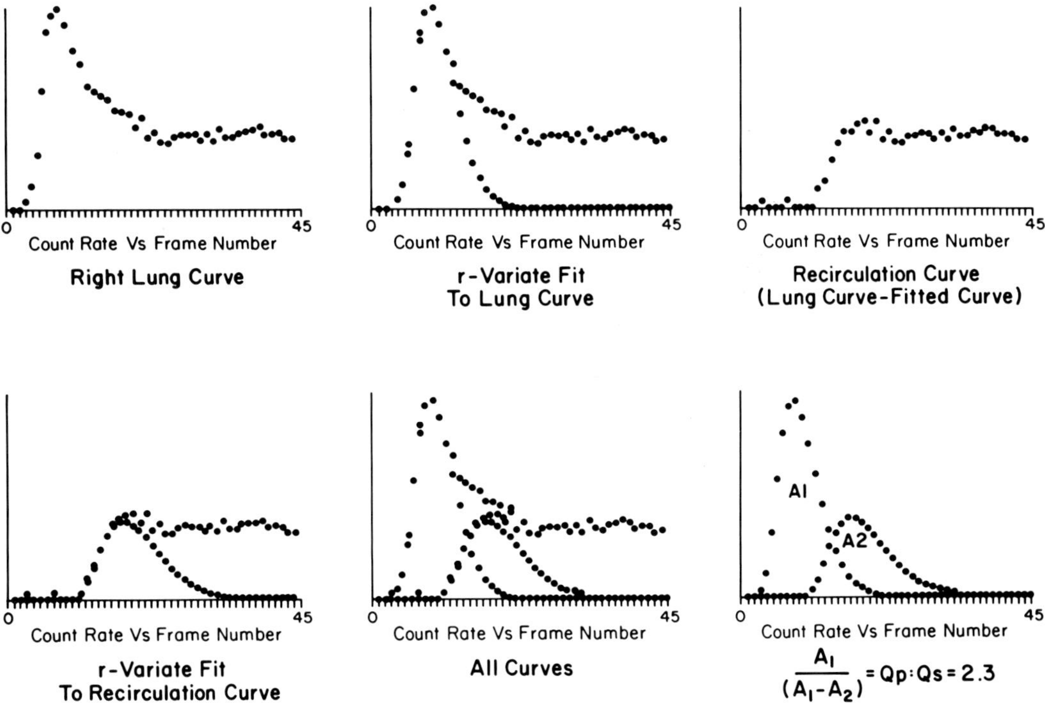

$$\frac{A_1}{(A_1 - A_2)} = Qp{:}Qs = 2.3$$

Fig. 4-12 Method for estimating pulmonary systemic flow $Q_p : Q_S$ ratios. Pulmonary time-activity histogram (upper left) is fit by a γ-variate (upper center). The derived histogram is then subtracted from the original pulmonary time-activity histogram with the resulting histogram representing the shunt and systemic recirculation (upper right). This latter, new histogram is fit by a γ-variate (lower left). The two areas are delimited: A_1, the proportion of pulmonary flow Q_p and area A_2, the proportion of shunted flow. Area A_1 minus A_2 is proportionate to systemic flow Q_S. A ratio of area A_1 divided by area A_1 minus A_2 provides an estimates of the $Q_p : Q_S$ ratio. (Modified from Askenazi et al.,[76] with permission.)

Quantitating Valvular Regurgitation

The first-transit and equilibrium radionuclide techniques have been reported to be excellent methods for detecting and quantitating the extent of valvular regurgitation in patients with aortic and mitral valve incompetence.[78–85] Rigo et al.[78] demonstrated that the ratio of left ventricular to right ventricular count output yielded stroke index ratios (count output ratios) in patients with left-sided valvular regurgitation that were proportionate to the angiographic assessment of valvular incompetence. Subsequently, Sorensen et al.[79] demonstrated that left ventricular minus right ventricular count output over left ventricular count output calculated a radionuclide regurgitant fraction that correlated with that obtained at catheterization in patients with mitral and aortic regurgitation (Fig. 4-13). Moreover, these investigators demonstrated that in patients who had valve replacement, the radionuclide regurgitant fraction calculation was very useful in assessing the adequacy of the surgical procedure, in that, the radionuclide regurgitant fractions fell within the normal range of ±20 percent.

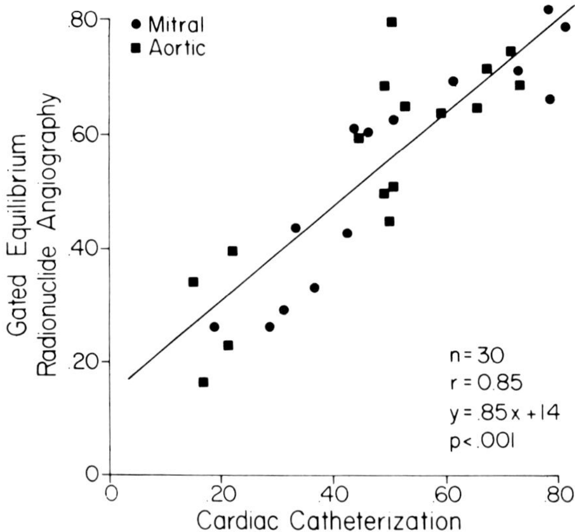

Fig. 4-13 Valvular regurgitant fractions calculated by equilibrium radionuclide angiography, on the ordinate, and at cardiac catheterization, on the abscissa, are compared for patients with mitral and aortic regurgitation. An excellent correlation is noted. (From Sorenson et al.,[79] with permission.)

Several potential pitfalls to the equilibrium radionuclide approach to quantitating left-sided valvular regurgitation have been raised.[82,84,85] First, this technique is predicated upon relative volume overload between the right and left ventricles, that is, the relative volume overload must exist only for the left ventricle. Thus, in patients with shunts or right-sided valvular incompetence, the radionuclide regurgitant index or fraction would be artificially underestimated and, therefore, not accurately quantitated. Second, the left-to-right ventricular stroke count ratio obtained using the equilibrium radionuclide approach is not accurate when left ventricular ejection fractions are depressed. Lam et al.[82] found that approximately 12 percent of patients had a regurgitant index calculated by the equilibrium radionuclide technique that was discordant from the clinical data; that is, the radionuclide technique either predicted severe regurgitation when no or trivial regurgitation was present or it predicted no or trivial regurgitation when clinically significant regurgitation was evident. In 8 of 10 patients with a left ventricular ejection fraction of less than 30 percent, there was a dis-

cordant regurgitant index calculated. Finally, the experience of some investigators has been that regurgitant fraction calculations using the equilibrium radionuclide technique may be spurious in patients in whom right atrial enlargement occurs. This is not surprising, since right atrial enlargement would lead to difficulties in defining right ventricular regions of interest and thereby alter right ventricular stroke count calculations. It is possible that the errors caused by right atrial enlargement may be the result of right ventricular dilation and triscupid regurgitation, which is often difficult to identify clinically. Therefore, the calculation and quantitation of left ventricular regurgitant fractions are difficult and should be done with great care and be interpreted with caution in patients with additional regurgitant lesions or shunts, left ventricular dysfunction (left ventricular ejection fraction of 30 percent or less), or severe right ventricular enlargement and right atrial dilatation.

Recently, Nusynowitz et al.[46] attempted to use the first-transit radionuclide technique to calculate right and left ventricular stroke volumes. They demonstrated that, using regions of interest over the right ventricle and lung, accurate right ventricular stroke volumes were obtained; and with regions of interest over the left ventricle, accurate left ventricular stroke volumes were obtained. Using this first-transit radionuclide technique, relative left-to-right ventricular stroke volume ratios were calculated that accurately detected the presence of valvular regurgitation. Thus, this first-transit radionuclide technique may provide a quantitative determination of left-sided valvular regurgitation in patients in whom the equilibrium radionuclide approach does not yield accurate regurgitant fraction determinations.

SUMMARY AND CONCLUSIONS

This chapter has highlighted some of the important developments in quantitative radionuclide imaging of the right and left ventricles at rest. The recent developments in calculating accurate radionuclide right and left ventricular volumes, which may be applied to sophisticated calculations of left ventricular contractile function, have been discussed. Moreover, both right and left ventricular ejection fractions have been demonstrated to be very important in determining prognosis in various cardiopulmonary pathologic conditions, particularly ischemic heart disease, valvular heart disease, congestive cardiomyopathy, and chronic obstructive pulmonary disease. Therefore, first-transit or equilibrium radionuclide techniques have over the past decade been established in many cases as the noninvasive imaging technique of choice for determining long-term prognosis in these disease states. Finally, first-transit and equilibrium radionuclide techniques have been demonstrated to be valuable methods for identifying and quantitating intracardiac left-to-right shunts and the extent of valvular regurgitation. Although there are limitations to these radionuclide approaches to quantitating left-to-right shunts or valvular regurgitation, they appear to be the noninvasive techniques of choice for this purpose.

ACKNOWLEDGMENTS

We appreciate the assistance in the preparation of this manuscript by Diane Bauer and Dorothy Budd.

REFERENCES

1. Massie BM, Kramer BL, Gertz EW, et al: Radionuclide measurement of left ventricular volume: Comparison of geometric and counts-based methods. Circulation 65:725, 1982
2. Dehmer GJ, Lewis SE, Hillis LD, et al: Nongeometric determination of left ventricular volumes from equilibrium blood pool scans. Am J Cardiol 45:293, 1980
3. Dehmer GJ, Firth BG, Lewis SE, et al: Direct measurement of cardiac output by gated equilibrium blood pool scintigraphy: Validation of scintigraphic volume measurements by a nongeometric technique. Am J Cardiol 47:1061, 1981
4. Links JM, Becker LC, Shindledecker JG, et al: Measurement of absolute left ventricular volume from gated blood pool studies. Circulation 65:82, 1982
5. Starling MR, Dell'Italia LF, Walsh RA, et al: Accurate estimates of absolute left ventricular volumes from equilibrium radionuclide angiographic count data using a simple geometric attenuation correction. J Am Coll Cardiol 3:789, 1984
6. Starling MR, Dell'Italia LJ, Nusynowitz ML, et al: Estimates of left ventricular volumes by equilibrium radionuclide angiography: Importance of attenuation correction. J Nucl Med 25:14, 1984
7. Burow RD, Wilson MF, Heath PW, et al: Influence of attenuation on radionuclide stroke volume determinations. J Nucl Med 23:781, 1982
8. Maurer AH, Siegel JA, Denenberg BS, et al: Absolute left ventricular volume from

gated blood pool imaging with use of esophageal transmission measurement. Am J Cardiol 51:853, 1983

9. Corbett JR, Jansen DE, Lewis SE, et al: Tomographic gated blood pool radionuclide ventriculography: Analysis of wall motion and left ventricular volumes in patients with coronary artery disease. J Am Coll Cardiol 6:349, 1985

10. Bunker SR, Hartshorne MF, Schmidt WP, et al: Left ventricular volume determination from single-photon emission computed tomography. AJR 144:295, 1985

11. Sagawa K: The end-systolic pressure-volume relation of the ventricle: Definition, modifications and clinical use. Circulation 63:1223, 1981

12. Kronenberg MW, Parrish MD, Jenkins DW, et al: Accuracy of radionuclide ventriculography for estimation of left ventricular volume changes and end-systolic pressure-volume relations. J Am Coll Cardiol 6:1064, 1985

13. Starling MR, Walsh RA, Dell'Italia LJ, et al: Maximum time-varying elastance and V_0 determined in man using equilibrium radionuclide angiography. Circulation 72:480, 1985

14. Folland ED, Hamilton GW, Larson SM, et al: The radionuclide ejection fraction: A comparison of three radionuclide techniques with contrast angiography. J Nucl Med 18:1159, 1977

15. Maddox DE, Wynne J, Uren R, et al: Regional ejection fraction: A quantitative radionuclide index of regional left ventricular performance. Circulation 59:1001, 1979

16. Papapietro SE, Yester MV, Logic JR, et al: Method for quantitative analysis of regional left ventricular function with first pass and gated blood pool scintigraphy. Am J Cardiol 47:618, 1981

17. Maddox DE, Holman BL, Wynne J, et al: Ejection fraction image: A noninvasive index of regional left ventricular wall motion. Am J Cardiol 41:1230, 1978

18. Holman BL, Wynne, J, Idoine J, et al: The paradox image: A noninvasive index of regional left ventricular dyskinesis. J Nucl Med 20:1237, 1979

19. Schelbert HR, Henning H, Ashburn WL, et al: Serial measurements of left ventricular ejection fraction by radionuclide angiography early and later after myocardial infarction. Am J Cardiol 30:407, 1976

20. Shah PK, Pichler M, Berman DS, et al: Left ventricular ejection fraction determined by radionuclide ventriculography in early stages of first transmural myocardial infarction. Am J Cardiol 45:542, 1980

21. Abrams DS, Starling MR, Crawford MH, et al: Value of noninvasive techniques for predicting early complications in patients with clinical class II acute myocardial infarction. J Am Coll Cardiol 8:818, 1983

22. Schulze RA Jr, Strauss HW, Pitt B: Sudden death in the year following myocardial infarction: Relation to ventricular premature contractions in the late hospital phase and left ventricular ejection fraction. Am J Med 62:192, 1977

23. The Multicenter Postinfarction Research Group: Risk stratification and survival after myocardial infarction. N Engl J Med 309:331, 1983

24. Starling MR, Crawford MH, Henry RL, et al: Prognostic value of electrocardiographic exercise testing and noninvasive assessment of left ventricular ejection fraction soon after acute myocardial infarction. Am J Cardiol 57:532, 1986

25. Hochreiter C, Niles N, Devereux RB, et al: Mitral regurgitation: Relationship of noninvasive descriptors of right and left ventricular performance to clinical and hemodynamic findings and to prognosis in medically and surgically treated patients. Circulation 73:900, 1987

26. Alexander J, Dainiak N, Berger HJ, et al: Serial assessment of doxorubicin cardiotoxicity with quantitative radionuclide angiocardiography. N Engl J Med 300:278, 1979

27. Gottdiener JS, Mathisen DJ, Borer JS, et al: Doxorubicin cardiotoxicity: Assessment of late left ventricular dysfunction by radionuclide cineangiography. Ann Intern Med 94:430, 1981

28. Bacharach SL, Green MV, Borer JS, et al: Left ventricular peak ejection rate, filling rate, and ejection fraction frame rate requirements at rest and exercise: concise communication. J Nucl Med 20:189, 1979

29. Bonow RO, Rosing DR, Bacharach SL, et al: Effects of verapamil on left ventricular systolic function and diastolic filling in patients

with hypertropic carciomyopathy. Circulation 64:787, 1981

30. Bonow RO, Bacharach SL, Green MV, et al: Impaired left ventricular diastolic filling in patients with coronary artery disease: Assessment with radionuclide angiography. Circulation 64:315, 1981

31. Bonow RO, Kent KM, Rosing DR, et al: Improved left ventricular diastolic filling in patients with coronary artery disease after percutaneous transluminal coronary angioplasty. Circulation 66:1159, 1982

32. Yamagishi T, Ozaki M, Kumada T, et al: Assynchronous left ventricular diastolic filling in patients with isolated disease of the left anterior descending coronary artery: Assessment with radionuclide ventriculography. Circulation 69:933, 1984

33. Magorien DJ, Shaffer P, Bush C, et al: Hemodynamic correlates for timing intervals, ejection rate and filling rate derived from the radionuclide angiographic volume curve. Am J Cardiol 53:567, 1984

34. Ishida Y, Meisner JS, Tsujioka K, et al: Left ventricular filling dynamics: Influence of left ventricular relaxation and left atrial pressure. Circulation 74:187, 1986

35. Iskandrian AS, Hakki A-H: Age-related changes in left ventricular diastolic performance. Am Heart J 112:75, 1986

36. Links JM, Douglass KH, Wagner HN Jr: Patterns of ventricular emptying by Fourier analysis of gated blood-pool studies. J Nucl Med 21:978, 1980

37. Frais MA, Botvinick EH, Shosa DW, et al: Phase image characterization of ventricular contraction in left and right bundle branch block. Am J Cardiol 50:95, 1982

38. Botvinick EH, Frais MA, Shosa DW, et al: An accurate means of detecting and characterizing abnormal patterns of ventricular activation by phase image analysis. Am J Cardiol 50:289, 1982

39. Nakajima K, Bunko H, Tada A, et al: Phase analysis in the Wolff-Parkinson-White syndrome with surgically proven accessory conduction pathways: Concise communication. J Nucl Med 25:7, 1984

40. Swiryn S, Pavel D, Byrom E, et al: Sequential regional phase mapping of radionuclide gated biventriculograms in patients with sustained ventricular tachycardia: Close correlation with electrophysiologic characteristics. Am Heart J 103:319, 1982

41. Vos PH, Vossepoel AM, Pauwels EKJ: Quantitative assessment of wall motion in multiple-gated studies using temporal Fourier analysis. J Nucl Med 24:388, 1983

42. Botvinick E, Dunn R, Frais M, et al: The phase image: Its relationship to patterns of contraction and conduction. Circulation 65:551, 1982

43. Starling MR, Walsh RA, Lasher JC, et al: Quantification of left ventricular regional dyssynergy by radionuclide angiography. J Nucl Med 28:1725, 1987

44. Parrish MD, Graham TP Jr, Born ML, et al: Radionuclide ventriculography for assessment of absolute right and left ventricular volumes in children. Circulation 66:811, 1982

45. Dell'Italia LJ, Starling MR, Walsh RA, et al: Validation of attenuation-corrected equilibrium radionuclide angiographic determinations of right ventricular volume: Comparison with cast-validated biplane cineventriculography. Circulation 72:317, 1985

46. Nusynowitz ML, Benedetto AR, Walsh RA, et al: First pass anger camera radiocardiography: Biventricular ejection fraction, flow, and volume measurements. J Nucl Med 28:950, 1987

47. Steele P, Kirch D, LeFree M, et al: Measurement of right and left ventricular ejection fractions by radionuclide angiocardiography in coronary artery disease. Chest 70:51, 1976

48. Maddahi J, Berman DS, Matsuoka DT, et al: A new technique for assessing right ventricular ejection fraction using rapid multiple-gated equilibrium cardiac blood pool scintigraphy: Description, validation and findings in chronic coronary artery disease. Circulation 60:581, 1979

49. Harolds JA, Grove RB, Bowen RD, et al: Right ventricular function as assessed by two radionuclide techniques: Concise communication. J Nucl Med 22:113, 1981

50. Holman BL, Wynne J, Zielonka JS, et al: A simplified technique for measuring right ventricular ejection fraction using the equilibrium radionuclide angiocardiogram and the slant-hole collimator. Radiology 138:429, 1981

51. Ham HR, Franken PR, Georges B, et al: Evaluation of the accuracy of steady-state kryptom-81m method for calculating right ven-

tricular ejection fraction. J Nucl Med 27:593, 1986

52. Caplin JL, Flatman WD, Dymond DS: Gated right ventricular studies using krypton-81m: Comparison with first-pass studies using gold-195m. J Nucl Med 27:602, 1986

53. Wong DF, Natarajan TK, Summer W, et al: Right ventricular ejection fraction measured by first-pass intravenous krypton-81m: Reproducibility and comparison with technetium-99m. Am J Cardiol 56:776, 1985

54. Mena I, Narahara KA, de Jong R, et al: Gold-195m, an ultra-short-lived generator-produced radionuclide: Clinical application in sequential first pass ventriculography. J Nucl Med 24:139, 1983

55. Treves S, Cheng C, Samuel A, et al: Iridium-191 angiocardiography for the detection and quantitation of left-to-right shunting. J Nucl Med 21:1151, 1980

56. Martin W, Tweddel AC, McGhie I, et al: Gated xenon scans for right ventricular function. J Nucl Med 27:609, 1986

57. Goldberg MJ, Mantel J, Friedin M; et al: Intravenous xenon-133 for the determination of radionuclide first pass right ventricular ejection fraction. Am J Cardiol 47:626, 1981

58. Korr KS, Gandsman EJ, Winkler ML, et al: Hemodynamic correlates of right ventricular ejection fraction measured with gated radionuclide angiography. Am J Cardiol 49:71, 1982

59. Brent BN, Berger HJ, Matthay RA, et al: Physiologic correlates of right ventricular ejection fraction in chronic obstructive pulmonary disease: A combined radionuclide and hemodynamic study. Am J Cardiol 50:255, 1982

60. Tobinick E, Schelbert HR, Henning H, et al: Right ventricular ejection fraction in patients with acute anterior and inferior myocardial infarction assessed by radionuclide angiography. Circulation 57:1078, 1978

61. Reduto LA, Berger JH, Cohen LS, et al: Sequential radionuclide assessment of left and right ventricular performance after acute transmural myocardial infarction. Ann Intern Med 89:441, 1978

62. Starling MR, Dell'Italia LJ, Chaudhuri TK, et al: First transit and equilibrium radionuclide angiography in patients with inferior transmural myocardial infarction: Criteria for the diagnosis of associated hemodynamically significant right ventricular infarction. J Am Coll Cardiol 4:923, 1984

63. Dell'Italia LJ, Starling MR, Crawford MH, et al: Right ventricular infarction: Identification by hemodynamic measurements before and after volume loading and correlation with noninvasive techniques. J Am Coll Cardiol 931, 1984

64. Dell'Italia LJ, Starling MR, Blumhardt R, et al: Comparative effects of volume loading, dobutamine, and nitroprusside in patients with predominant right ventricular infarction. Circulation 72:1327, 1985

65. Polak JF, Holman BL, Wynne J, et al: Right ventricular ejection fraction: An indicator of increased mortality in patients with congestive heart failure associated with coronary artery disease. J Am Coll Cardiol 2:217, 1983

66. Baker BJ, Wilen MM, Boyd CM, et al: Relation of right ventricular ejection fraction to exercise capacity in chronic left ventricular failure. Am J Cardiol 54:596, 1984

67. Franciosa JA, Baker BJ, Seth L: Pulmonary versus systemic hemodynamics in determining exercise capacity in patients with chronic left ventricular failure. Am Heart J 110:807, 1985

68. Colucci WS, Holman BL, Wynne J, et al: Improved right ventricular function and reduced pulmonary vascular resistance during prazosin therapy of congestive heart failure. Am J Med 71:75, 1981

69. Konstam MA, Cohen SR, Salem DN, et al: Effect of amrinone on right ventricular function: Predominance of afterload reduction. Circulation 74:359, 1986

70. Berger HJ, Matthay RA, Loke J, et al: Assessment of cardiac performance with quantitative radionuclide angiocardiography: Right ventricular ejection fraction with reference to findings in chronic obstructive pulmonary disease. Am J Cardiol 41:897, 1978

71. Olvey SK, Reduto LA, Stevens PM, et al: First pass radionuclide assessment of right and left ventricular ejection fraction in chronic pulmonary disease: Effect of oxygen upon exercise response. Chest 78:4, 1980

72. Mathur PN, Powles P, Pugsley SO, et al: Effect of digoxin on right ventricular function in severe chronic airflow obstruction: A controlled clinical trial. Ann Intern Med 95:283, 1981

73. Matthay RA, Berger HJ, Loke J, et al: Effects

of aminophylline upon right and left ventricular performance in chronic obstructive pulmonary disease: Noninvasive assessment by radionuclide angiocardiography. Am J Med 65:903, 1978

74. Brent BN, Mahler D, Berger HJ, et al: Augmentation of right ventricular performance in chronic obstructive pulmonary disease by terbutaline: A combined radionuclide and hemodynamic study. Am J Cardiol 50:313, 1982

75. Brent BN, Berger HJ, Matthay RA, et al: Contrasting acute effects of vasodilators (nitroglycerin, nitroprusside, and hydralazine) on right ventricular performance in patients with chronic obstructive pulmonary disease and pulmonary hypertension: A combined radionuclide-hemodynamic study. Am J Cardiol 51:1682, 1983

76. Askenazi J, Ahnberg DS, Korngold E, et al: Quantitative radionuclide angiocardiography: Detection and quantitation of left-to-right shunts. Am J Cardiol 37:382, 1976

77. Sorensen SG, Starling MR, Chaudhuri TK, et al: Non-invasive quantitation of right ventricular volume overload in adults by gated equilibrium radionuclide angiography. J Nucl Med 23:957, 1982

78. Rigo P, Alderson PO, Robertson RM, et al: Measurement of aortic and mitral regurgitation by gated cardiac blood pool scans. Circulation 60:306, 1979

79. Sorensen SG, O'Rourke RA, Chaudhuri TK: Noninvasive quantitation of valvular regurgitation by gated equilibrium radionuclide angiography. Circulation 62:1089, 1980

80. Bough EW, Gandsman EJ, North DL, et al: Gated radionuclide angiographic evaluation of valve regurgitation. Am J Cardiol 46:423, 1980

81. Urquhart J, Patterson RE, Packer M, et al: Quantification of valve regurgitation by radionuclide angiography before and after valve replacement surgery. Am J Cardiol 47:287, 1981

82. Lam W, Pavel D, Byrom E, et al: Radionuclide regurgitant index: Value and limitations. Am J Cardiol 47:292, 1981

83. Konstam MA, Wynne J, Holman BL, et al: Use of equilibrium (gated) radionuclide ventriculography to quantitate left ventricular output in patients with and without left-sided valvular regurgitation. Circulation 64:578, 1981

84. Nicod P, Corbett JR, Firth BG, et al: Radionuclide techniques for valvular regurgitant index: Comparison in patients with normal and depressed ventricular function. J Nucl Med 23:763, 1982

85. Alderson PO: Radionuclide quantification of valvular regurgitation. J Nucl Med 23:851, 1982

5

Cardiac Evaluation by Nuclear First-Pass Techniques

Martin L. Nusynowitz
Anthony R. Benedetto

Cardiovascular nuclear medicine techniques are valuable in assessing the presence and extent of myocardial infarction and myocardial ischemia, the integrity of the septa between the various chambers of the heart, the competence of the mitral and aortic valves, and the pumping performance of the heart. First-pass radiocardiographic techniques may be the preferred methods for detecting and quantifying shunts, detecting and quantifying valvular regurgitation, assessing the pumping performance of the right ventricle, and measuring right ventricular volumes and cardiac output.

The principal advantages of first-pass methods, compared with gated equilibrium methods, are the minimization of difficulties associated with overlapping cardiac chambers and the avoidance of generalized total body background. First-pass techniques employing radionuclide tracers also have advantages over other techniques used in cardiovascular laboratories, such as dilution methods using nonradioactive tracers, oximetry, and cineangiography. It is important for the nuclear medicine physician to have some understanding of these methods in order to recognize the relative advantages offered by first-pass angiocardiography.

EJECTION FRACTION, VOLUME, AND FLOW MEASUREMENTS: THEORETICAL OVERVIEW

First-pass radionuclide angiocardiography may be performed for the assessment of right ventricular ejection fraction (RVEF) or for the comprehensive evaluation of RV and LV cardiac outputs, volumes, and ejection fractions. If only RVEF is desired, any technetium-labeled radiopharmaceutical can be used. A rapidly excreted agent such as technetium-99m DTPA should be used if LV evaluation by subsequent gated equilibrium technique is not needed. The right anterior oblique (RAO) projection is used, since it gives optimal spatial and temporal separation between right atrium and right ventricle and adequate temporal separation between the right and left sides of the heart. If an equilibrium-gated study to assess LV function is also to be performed, the RVEF can be determined from the injection of technetium-99m pertechnetate used to label erythrocytes in vivo. Since RVEF is only one of the many parameters that can be measured by the first-pass study of both ventricles, a thorough discussion of the clinical applications of the first-pass method requires a detailed analysis of its uses in deriving a variety of important cardiac functional parameters.

Right Ventricular and Left Ventricular Ejection Fractions

Ejection fraction is defined as the fractional amount of end-diastolic volume (EDV) leaving the ventricle during a contraction, that is

$$EF = \frac{\text{stroke volume (SV)}}{EDV} = \frac{EDV - ESV}{EDV} \quad (1a)$$

Since the ventricular volume is proportional to the count rate emanating from the ventricle,

$$EDV = kEDC \text{ (end-diastolic counts)}$$
$$ESV = kESC \text{ (end-systolic counts)}$$

and

$$EF = \frac{kEDC - kESC}{kEDC} = \frac{EDC - ESC}{EDC} \quad (1b)$$

A bolus of radiopharmaceutical passing through a ventricular chamber will yield a count rate-versus-time curve of high fidelity if the framing rate is at least 25 images/sec, or 40 msec/image (Fig. 5-1). The peaks on the curve represent end-diastole, and the valleys represent end-systole for the series of beats during which the radionuclide bolus passes through the ventricular chamber. The ejection fraction for each beat can be calculated as in equation 1b and an average obtained.

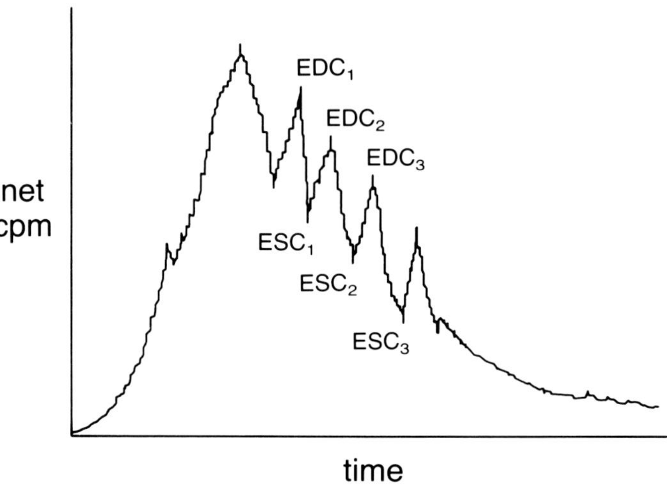

Fig. 5-1 First-pass radiocardiogram recorded at 25 frames/sec. Ejection fraction is calculated beat by beat as $(EDC_n - ESC_n)/(EDC_n)$; individual beat EF then averaged. Curve has been corrected for background, if appropriate.

For a tight-bolus peripheral venous injection (e.g., jugular vein), it is usually possible to identify 3 to 5 beats for the RV and 5 to 7 beats for the LV (due to bolus spreading during transit through the RV and lungs).

Note that the ordinate in Figure 5-1 is net count rate, that is, corrected for background. Assuming the patient has not recently received radioactive material that localizes in the bloodstream or thorax, there will be no background counts for the RV. For the LV, however, it is necessary to correct for the background γ rays arising from the lungs as the bolus enters the LV and for counts arising from the descending aorta (if it lies behind the LV) as the bolus leaves the LV.

Cardiac Output

First-pass radionuclide techniques for measurement of cardiac output are based on well-established indicator dilution methods previously validated with nonradioactive indicators, including indocyanine green dye, chilled saline, and various gases.[1]

If a radioactive indicator is not removed from the bloodstream between the point of bolus injection and the point of sampling, the blood flow (in this case, cardiac output) through a defined region of interest (ventricular chamber) can be calculated by dividing the total dosage injected by the area under the time-activity curve obtained over the ROI:

$$
\begin{aligned}
&\text{Flow or Cardiac Output (ml/min)} \\
&= \frac{\text{total dose injected } (\mu\text{Ci})}{\text{area under curve } (\mu\text{Ci} \cdot \text{min} \cdot \text{ml}^{-1})}
\end{aligned} \tag{2a}
$$

A bolus of radiopharmaceutical administered in a peripheral vein will yield a count rate-versus-time curve such as that shown in Figure 5-2, if the framing rate is 2 images/sec, or 0.5 sec/image. Resolution of the individual beats is unnecessary for determination of cardiac output. If the activity (μCi) injected is known and the ordinate of Figure 5-2 is also activity, which would permit calculation of the area under the curve in units of activity versus time, equation 2a can easily be solved for cardiac output.

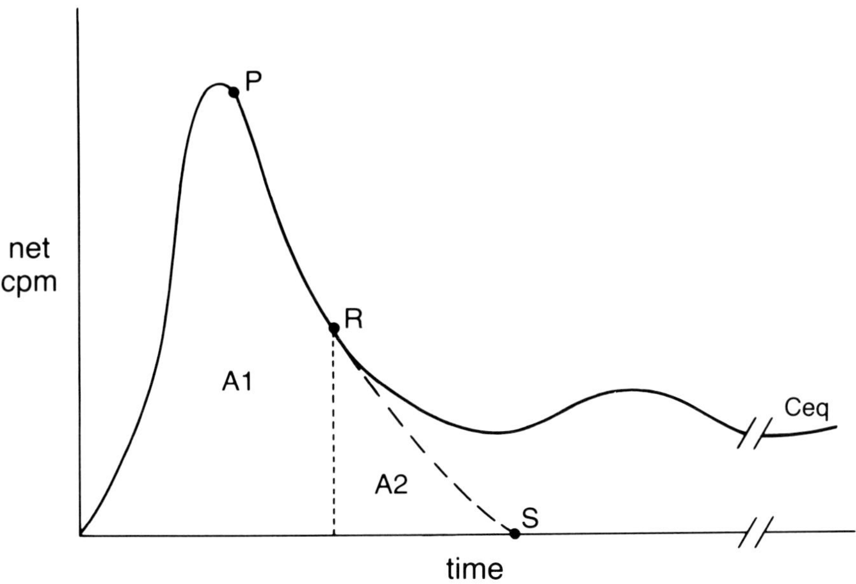

Fig. 5-2 First-pass radiocardiogram recorded at 2 frames/sec. Curve has been corrected for background, if appropriate.

Although activity (μCi) cannot be measured directly using a gamma camera, the count rate obtained by the camera is directly proportional to activity, with the proportionality constant taking into account geometry, sensitivity, and attenuation from overlying tissues. If the patient is not moved throughout the study, the proportionality constant relating microcuries and counts per minute in equation 2a will be identical to the proportionality constant in the denominator, and the two will cancel. Equation 2a may then be rewritten as follows:

Flow or Cardiac Output (ml/min)

$$= \frac{\text{total dosage injected (cpm)}}{\text{area under curve (cpm} \cdot \text{min} \cdot \text{ml}^{-1})} \quad (2b)$$

At equilibrium (5 to 15 minutes postinjection), the total injected dosage will be diluted in the total blood volume (TBV). Therefore, the concentration of the tracer at equilibrium, C_{eq}, expressed as a count rate per unit volume, will be

$$C_{eq}\,(\text{cpm/ml}) = \frac{\text{total injected dosage (cpm)}}{\text{TBV (ml)}}$$
$$(3a)$$

or

$$\text{Total injected dosage (cpm)} = C_{eq} \times \text{TBV}$$
$$(3b)$$

The area under the tracer-dilution curve can be calculated by either of two methods: the Stewart-Hamilton curve extrapolation method, or the gamma-variate method.

STEWART-HAMILTON CURVE EXTRAPOLATION METHOD

Because recirculation of activity through the heart from the systemic circulation occurs before the radionuclide bolus completely leaves the ventricle, it is necessary to extrapolate the downslope of the curve (Fig. 5-2) to 0 counts to define the first pass curve. Since the washout of tracer from the ventricle is a monoexponential function,[2] we can readily use the portion of the downslope prior to recirculation (PR) to calculate the equation

of the exponential curve (PRS), hence of the latter portion of the curve (RS). Area A_1 is calculated by simply summing all the individual data points from the time of injection up to R. Area (A_2) under the exponential curve RS is calculated as follows:

$$A_2 = \frac{\text{R}}{\text{slope}} \quad (4)$$

where the slope is obtained from a log–linear regression, using the data points in the segment PR.

Therefore, the denominator of equation 2b is simply

$$A = A_1 + A_2$$

Equation 2b now becomes

Flow or Cardiac Output (ml/min)

$$= \frac{C_{eq}\,(\text{cpm} \cdot \text{ml}^{-1}) \cdot \text{TBV (ml)}}{A\,(\text{cpm} \cdot \text{min} \cdot \text{ml}^{-1})} \quad (5)$$

Before the first-pass portion of the study, TBV is measured using Iodine-125 human serum albumin (HSA)[3]; correction for the difference between central and peripheral hematocrit (Hct) is incorporated into the calculation of red blood cell (RBC) volume from the measured plasma volume.[4]

The equilibrium count rate C_{eq} is obtained by collecting images 5 to 15 minutes after injection of the bolus; since the tracer disappears from the bloodstream monoexponentially during the 5- to 15-minute equilibrium period,[3] it is necessary to extrapolate the 5- to 15-minute segment of the count-rate curve logarithmically back to the injection time.

GAMMA-VARIATE METHOD

Thompson et al.[5] noted that the indicator dilution curve (Fig. 5-2) could be approximated by the gamma–variate curve described as follows:

$$C(t) = K(t - AT)^{\alpha} e^{-(t - AT)/\beta} \quad (6)$$

where $C(t)$ = indicator concentration at time t postinjection

AT = appearance time of the bolus in the region of interest (ROI)

K, α, β = scaling and fitting parameters

When scaling and curve-fitting parameters are selected properly, this gamma-variate curve closely approximates the shape of the curve in Figure 5-2 and carries itself to the 0 count-rate axis, thereby correcting for recirculation. This allows for the calculation of the area under the curve—the denominator of equation 5 for cardiac output. The calculation of the numerator of equation 5 for the gamma-variate is identical to that described in the preceding section for the Stewart-Hamilton cardiac output. The gamma-variate method slightly underestimates the area of the count rate curve (Fig. 2) compared with the Stewart-Hamilton logarithmic extrapolation area, yielding a slightly higher gamma-variate cardiac output result.

COMPARISON OF ALTERNATIVE DILUTION METHODS FOR CARDIAC OUTPUT DETERMINATION

Cardiac output can be measured by nonradionuclide dilution techniques using indocyanine green dye and by thermodilution methods. Measurements of cardiac output by the indocyanine green dye method are usually performed during a cardiac catheterization procedure.[1] For measurements of right-sided cardiac output, a catheter is placed in the right atrium for injection, and another catheter is inserted in the pulmonary artery for dye sampling; left-sided measurements use catheter placements in the pulmonary artery (injection) and a systemic artery, usually aorta (sampling).

Indocyanine green dye concentration is measured spectrophotometrically as blood is automatically sampled at a rapid constant rate. Since the amount of dye is known, cardiac output is readily calculated by dividing the amount of dye injected by the area under the dye concentration-versus-time curve.

Thermodilution cardiac output generally uses ice-cold (0° to 4°C) saline. Blood flow disperses the cold saline into the bloodstream, reducing the normal 37°C blood temperature by 1° to 2°C at the sampling site. A Swan-Ganz catheter with a thermistor (heat sensor) in its distal tip measures the temperature continuously and a temperature-versus-time curve is obtained. The amount of indicator injected in thermodilution is the heat energy added to the blood by the injected cold saline. Cardiac output is calculated by a dedicated microprocessor and displayed digitally. A recording of the temperature-time curve is made to verify technical adequacy of the procedure.

Many advantages and disadvantages are shared by the first-pass radionuclide, indocyanine green dye, and thermodilution techniques, since they are all indicator dilution methods. Recirculation occurs to a significant degree in both the radionuclide and indocyanine green dye measurements, which complicates calculation of the area under the indicator dilution curve; recirculation is negligible in thermodilution. All the tracers (technetium-99m HSA, indocyanine green dye, chilled saline) must be carefully and meticulously prepared and handled. Invasive catheterization is required for the indocyanine green dye and thermodilution methods, while the radionuclide method can be performed with a peripheral venous injection. The indocyanine green dye is rapidly removed from the bloodstream, and the chilled saline is rapidly warmed to the bulk blood temperature, such that repeat measurements can be made after about 10 to 15 minutes; when technetium-99m HSA has been used, multiple repeat radionuclide measurements are difficult, since technetium-99m HSA stays in the bloodstream for hours. Indicator dilution cardiac outputs by all three methods tend to be somewhat smaller than those calculated by Fick oximetry.

COMPARISON WITH NONDILUTION TECHNIQUES

Fick oximetry and cardiac cineangiography can also be used to obtain cardiac output; cardiac cineangiography can be used to calculate chamber volumes and ejection fractions and to estimate the severity of regurgitation. Both require invasive catheterization, and the sedation and anesthesia administered during catheterization may cause the data obtained not to be representative of the patient's basal state.

In cardiac output determination by Fick oximetry, oxygen consumption is measured from expired air collected into a Douglas bag over a 3- to 5-minute period. Aliquots of blood are withdrawn from the pulmonary artery and a systemic artery during the middle portion of breath collection, and the oxygen content is measured spectrophotometrically.

Fick oximetry requires meticulous attention to detail. Collection of air must be complete, and the respiratory pattern should be stable throughout collection of expired air. Estimation of oxygen consumption from nomograms can give unacceptable values when the patient is sedated, under anesthesia, uncooperative, or has valvular heart disease. Hypothyroidism and hyperthyroidism, valvular heart disease, and nonbasal states can all contribute to erroneous measurement of oxygen consumption. Hyperthyroidism and left-to-right shunts cause narrowed arteriovenous (A-V) difference, while low-output states lead to widened A-V differences. Since indocyanine green dye interferes with the spectrophotometric measurement of oxygen content, oximetry must be performed first and cannot be readily repeated after green dye has been injected.

Because of their difficulty, cineangiography techniques are applied primarily to the left ventricle. During cardiac catheterization, radiographic contrast material is injected into the LV, and image intensifier images are collected on cine-film at high framing rates. Using beats visually determined to be representative, the LV silhouettes at end-diastole and end-systole are enlarged and traced onto a clear plastic sheet or a piece of opaque paper, or they are digitized into a minicomputer or powerful microcomputer. If biplane angiography is performed, the LV is assumed to be represented mathematically as an ellipsoid rotated in space; the mathematical model is a prolate spheroid in the case of single-plane angiography. These models permit calculation of end-diastolic and end-systolic volumes, from which ejection fraction, stroke volume, and cardiac output may be determined in turn.

Cardiac cineangiography is regarded as the gold standard, yet it is fraught with difficulties, disadvantages, and tenuous assumptions. Contrast material is inotropic, so only a few beats may be used post injection. Contrast material may be toxic to the kidneys, so the total volume employed must be kept small. This limits the number of runs that can be recorded; it also limits the ability to define the LV silhouette accurately due to low visual contrast between the wall and contents of the LV.

Furthermore, the mathematical models employed are not exact, even in normal patients, and they become increasingly inaccurate with deranged ventricular morphology and with abnormal wall motion. Single-plane angiography is less accurate than biplane methods, especially in ventricles of abnormal shape. Radiographic magnification at the midplane of the LV must be measured, and correction for pincushion distortion should be performed. Improper placement of the catheter can cause dysrhythmias and can interfere with mitral valve function. Delineation of the LV silhouette should include the papillary muscles and trabeculations; this is currently more art than science and requires operator skill for accuracy and reproducibility. Angiographic methods overestimate LV volumes compared with postmortem casts. Regression equations must be used to adjust the resultant geometric volumes.

Parameters Derived from Ejection Fraction and Cardiac Output

Let us assume that ejection fraction (RV, LV) and cardiac output (RV, lungs, LV) have been determined. Since bolus streaming in the RV yields a cardiac output that is artifactually high, and the use of a lung ROI to estimate RV cardiac output has consistently resulted in more realistic cardiac output values, we prefer to use the lung flow as representative of RV cardiac output and, in conjunction with measured RVEF, to calculate RV volumes and left-sided valvular regurgitation. Parameters derived from EF and cardiac output (F) so determined are as follows:

Stroke Volume (SV):

$$SV \text{ (ml)} = \frac{F \text{ (ml} \cdot \text{min}^{-1})}{HR \text{ (beats} \cdot \text{min}^{-1})} \qquad (7)$$

where HR = heart rate (bpm).

RV End-diastolic and End-systolic Volumes (EDV, ESV):

$$RVEDV \text{ (ml)} = \frac{RVSV \text{ (ml)}}{RVEF} \qquad (8)$$

$$RVESV \text{ (ml)} = (RVEDV - RVSV) \qquad (9)$$

Left Ventricle Volumes and Regurgitant Fraction:

If bolus smearing does not occur and the patient does not have valvular regurgitation, LVEDV and LVESV can be calculated using equations 8 and 9 and using LVEF rather than RVEF. The mathematical effect of both bolus smearing and regurgitation is to increase the area under the indicator dilution curve (equation 2b) and thereby to apparently reduce the cardiac output. Since cardiac output *F* is used to calculate SV (equation 7) and then EDV and ESV (equations 8 and 9), bolus smearing and regurgitation cause all three parameters (SV, EDV, ESV) to be artifactually low.

If we assume that the patient does not have right-sided valvular regurgitation, we may estimate the magnitude of left-sided valvular regurgitation (if present) in the following manner. The uncorrected stroke volume (equation 7) is the algebraic summation of the forward flow ejected into the aorta (FF) and the backward flow (BF), which is the regurgitant flow (if present), plus the apparent decreased flow due to bolus smearing.[7] If there is no right-sided regurgitation, the RVSV estimated from the lung ROI, $RVSV_{LU}$, must be equal to the LV forward flow, LVFF, that is

$$LVFF = RVSV_{LU} \qquad (10a)$$

Since

$$LVSV_{uncorr} = LVFF - BF, \qquad (10b)$$

$$BF = RVSV_{LU} - LVSV_{uncorr}$$

But the total LV flow $LVSV_{corr}$ is the forward flow plus the back flow:

$$LVSV_{corr} = LVFF + BF \qquad (10c)$$

Thus

$$LVSV_{corr} = RVSV_{LU} + BF \qquad (10d)$$

The regurgitant fraction RF is the ratio of the back flow to the total LV flow:

$$RF = \frac{BF}{LVSV_{corr}} \qquad (11)$$

In our experience, RF is in the range of 0 to 18 percent for patients without valvular regurgitation, due to bolus smearing. Values of RF greater than 18 percent are strongly suggestive of regurgitation.[7]

Clinical Acquisition Methodology

In first-pass radionuclide angiocardiography, no special patient preparation is required. Prior to imaging, the patient's total blood volume (equation 6) is measured using 0.2 MBq (5- to 10-μCi) iodine-125 HSA, and the patient's height and weight are recorded for calculation of body surface area (BSA), which is used for the derivation of the cardiac index (CI). The patient is positioned supine under a large crystal gamma camera equipped with a general purpose low-energy collimator, with the camera centered on the heart and oriented for a 45-degree LAO, 10-degree caudal (toward the feet) tilt. A modest zoom of about 1.2 to 1.4 times is used. This LAO projection optimizes the spatial and temporal separation of the right and left ventricles. ECG electrodes are placed in the standard configuration for an equilibrium-gated study.

A dosage of 370 MBq (10 mCi) of technetium-99m HSA is rapidly injected as a tight bolus into the right external jugular vein. This dosage is not large enough to cause significant deadtime losses, yet it provides adequate count statistics. The neck vein is used to avoid excessive bolus smearing. Patients accept the neck injection well, when it is explained to them that a neck injection is technically necessary and that the pain is actually less than for an arm injection.

Three seconds prior to injection, the ECG recorder and computer are started and allowed to run for 60 seconds. The patient's heart rate (equation 7) is calculated from the full 60-second strip; a resting HR taken before the study or during a subsequent equilibrium-gated study cannot be used, since the HR is usually elevated during the first-pass study. We usually perform first-pass studies on a computer that is capable of acquiring data in serial (list) mode, since EF analysis requires 25 frames/sec and cardiac output analysis requires only 2 frames/sec. If serial mode is not available, a framing rate of 24 frames/sec would be acceptable for EF analysis; the cardiac output calculations can then be based on a reformatted series of images formed by adding 8 of the 24-frame/sec images together, thereby creating 3-frame/sec images. Either the camera timer or a stopwatch is started at the time of injection.

At the end of the first 60 seconds, the computer is quickly reset to collect 10-second static images with the same matrix, zoom, and high count-rate parameters and switch settings used for the initial flow acquisition. The patient and the camera must not be moved. Static images are collected at 5, 7.5, 10, 12.5, and 15 minutes elapsed time. These images will be used to calculate the equilibrium count rate (Ceq) (equation 3a), correcting for the disappearance rate of technetium-99m HSA from the bloodstream.

Since the positioning of the camera for the first-pass study does not always permit careful separation of the RV and LV, and since the descending aorta may lie behind the LV, it has been our experience that first-pass LVEF is occasionally artifactually low. Therefore, we routinely inject a second dosage of 370 MBq of technetium-99m HSA, allow it to mix in the patient's bloodstream for 10 to 15 minutes, and then perform a routine equilibrium-gated study to assess RV and LV wall motion and LVEF.

DATA ANALYSIS

In a typical first-pass study, the total counts in each of the 25 frames/sec images obtained are too low to permit accurate delineation of the various ROI that must be flagged. Therefore, we use the 2-frame/sec images as the primary basis for flagging ROI, supplementing them with summed images as necessary. ROI are created for the superior vena cava (SVC), RV, lungs (excluding major vessels), LV, and LV background (BKGD). These ROI and the 2-frame/sec images are used to generate a set of curves that provide data for the calculation of the area under the count rate-versus-time curve (A_1) and the logarithmic extrapolation for A_2 (equation 4). The SVC curve permits assessment of the quality of the bolus. These ROI (minus SVC) are also used to determine the count rate in each region from the five static images to measure the equilibrium count rate (C_{eq}).

Reformatting all 60 seconds of the flow study into 25-frame/sec images would create 1,500 images. The time and disk storage space needed to deal with so many images is unwarranted, since the only purpose of these images is the calculation of RVEF and LVEF. We use the 2-frame/sec curves and images to define the appearance time of the bolus in the RV and the time when most of the bolus has left the LV, then reformat at 25 frames/sec only between these two times. The total number of images is usually 500 to 750.

The RV, LV, and LV BKGD ROI are used in conjunction with the 25-frame/sec images to generate curves. In order to correct for LV background, the ratio of LV pixels divided by LV BKGD pixels is multiplied by the LV BKGD curve. We then perform 10 sequential 3-point 1-2-1 temporal smooths of the multiplied LV BKGD curve in order to minimize statistical fluctuations. The smoothed LV BKGD curve is subtracted from the gross LV curve to obtain the LV NET curve. The RV and LV NET curves are then smoothed once and used to calculate RVEF and LVEF (equation 1b).

The RV, lungs, LV, and LV BKGD ROI, the 2-frame/sec images, and the five static equilibrium images are used to obtain input data for the calculation of cardiac output

(equation 5). An LV NET curve is generated in the same manner as described in the preceding paragraph. For the RV, lungs, and LV NET curves, the computer is told where point R occurs. The area A_1 is obtained by adding all the individual points from the beginning of the upslope to and including point R. The segment PR is used in a log-linear regression to calculate the slope of the segment PRS and to calculate A_2 using equation 4. The denominator of equation 5 is simply $A_1 + A_2$.

The equilibrium concentration C_{eq} is derived from the RV, lungs, and LV NET data from the five static equilibrium images. Since technetium-99m HSA disappears significantly from the bloodstream during the first 15 minutes, the five points for each ROI are entered into a log-linear regression program to calculate the value at $t = 0$ (C_{eq}). The corrected total blood volume is calculated from the iodine-125 HSA study.[4] The numerator of equation 5 is the injected activity,

$$\text{TBV} \times C_{eq} \qquad (3b)$$

The heart rate during the first 60 seconds is calculated and manually entered into the computer. Equations 7 to 9 are used to calculate RV and lung SV, EDV, and ESV. The regurgitant fraction (RF) is calculated using equation 11, and the corrected LV SV (equation 10) is used to adjust F, cardiac index, EDV, and ESV for the effects of regurgitation and bolus smearing.

CLINICAL EXPERIENCE AND VALIDATION

First-Pass Ejection Fraction

There is excellent correlation and almost identical results between first-pass (FP) LVEF and LVEF measured from equilibrium radiocardiographic (EQ) images:[7]

$$EQ\ LVEF = 0.99\ FP\ LVEF + 1.4,\ p < 0.001$$

In an occasional patient, however, the FP LVEF may be lower than the EQ LVEF due to malpositioning of the interventricular septum and/or to superimposition of the LV over the descending aorta. In these uncommon instances, we use the EQ LVEF to calculate end-systolic and end-diastolic volumes (equations 8 and 9).

Correlation of EQ and FP LVEF with biplane cineangiographic LVEF is excellent and well established. However, RVEF is not readily measured using cineangiography. We have shown that FP RVEF correlates highly with FP LVEF in patients without regurgitant valvular disease, and that the values obtained are reasonable.[8]

First-Pass Cardiac Output

The use of an RV curve to calculate cardiac output results in artifactually high values, probably due to inadequate mixing.[7]

Therefore we use the lung curve, since the SV calculated for the lung ROI correlates very well with SV determined by the Fick and indocyanine green methods.[1] Thus, in equations 8 and 9 we use the measured RVEF and the lung SV to calculate RVEDV and RVESV. LVEDV and LVESV are based on the measured LVSV, corrected for bolus smearing and regurgitation, and the FP LVEF; if the FP LVEF is technically inadequate, the EQ LVEF is used.

The regurgitant fraction (equation 11) was observed to correspond very closely to the degree of regurgitation estimated visually during contrast angiocardiography.[7] A gross RF of 18 percent or greater was strongly predictive of the presence of valvular regurgitation. Bolus smearing through the right side of the heart and the lungs contributes to the 0 to 18 percent range of results obtained in patients without regurgitation.

SHUNTS

Left-to-Right Shunt

In the procedure for left-to-right shunt quantification, the patient is positioned for an anterior heart-lung acquisition, and the computer is set to acquire 4 frames/sec for 30 seconds. A tight rapid bolus of technetium-99m DTPA is injected into an external jugular vein. Peripheral vein injections frequently cause unacceptable bolus smearing and should be avoided.[9] An ROI is delineated over the lungs, and a pulmonary activity-time curve is generated.

In a normal patient (Fig. 5-3A), the downslope of the primary curve is rapid and uninterrupted; the normal (late) recirculation of the radionuclide appears as a small second peak, clearly separated from the first peak. In a patient with a left-to-right shunt (Fig. 5-3B), a portion of the radiopharmaceutical returns prematurely to the lungs via the shunt, causing an early recirculation peak; the late recirculation peak may occur close in time to the shunt peak, and they may be difficult to distinguish from each other.

The flow through the shunt is proportional to the area under the secondary peak A_2 in Figure 5-3B.[9] If the total area under the extrapolated initial portion of the curve is designated A_1, the systemic flow Q_s is proportional to the area A_1-A_2. Thus

$$\frac{Q_p}{Q_s} = \frac{A_1}{A_1 - A_2} \qquad (12)$$

The A_1 curve is estimated either by logarithmically extrapolating the downslope of the primary peak or by fitting a gamma-variate curve to the upslope of the primary peak. Most commercial computer software uses the gamma-variate method, since the downslope is frequently too brief to permit accurate extrapolation, especially in moderate and severe

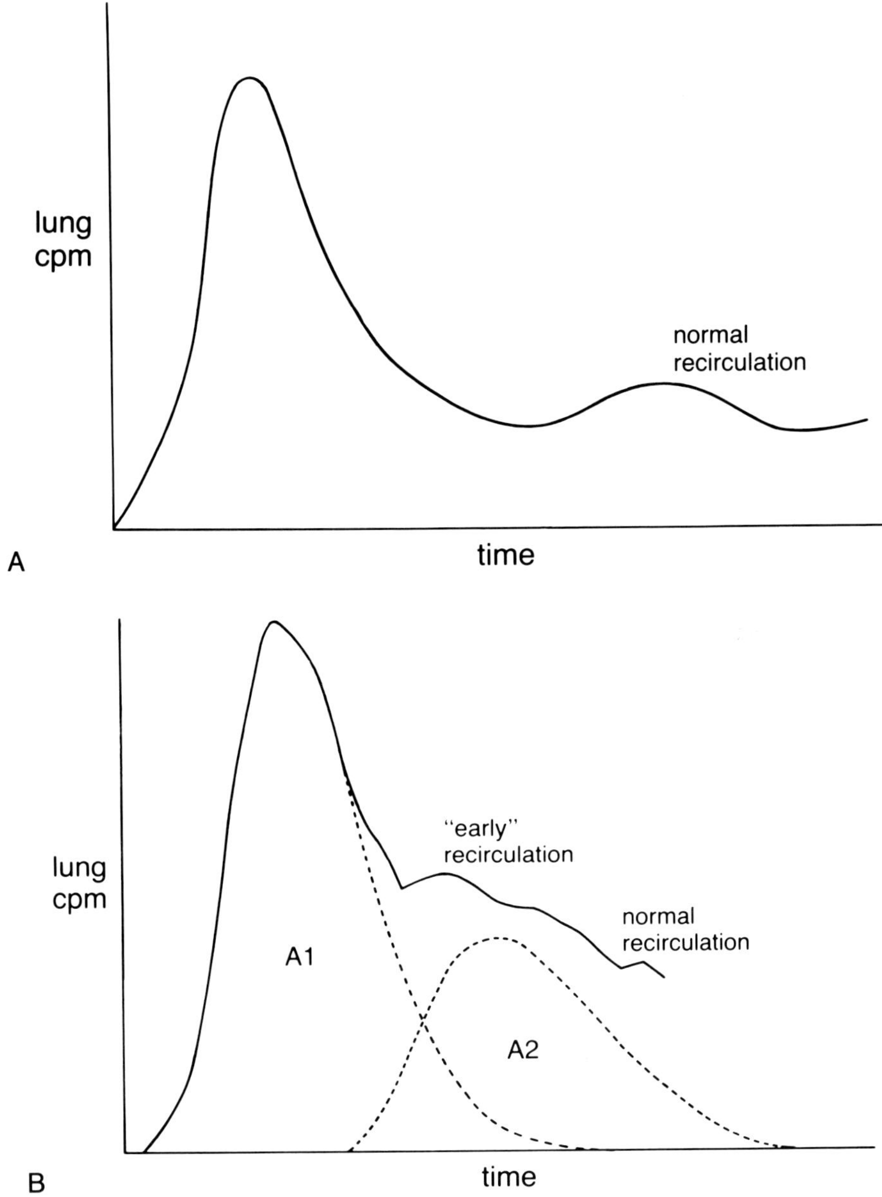

Fig. 5-3 (A) First-pass radiocardiogram using lung region of interest in a patient without left-to-right shunt. **(B)** Patient with left-to-right shunt, as evidenced by early return of radiopharmaceutical to the lung via the shunt.

shunting. If the derived A_1 curve is then subtracted from the gross count rate-versus-time (solid line), the upslope portion of the shunt curve will be obtained. The gamma-variate method is used a second time to fit the upslope of the shunt curve and to obtain the complete shunt curve A_2. The shunt severity is then calculated from equation 12. Minimum detectable values are about 1.3.

All the non-nuclear techniques for detecting or quantitating left-to-right shunts require the invasive placement of catheters. Qualitative detection of a shunt is performed by passing a catheter through the defect. Contrast angiocardiography yields a semiquantitative assessment of the amount of contrast material passing through the defect (i.e., mild, moderate, severe). The quantitative techniques (oximetry and indicator dilution) are similar in concept to those described earlier in this chapter.

The minimum detectable Q_p/Q_s ratio for oximetry is also about 1.3, provided that the cardiac index is in the lower range of normal, that is, up to 3 L·min^{-1}·m^{-2} (normal: 2.5 to 4.5 L·min^{-1}·m^{-2}). Oxygen consumption, hemoglobin, and arterial oxygen saturation must also be normal.

Using indocyanine green dye dilution, a left-to-right shunt yields an early peak in the downslope of the dye curve when the dye is injected in the right side of the heart and sampled in a systemic artery. As in the radiocardiographic technique, the early peak may be difficult to distinguish from normal recirculation, especially if the shunt is not severe. Q_p/Q_s must be greater than 1.33, there must be no valvular regurgitation, and shunting can only be unidirectional.

Right-to-Left Shunt

Radionuclide methods have been devised for right-to-left shunts,[9] but they are infrequently used, as techniques not requiring radioactive materials are readily available.

REFERENCES

1. Saksena FB: Hemodynamics in Cardiology: Calculations and Interpretations. Praeger, New York, 1983
2. Lassen NA, Perl W: Tracer Kinetic Methods in Medical Physiology. Raven Press, New York, 1979
3. Nusynowitz ML, Straw JD, Benedetto AR, Dixon RS: Blood clearance rates of technetium-99m albumin preparations. J Nucl Med 19:1142, 1978
4. Nusynowitz ML, Blumhardt R: Estimation of true red cell volume from RISA red cell volume. AJR 120:549, 1974
5. Thompson HK Jr, Starmer CF, Whalen RE, McIntosh HD: Indicator transit time considered as a gamma variate. Circ Res 14:502, 1964
6. Yoder RD, Swan EA: Cardiac output: Comparison of Stewart-Hamilton and gamma-function techniques. J Appl Physiol 31:318, 1971
7. Nusynowitz ML, Benedetto AR, Walsh RA, Starling MR: First-pass Anger camera radiocardiography: Biventricular ejection fraction, flow, and volume measurements. J Nucl Med 28:950, 1987
8. Benedetto AR, Nusynowitz ML: Correlation of right and left ventricular ejection fraction and volume measurements. J Nucl Med 29:1114, 1988
9. Treves T, Parker JA: Detection and quantification of intracardiac shunts. p. 148 in Strauss HW, Pitt B (eds): *Cardiovascular Nuclear Medicine*. 2nd Ed. CV Mosby, St. Louis, 1979

6

Exercise Radionuclide Angiography

Ian P. Clements

Modern radionuclide left ventriculography developed during the 1970s as computer and imaging technology combined to enable the study of cardiac volume changes at rest and with exercise. This technology permitted the study of either the passage of a bolus of isotope through the heart or the blood-pool activity in the heart. Importantly, in patients with significant coronary artery disease, studies using contrast angiography demonstrated that left ventricular ejection fraction may decrease and left ventricular wall motion may worsen with exercise.[1,2] Radionuclide ventriculography permitted noninvasive assessment of such exercise-induced changes in the left ventricle.

Initial studies showed a remarkably consistent response in the left ventricle.[3–6] Patients with coronary artery disease almost invariably showed a decrease in ejection fraction or a worsening in wall motion with exercise. If a patient did not have cardiac disease, ejec-

tion fraction rose and wall motion remained normal.

As experience with the technique broadened during the late 1970s, two observations were noted. First, radionuclide ventriculography permitted the most accurate noninvasive means of studying left ventricular ejection fraction and volume during interventions, including exercise. Second, the division between a normal and an abnormal response to exercise was not as clear cut[7,8] as first anticipated. This latter finding entailed a diminished ability of exercise radionuclide ventriculography to identify underlying pathology, in particular, coronary artery disease.

This chapter reviews the current application of exercise radionuclide ventriculography in cardiology. Initially, the exercise response of the normal heart will be reviewed. Subsequently, the ability of exercise radionuclide ventriculography to detect disease and determine prognosis in cardiac disease states is analyzed.

NORMAL EXERCISE RADIONUCLIDE ANGIOGRAM

Reproducibility

Before understanding the significance of an abnormal response of the left ventricle to exercise, we should consider the nature of a normal response. The radionuclide ventriculogram focuses on the measurement of ejection fraction and its response to exercise.

Although radionuclide angiography is the most accurate and reproducible method of measuring left ventricular ejection fraction, this measurement has a certain error. Wackers and co-workers[9] described an average error of 3.9 ± 3.1 percent between consecutive measurements of left ventricular ejection fraction and noted that this error was related to ejection fraction. An error of 5.4 ± 4.4 percent was noted in repeated ejection fraction measurements when resting ejection fraction was greater than or equal to 55 percent and of 2.1 ± 2.0 percent when resting ejection fraction was less than 55 percent.

This variability was confirmed[10] and led to the acceptance of a change of five ejection fraction units as representing a measurable change in ejection fraction after an intervention such as exercise. However, when resting ejection fraction was high, a greater change was required to be considered a measurable change. Ejection fraction response to exercise is highly reproducible if obtained on two occasions under similar hemodynamic conditions.[10]

Normal Exercise Ejection Fraction Response

The accuracy of the radionuclide method has led to difficulty in defining the normal exercise ejection fraction. Differences in the cardiac response from rest to exercise in normal subjects are dependent on age, gender, resting ejection fraction, work load achieved, exercise position, exercise protocol, and fitness level. Patients without angiographic cardiac disease and clearly normal coronary arteries also form a subset in which the exercise ejection fraction response has been measured and used to define a "normal" value. However, these patients have certain unique characteristics that preclude the general application of the exercise ejection fraction response in this subset as a "normal" value.

Ejection fraction response to exercise was decreased in normal subjects above 60 years of age.[11] In these older subjects, ejection fraction either increased by less than 5 percent with exercise or actually decreased. Such a trend was noted by others[12] and more detailed analysis of ventricular function demonstrated a greater increase in end-systolic and end-diastolic left ventricular volume with exercise in older compared with younger subjects. These findings suggested a greater use of the Frank-Starling mechanism to increase cardiac output in older individuals. These results[12] and other studies[13] confirmed the anticipated blunting of exercise heart rate response in older subjects. Recently, the exercise ejection fraction response in older subjects was shown to be related to work load.[13] When older and younger subjects were compared at similar work loads, exercise ejection fraction responses were comparable and, at high work loads, ejection fraction with exercise increased by at least 5 percent.

Ejection fraction response to exercise in women thought to be without cardiac disease was less likely to increase from rest to peak exercise by 5 percent or more compared to a similar group of men.[13] Work load was less at maximal exercise in women than in men. Thus, it was unclear whether this difference would be maintained if women and men exercise to a similar maximal work load.

Normal subjects with high resting ejection fractions (greater than or equal to 0.65) may not increase their ejection fractions with exercise.[13,14] Under these circumstances, left ventricular ejection fraction at peak exercise remains similar or decreases relative to resting level. Thus, maintenance of or a slight decrease in a high resting left ventricular ejection fraction with exercise must be considered normal. It has been my experience that a drop in ejection fraction in excess of the interobservation error margin for a high ejection fraction should be considered abnormal. Such a drop, if associated with angina of effort or ischemic electrocardiographic (ECG) changes at a low work load, is likely to represent coronary artery disease.

The data from these studies emphasize that when considering an exercise radionuclide angiogram, it is important to note whether maximal exercise was attained by the patient. This usually means that the patient has achieved 85 percent of the age-related maximal heart rate with exercise. At submaximal levels of exercise and heart rate response, left ventricular ejection fraction may not increase in a significant number of normal subjects.[13] If a maximal exercise is attained, an increase in left ventricular ejection fraction from rest to exercise of at least 5 percent usually is associated with the absence of coronary artery disease (Fig. 6-1).

Studies of volume and ejection fraction response have been done in normal subjects both in the upright and in the supine position.[15–18] When subjects exercised maximally, ejection fraction increased by at least 5 percent from rest to exercise with upright and supine exercise. However, it has been observed that volume responses with exercise depend on position. At rest in the upright position, end-diastolic and end-systolic volumes were less than in the supine position, but with exercise there was a greater increase in end-diastolic volume and a lesser decrease in end-systolic volume in the upright position than in the supine position.[15] These subtle changes indicate the dynamic nature of cardiac loading conditions and the importance of defining the exercise condition of any exercise protocol.

The exercise protocol itself must be carefully designed so as not to influence exercise ejec-

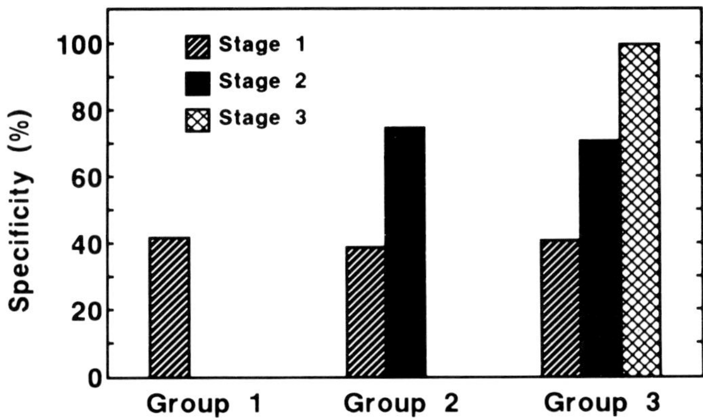

Fig. 6-1 Specificity of ejection fraction response in relation to work load achieved. Increase in ejection fraction by ≥0.05 from rest to exercise was considered a normal response. Groups 1, 2, and 3 indicate 12, 28, and 17 patients, respectively, who exercised one, two, or three exercise stages. All patients had normal coronary angiograms. Specificity increases as stage of exercise achieved increases. (From Kuo et al.,[13] with permission.)

tion fraction response adversely. This point was strikingly made when normal subjects were asked to exercise in a protocol in which work load increased markedly in the initial stage of the protocol.[19] This produced a marked decrease in ejection fraction. By contrast, when the work load increments were more gradual, the normal increase in left ventricular ejection at maximal exercise was observed.

It may be useful to generate an anticipated exercise work load for each patient being tested during exercise. This may be approximated from existing bicycle exercise data in normal subjects that relates work load, age, and weight.[20–22] By generating such an anticipated work load, an exercise protocol may be modified to avoid too great an initial increment in work load in a particular patient. This can be particularly important in elderly patients for whom an increment of 300 kg/min (50 watts) at the first stage of exercise may represent 100 percent of maximal exercise.

In normal subjects, the cardiovascular response to exercise depended on the level of physical fitness.[23] Physically fit subjects increased stroke volume with exercise and ex-hibited a marked decrease in end-systolic volume, whereas in sedentary subjects an increase in stroke volume was associated with an increase in end-diastolic volume. However, fitness did not alter the left ventricular ejection fraction response to exercise.

Insight into the normal response of the left ventricle to exercise has been obtained from studies of patients with normal coronary arteries and normal resting ventricular function. In such patients, there was clearly a wide spectrum of ejection fraction response to exercise that ranged from a decrease of 23 percent to an increase of 24 percent[24] (Fig. 6-2). Up to one-third of these patients had a blunted ejection fraction response (increase of up to 0.05 over rest) to exercise.[25] Rozanski and colleagues [26,27] pointed out that such patients were often referred for angiography because of unusual chest pain or other borderline abnormalities and therefore did not represent a normal population. These investigators indicated that, within this group, patients with a low probability of coronary disease based on clinical factors were the patients who increased their ejection fraction with exercise by the more normal 5 percent[26] (Fig. 6-3). Others have stressed the importance of exercise duration in this patient

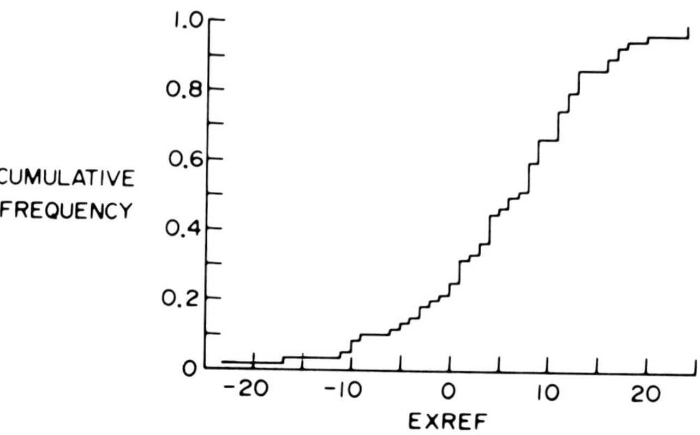

Fig. 6-2 Cumulative frequency of ejection fraction response to exercise (EXREF) in 60 patients with chest pain and normal coronary angiograms. Range of response was from −23 percent to +24 percent. (From Gibbons et al.,[24] with permission.)

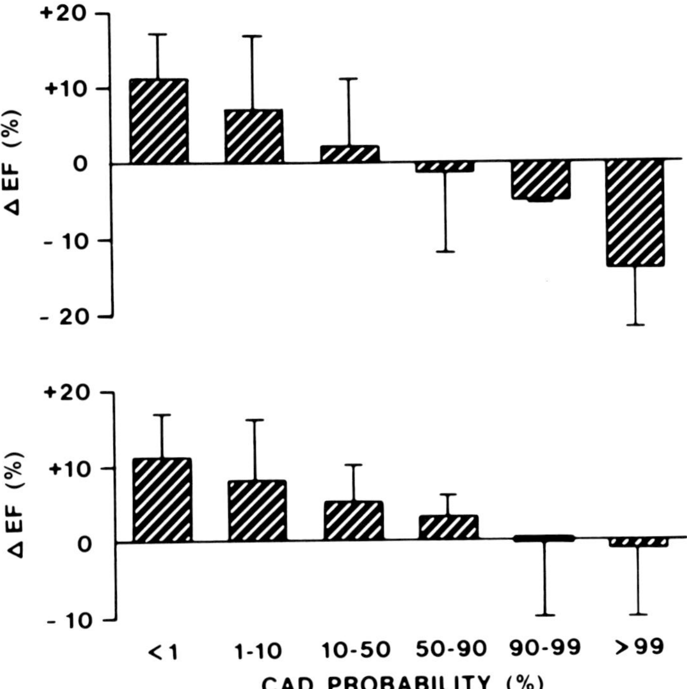

Fig. 6-3 Mean change in left ventricular ejection fraction from rest to exercise in patients with normal coronary arteries (*top*) and in uncatheterized patients (*bottom*) related to coronary artery disease probability. Patients with a low probability of coronary artery disease showed a marked increase in ejection fraction with exercise independent of whether or not the absence of coronary disease was confirmed by catheterization. (From Rozanski et al.,[26] wtih permission.)

group.[13] Subjects who achieve 85 percent of their maximal heart rate are likely to increase ejection fraction by at least 5 percent, whereas submaximal exercise was associated with a blunted ejection fraction response.

From this collected information, it is clear that to obtain an adequate exercise radionuclide angiogram, patients must exercise to a high work load, that is, to 85 percent of their maximal heart rate. Also, the exercise protocol should be graduated in relationship to the anticipated maximal work load of the patient. If such conditions are adhered to, even in the older patient, an increase in ejection fraction by 5 percent over rest would be considered an ejection fraction response to exercise of a left ventricle without significant coronary artery or myocardial disease.

In addition, left ventricular wall motion should be normal at rest and should not worsen with exercise; if measured, end-systolic volume should not increase. However, in the hyperdynamic left ventricle (ejection fraction of at least 0.65), ejection fraction may not increase, and could decrease by up to 0.05. In the latter circumstance, the likelihood that coronary disease is absent is enhanced if the patient achieves the anticipated work load or a double product of at least 21,000 beats/min × mmHg[28] (Fig. 6-4).

Role of Patient Characteristics

The sensitivity and specificity of the exercise radionuclide angiogram have been claimed to be changing dramatically with time.[27] In

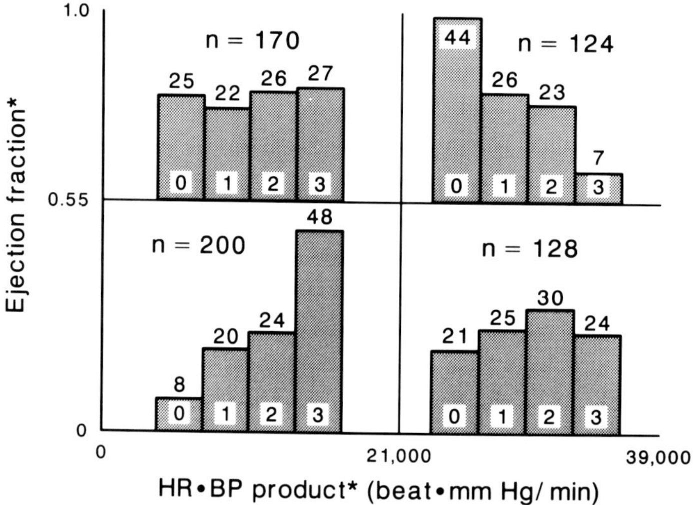

Fig. 6-4 Percentage of patients (vertical bars) with zero-, one-, two-, or three-vessel coronary artery disease related to four quadrants of maximal exercise ejection fraction and heart rate × blood pressure product. Patients with a high exercise left ventricular ejection fraction were more likely to have no coronary artery disease if a heart rate × blood pressure product in excess of 21,000 beats × mmHg/min was achieved. (*At maximal exercise.) (From Clements et al.,[41] with permission.)

particular, the specificity of the test has decreased markedly. Initial studies with exercise radionuclide angiography demonstrated that in normal subjects ejection fraction increased and in patients with coronary artery disease ejection fraction decreased.[4,6,29] Sensitivity and specificity approached 100 percent. However, later assessment of sensitivity and specificity demonstrated a decline in both measures,[30] particularly in specificity. By multivariate analysis, a group of radionuclide variables was defined that best predicted the presence or absence of coronary artery disease in a group of patients who underwent cardiac catheterization in 1980.[31,32] This approach yielded a sensitivity of just under 0.90 and a specificity of almost 0.60. Analysis of this information indicated that this apparent changing of specificity and of sensitivity was a consequence of patient selection. This phenomenon was seen particularly in patients who had undergone coronary arteriography and had normal or near-normal coronary arteries (Fig. 6-5). Often contrast angiography

was performed in these patients because of an abnormal radionuclide angiogram. Thus, these patients were preselected to have an abnormal radionuclide angiogram and, on the basis of the abnormal radionuclide angiogram, were referred for angiography. Limited exercise tolerance, age, gender, and small vessel coronary artery disease may be contributing factors producing the abnormal exercise radionuclide angiogram. When patients with normal coronary arteries by contrast angiography had a low probability of coronary artery disease, a normal exercise ejection fraction response to exercise was usual, particularly if the patients exercised to a high level[13,26] (85 percent or more of maximal heart rate). Specificity was 42 percent in patients with normal coronary arteries who exercised only to one level, whereas it was 100 percent when similar patients exercised to three stages or to 85 percent of maximal heart rate.[26] These findings stress again the importance of an adequate work load in exercise radionuclide angiography.

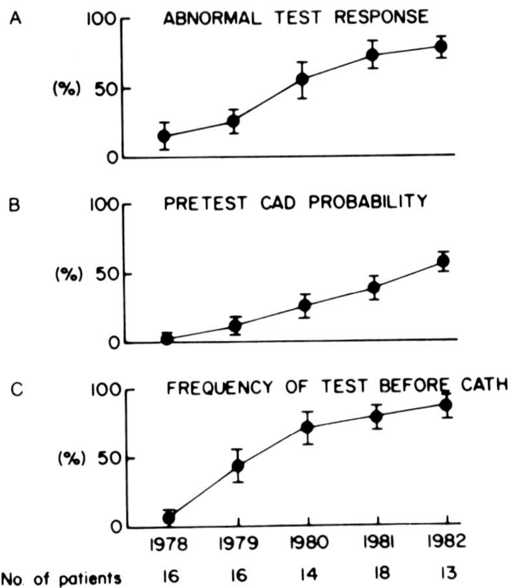

Fig. 6-5 Patterns in 77 angiographically normal patients during 1978 to 1982. (*A*) Increasing frequency of abnormal ejection fraction or wall motion responses. (*B*) Increasing pretest likelihood of coronary artery disease (CAD). (*C*) Increasing frequency of radionuclide angiography preceding cardiac catheterization (CATH). (From Rozanski et al.,[27] with permission.)

RADIONUCLIDE ANGIOGRAPHY IN CORONARY ARTERY DISEASE

The initial approach to the use of radionuclide angiography in coronary artery disease was for diagnostic purposes. Because exercise radionuclide angiography was demonstrated to have a high sensitivity and specificity, this approach appeared both reasonable and useful. However, several concerns have modified this approach. The first of these concerns is based on bayesian rules. Because exercise radionuclide angiography is neither 100 percent sensitive nor specific, false-negative and false-positive results occur. In addition, the prevalence of coronary artery disease varies depending on the patient population studied. The statistical importance of the aspects of bayesian probability in the noninvasive diag-

nosis of coronary artery disease has been outlined elsewhere[33–35] and is not detailed in this chapter. It is sufficient to indicate that the performance of exercise radionuclide angiography did little to enhance the diagnosis of coronary artery disease in patients with a high likelihood (80 percent or more) of coronary artery disease (i.e., patients with typical angina). Also, in patients with a low likelihood (up to 20 percent) of coronary disease (i.e., young women with noncardiac chest pain), a positive exercise radionuclide angiogram was misleading and was usually associated with the absence of coronary artery disease. Exercise radionuclide angiography added the most to clinical diagnosis in patients in whom the likelihood of coronary artery disease was moderate (i.e., middle-aged men with atypical chest pain). In these circumstances, a positive or a negative test added significantly to the likelihood of the presence or absence of coronary artery disease, respectively.

The remaining concerns that impinge on the use of exercise radionuclide ventriculography to diagnose coronary disease are related to aspects of the test already discussed and to additional patient characteristics. Sensitivity and specificity are lower than initially expected. The reasons for this diminished sensitivity and specificity were outlined previously; clearly, to achieve maximum sensitivity and specificity, a patient had to exercise to a high work load (heart rate at peak exercise at 85 percent maximal anticipated heart rate). Even if criteria for a satisfactory exercise test were achieved, intrinsic patient and cardiac factors remained that diminished sensitivity and specificity. The exercise ejection fraction response can be diminished in patients with normal coronary arteries but decreased coronary artery flow reserve.[36] This effect will decrease specificity of the test. β-blocking agents have variable effects on exercise changes in ejection fraction. In patients or subjects without coronary disease, propranolol may diminish the exercise ejection fraction response,[37] thereby tending to decrease specificity. The presence of hypertension is associated with a blunted ejection fraction response to exercise,[38] which may decrease the sensitivity of exercise radionuclide angiography to detect coronary artery disease.

Depending on test and patient conditions, sensitivity, and particularly specificity, of exercise radionuclide angiography may have different values. Both sensitivity and specificity are maximum when the patient exercises to a high work load and achieves 85 percent of maximal heart rate. Thus, if the exercise radionuclide angiogram is performed for diagnostic purposes, it is important to achieve this condition.

A different approach to the use of the exercise radionuclide angiogram in coronary artery disease is to attempt to predict the extent of coronary artery disease. A further extension of this approach is to predict low-risk or high-risk groups for three-vessel disease or for left main coronary artery disease.

In patients undergoing exercise radionuclide angiography for assessment of chest pain syndromes, there is a relationship between extent of coronary artery disease and several exercise radionuclide factors. DePace and co-workers[39] used multivariate analysis and examined the presence or absence of Q-wave infarction, exercise left ventricular ejection fraction, and change in systolic blood pressure from rest to exercise; these investigators identified 83 percent of patients with severe coronary artery disease and 85 percent of patients with mild coronary artery disease based on the Gensini score. In an extension of this method,[40] exercise left ventricular ejection fraction correlated negatively ($r = -0.70$) with disease severity (Fig. 6-6) based on a coronary artery disease score. A better correlation between these two measures ($r = -0.82$) was seen in patients under 50 years of age (Fig. 6-7). Studies at the Mayo Clinic have also demonstrated the predictive value

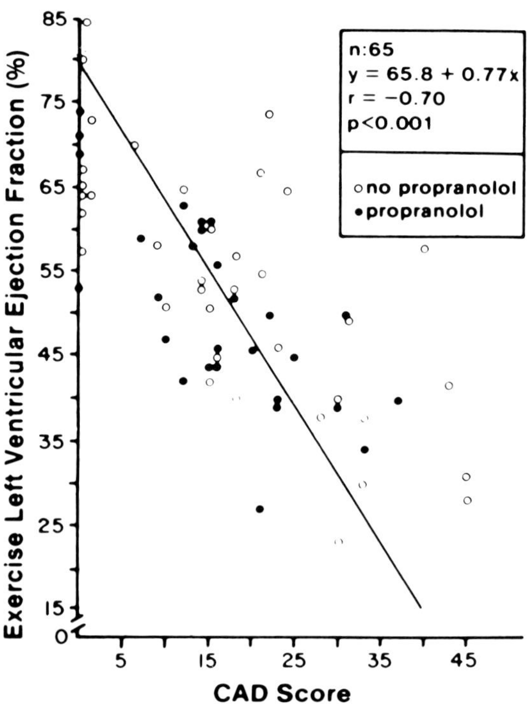

Fig. 6-6 Correlation between exercise left ventricular ejection fraction and coronary artery disease (CAD) score in 65 patients. (From DePace et al,[40] with permission.)

of exercise ejection fraction.[28] Of 22 radionuclide variables, exercise left ventricular ejection fraction was the second most significant variable, by discriminant analysis, in predicting the number of diseased coronary arteries in a group of 296 patients who had undergone cardiac catheterization and exercise radionuclide angiography for assessment of chest pain. Exercise ejection fraction was considerably more significant than rest ejection fraction but was less significant than exercise rate × pressure product; the latter factor correlated best with number of diseased coronary arteries. Thus, it was possible to combine exercise left ventricular ejection fraction and rate × pressure product and to predict the probability of zero, one, two, or three diseased coronary arteries[41] (Fig. 6-8). This analysis indicated that, if exercise rate × pressure was greater than 21,000 beats/min ×

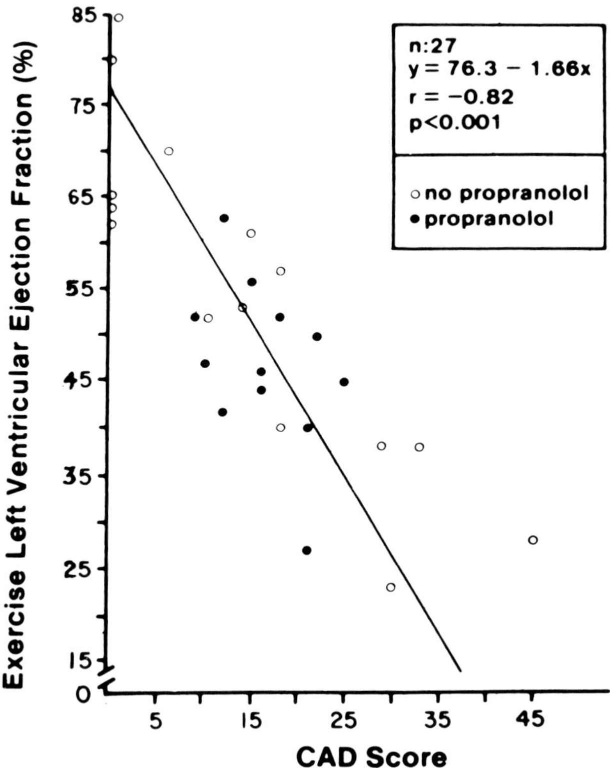

Fig. 6-7 Correlation between exercise left ventricular ejection fraction and coronary artery disease (CAD) score in 27 patients under 50 years of age. (From DePace et al.,[40] with permission.)

mmHg and ejection fraction was greater than 0.55, mild coronary disease was likely (70 percent). If these measurements were less than 21,000 beats/min × mmHg and 0.55, respectively, multivessel disease was usual (72 percent likely). Weintraub and co-workers[42] also used a discriminant analysis approach and identified maximal exercise ejection fraction, ST-segment depression, and heart rate as independent predictors of the number of stenosed major coronary arteries. These variables generated equations that predicted those patients who would not have stenosis and three-vessel disease on 71 percent and 80 percent of occasions, respectively. Inclusion of the clinical parameters of gender and exercise ST-segment changes with exercise ejection fraction and rate × pressure product can also provide informa-

tion as to the likelihood of left main or three-vessel coronary artery disease.[43] It was not possible to distinguish between three-vessel disease and left main coronary disease.[44]

This approach is useful in that it moves away from what is considered a normal ejection fraction response to exercise. It looks at the absolute exercise ejection fraction response and at the extent of exercise based on rate × pressure product. This is useful in understanding the likelihood of disease in patients with little change in ejection fraction with exercise, particularly those patients with higher ejection fractions. However, this approach would probably be more accurate if patients were to exercise to a high work load and to achieve 85 percent of their maximal heart rate.

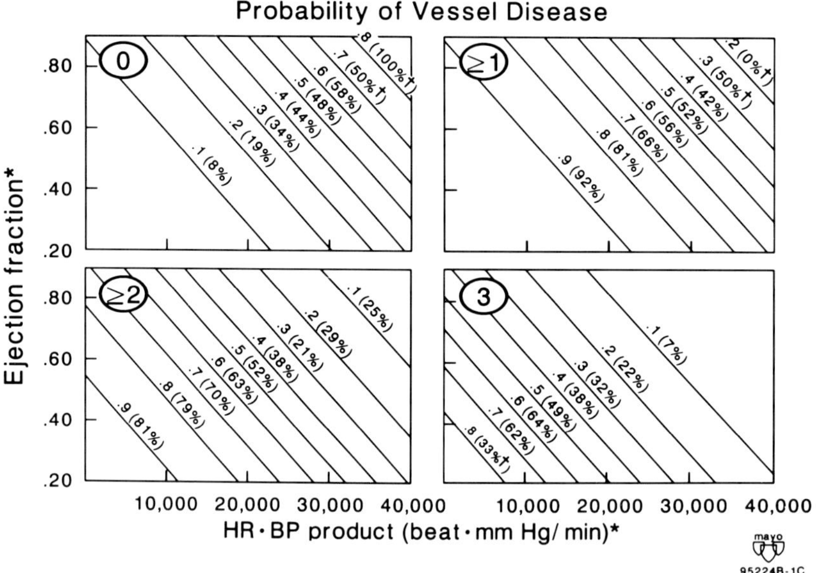

Fig. 6-8 Probability contours (solid diagonal lines) of no significant coronary artery disease (CAD) (upper left), one-vessel or more CAD (upper right), multivessel CAD (lower left), and three-vessel CAD (lower right) in relation to the distribution of left ventricular ejection fraction (LVEF) and heart rate × blood pressure (HR × BP) product at maximal exercise. The specific probability is indicated on each contour with the actual proportion of patients in a ±0.05 band around each probability contour in parentheses. (*At maximal exercise. †Data based on less than 10 patients.) (From Clements et al.,[41] with permission.)

Prediction of Prognosis

Another avenue for considering the value of exercise radionuclide angiography is to consider its effectiveness in predicting prognosis in patients with coronary artery disease. Resting left ventricular ejection fraction is related to prognosis on the basis of both contrast[45] and radionuclide angiography[46] (Fig. 6-9). Studies have addressed whether exercise radionuclide ejection fraction added any additional prognostic information to resting ejection fraction. Medically treated patients with coronary artery disease who had an abnormal ejection fraction response to exercise had a poorer 3-year survival than did patients who had a normal exercise ejection fraction response.[47] A further study indicated that exercise ejection fraction contributed prognostic information in addition to resting ejection fraction.[48] Furthermore, Bonow and co-workers[49] demonstrated that exercise radionuclide variables distinguished high- and low-risk groups among patients with three-vessel coronary disease, preserved left ventricular function, and minimal angina (Fig. 6-10). Forty-three such patients were identified. There were five sudden deaths over a follow-up period of 4 years in 19 patients of the high-risk group who had a decrease in ejection fraction with exercise, a low peak work load, and an abnormal exercise ECG. No deaths occurred in the remaining 24 patients. By contrast, a study[50] of 53 patients with three-vessel coronary artery disease with resting radionuclide left ventricular ejection fraction of at least 0.40 failed to identify a high-risk subgroup based on the criteria of Bonow and colleagues. Mortality in the National Institutes of Health (NIH) study was double that of the Mayo Clinic study (12 percent versus 6 percent) for these sub-

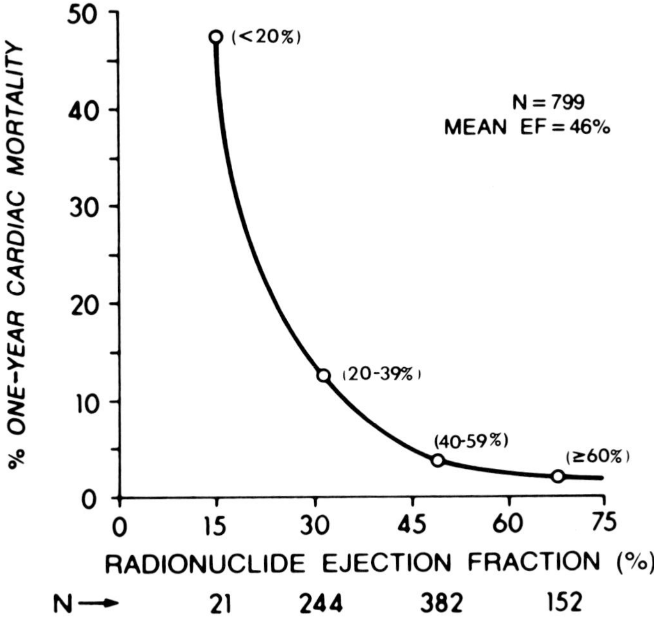

Fig. 6-9 Cardiac mortality (vertical axis) after myocardial infarction related to resting left ventricular ejection fraction (horizontal axis). (From the Multicenter Postinfarction Research Group,[46] with permission.)

groups of patients with three-vessel disease and preserved ejection fraction. The distribution of deaths between the high- and low-risk groups was five and 0, respectively, in the NIH study and one and two in the Mayo study. Because of the low numbers involved, it is clear that a slight variation in deaths between the high- and low-risk groups could alter the final conclusions of either study considerably. Thus, to understand whether exercise radionuclide angiography can be useful in determining prognosis in patients with coronary artery disease once coronary artery anatomy is known, studies in much larger groups of patients must be performed.

Until more definitive studies are available, it would be prudent to advise coronary artery revascularization in patients with three-vessel disease and preserved ventricular function who have the three high-risk characteristics as defined by the NIH group.

EXERCISE RADIONUCLIDE ANGIOGRAPHY IN MYOCARDIAL INFARCTION

There are data to support the prognostic value of exercise duration and ST-segment changes induced with exercise early after myocardial infarction. Patients with recent myocardial infarction and ST-segment depression with exercise had a 25 percent 1-year mortality.[51] The additional prognostic value of exercise radionuclide angiography in this condition needs exploration.[52] Certainly, resting left ventricular ejection fraction determined by radionuclide angiography contains valuable prognostic information (see Fig. 6-9). Patients with a normal ejection fraction at rest after myocardial infarction had a 1-year mortality of less than 5 percent; by contrast, if rest ejection fraction was 20 percent, mortality after 1 year approached 40 percent.[46] However, the additional prog-

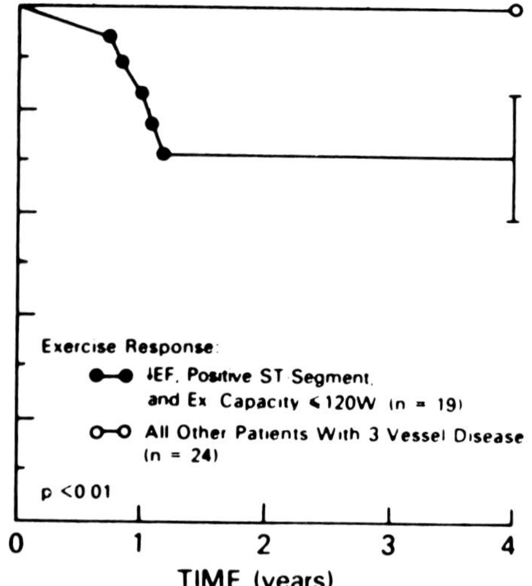

Fig. 6-10 Mortality in patients with three-vessel coronary disease and preserved ejection fraction (greater than or equal to 0.40). High-risk patient group (lower line) with decrease in exercise ejection fraction, low-peak work load, and abnormal stress electrocardiogram. Low-risk group (upper line) without the three noted risk factors. Five of 19 patients in the high-risk group suddenly died over the follow-up period, whereas none of the patients in the low-risk group died. (From Bonow et al,[49] with permission.)

nostic value of an exercise left ventricular ejection fraction determination remains unclear in these circumstances. Exercise early after myocardial infarction is usually performed to a submaximal level. This constraint may well influence the value of exercise ejection fraction determination early after recovery from myocardial infarction.

Borer and colleagues[53] found little change from rest in exercise ejection fraction in patients recovering from acute myocardial infarction; only 8 of 45 patients showed a change in ejection fraction of greater than or equal to 5 percent. Thus, these investigators could make no statement as to the value of exercise radionuclide angiography after acute myocardial infarction. A failure to increase ejection fraction from rest to exercise

by 0.05 was highly sensitive in predicting major cardiac events (death, recurrent infarction, and severe angina) during the 9 months after myocardial infarction.[54] This measure was more sensitive than ST-segment changes on the exercise ECG.[54] In a larger group of patients recovering from myocardial infarction with preserved left ventricular function, a decrease in ejection fraction of at least 5 percent from rest to peak exercise identified a high-risk group of 22 patients; of this group, 23 percent experienced either nonfatal ventricular fibrillation or recurrent myocardial infarction or died during the first year postinfarction.[55] Exercise ejection fraction was related to mortality, whereas the change in ejection fraction from rest to exercise was associated with the timing of coronary bypass surgery for refractory angina.[56] In this study, resting ejection fraction was also related to mortality, and both rest and exercise ejection fraction were better predictors of mortality than were clinical variables. An exercise ejection fraction up to 0.40 was associated with a mortality at 2 years of at least 20 percent; mortality worsened as exercise ejection fraction decreased.[56]

There is some evidence that patients with a recent inferior infarction who show a decrease in ejection fraction with exercise are more likely to have multivessel coronary artery disease. However, in patients with anterior infarction, a decrease in ejection fraction with exercise may not distinguish between single-vessel and multivessel coronary artery disease.[57]

Thus, radionuclide angiography may have considerable prognostic value in patients with suspected coronary artery disease. The ability of exercise radionuclide angiography to measure rest and exercise ejection fraction and the importance of these measurements in determining prognosis after myocardial infarction argue strongly for exercise radionuclide angiography as a routine test after acute myocardial infarction. If such a test were combined with ECG monitoring, it would add considerably to determining prognosis after myocardial infarction and the need for coronary angiography. This could be particularly useful in patients without clinical evidence of left ventricular dysfunction.

EXERCISE RADIONUCLIDE ANGIOGRAPHY IN VALVULAR HEART DISEASE

Determination of left ventricular function at rest and with exercise has been investigated as a method for predicting deterioration in cardiac function with chronic valvular heart disease, particularly aortic regurgitation.[58–60] It was evident that ejection fraction in valvular regurgitation is a complex interaction of heart rate, diastolic intervals, regurgitant fraction, and afterload[61]—so much so that ejection fraction measures reflected loading conditions in aortic regurgitation rather than left ventricular myocardial function. There was some evidence that indicated end-systolic volume may be a better estimate of left ventricular function than ejection fraction in aortic regurgitation.[58,62] The data suggested that a decreased resting and exercise ejection fraction (less than 0.45) with an enlarged end-systolic volume represented a deterioration in left ventricular function.[63] However, if the patient was asymptomatic (i.e., without significant exercise limitation, dyspnea, or angina), it was not necessary to advise aortic valve replacement because of resting or exercise radionuclide abnormalities.[64–67] Often, despite decreased left ventricular function, patients demonstrated an improvement in ejection fraction and a decrease in cardiac volume after valve replacement.[63] Thus, despite abnormal rest and exercise function, symptomatic management remains pre-eminent for the timing of valve replacement. If, however, serial deterioration in rest or exercise function occurs over a period of years despite lack of symptoms, it may be prudent to advise aortic valve replacement. Thus, serial radionuclide angiography at rest

and with exercise may be of value in determining the appropriate timing of operation in patients with aortic valve regurgitation and no or minimal cardiac symptoms.

EXERCISE RADIONUCLIDE ANGIOGRAPHY AND ASSESSMENT OF REVASCULARIZATION

Exercise radionuclide angiography has demonstrated an improvement in the exercise response of the left ventricle in patients who have undergone successful revascularization after either coronary bypass surgery[68,69] or balloon angioplasty.[70] These studies demonstrated that prerevascularization abnormalities in wall motion and ejection fraction response to exercise were normalized by a successful revascularization procedure. If the revascularization procedure proved unsuccessful, these abnormalities were not changed after the intervention. Exercise radionuclide angiography was useful in following patients for occlusion of coronary bypass grafts and restenosis of dilated coronary arteries.[71]

SUMMARY

Exercise radionuclide angiography using blood-pool imaging gives an unparalleled noninvasive assessment of ventricular contraction and volume with exercise. The studies of the 1980s have created important guidelines in the interpretation of these studies, in the light of acute and chronic coronary disease and valvular disease. This includes knowledge of the exercise protocol, exercise duration, and clinical data. The interpretation of the result of the test should also be placed within the context of whether the test is used to diagnose coronary disease, quantify coronary disease, or provide prognostic information. In aortic regurgitation, serial radionuclide studies may be useful in predicting left ventricular deterioration and may indicate aortic valve replacement in asymptomatic patients. Exercise radionuclide angiography may also be useful for assessing patency of coronary bypass grafts and dilated coronary arteries, particularly if serial studies are available. Exercise radionuclide angiography plays an important role in the noninvasive assessment of patients with cardiac disease.

REFERENCES

1. Sharma B. Goodwin JF, Raphael MJ, et al: Left ventricular angiography on exercise: A new method of assessing left ventricular function in ischaemic heart disease. Br Heart J 38:59, 1976
2. Sharma B, Taylor SH: Localization of left ventricular ischaemia in angina pectoris by cineangiography during exercise. Br Heart J 37:963, 1975
3. Borer JS, Kent KM, Bacharach SL, et al: Sensitivity, specificity and predictive accuracy of radionuclide cineangiography during exercise in patients with coronary artery disease: Comparison with exercise electrocardiography. Circulation 60:572, 1979
4. Borer JS, Bacharach SL, Green MV, et al: Real-time radionuclide cineangiography in the noninvasive evaluation of global and regional left ventricular function at rest and during exercise in patients with coronary-artery disease. N Engl J Med 296:839, 1977
5. Jengo JA, Freeman R, Brizendine M, Mena I: Detection of coronary artery disease: Comparison of exercise stress radionuclide angiocardiography and thallium stress perfusion scanning. Am J Cardiol 45:535, 1980
6. Rerych SK, Scholz PM, Newman GE, et al: Cardiac function at rest and during exercise in normals and in patients with coronary heart disease: Evaluation by radionuclide angiocardiography. Ann Surg 187:449, 1978
7. Berger HJ, Reduto LA, Johnstone DE, et al: Global and regional left ventricular response to bicycle exercise in coronary artery disease: Assessment by quantitative radionuclide angiocardiography. Am J Med 66:13, 1979
8. Brady TJ, Thrall JH, Lo K, Pitt B: The importance of adequate exercise in the detection of coronary heart disease by radionuclide ventriculography. J Nucl Med 21:1125, 1980
9. Wackers FJT, Berger HJ, Johnstone DE, et al: Multiple gated cardiac blood pool imaging for left ventricular ejection fraction: Validation of the technique and assessment of variability. Am J Cardiol 43:1159, 1979
10. Upton MT, Rerych SK, Newman GE, et al: The reproducibility of radionuclide angiographic measurements of left ventricular function in normal subjects at rest and during exercise. Circulation 62:126, 1980
11. Port S, Cobb FR, Coleman RE, Jones RH: Effect of age on the response of the left ventricular ejection fraction to exercise. N Engl J Med 303:1133, 1980
12. Rodeheffer RJ, Gerstenblith G, Becker LC, et al: Exercise cardiac output is maintained with advancing age in healthy human subjects: Cardiac dilatation and increased stroke volume compensate for a diminished heart rate. Circulation 69:203, 1984
13. Kuo LC, Bolli R, Thornby J, et al: Effects of exercise tolerance, age, and gender on the specificity of radionuclide angiography: Sequential ejection fraction analysis during multistage exercise. Am Heart J 113:1180, 1987
14. Rozanski A, Diamond GA, Jones R, et al: A format for integrating the interpretation of exercise ejection fraction and wall motion and its application in identifying equivocal responses. J Am Coll Cardiol 5:238, 1985
15. Clements IP, Offord KP, Baron DW, et al: Cardiovascular hemodynamics of bicycle and handgrip exercise in normal subjects before and after administration of propranolol. Mayo Clin Proc 59:604, 1984
16. Freeman MR, Berman DS, Staniloff H, et al: Comparison of upright and supine bicycle exercise in the detection and evaluation of extent of coronary artery disease by equilibrium radionuclide ventriculography. Am Heart J 102:182, 1981
17. Manyari DE, Kostuk WJ: Left and right ventricular function at rest and during bicycle exercise in the supine and sitting positions in normal subjects and patients with coronary artery disease: Assessment by radionuclide ventriculography. Am J Cardiol 51:36, 1983
18. Poliner LR, Dehmer GJ, Lewis SE, et al: Left ventricular performance in normal subjects: A comparison of the responses to exercise in the upright and supine positions. Circulation 62:528, 1980

19. Foster C, Anholm JD, Hellman CK, et al: Left ventricular function during sudden strenuous exercise. Circulation 63:592, 1981
20. Bruce RA: Principles of exercise testing. p. 45. In Naughton J, Hellerstein HK, Mohler IC (eds): Exercise Testing and Exercise Training in Coronary Heart Disease. Academic Press, New York, 1973
21. Astrand P-O, Rodahl K: Textbook of Work Physiology. 3rd Ed. McGraw-Hill, New York, 1986
22. American College of Sports Medicine: Guidelines for Graded Exercise Testing and Exercise Prescription. 2nd Ed. Lea & Febiger, Philadelphia, 1980
23. Bar-Shlomo B-Z, Druck MN, Morch JE, et al: Left ventricular function in trained and untrained healthy subjects. Circulation 65:484, 1982
24. Gibbons RJ, Lee KL, Cobb F, Jones RH: Ejection fraction response to exercise in patients with chest pain and normal coronary arteriograms. Circulation 64:952, 1981
25. Berger HJ, Sands MJ, Davies RA, et al: Exercise left ventricular performance in patients with chest pain, ischemic-appearing exercise electrocardiograms, and angiographically normal coronary arteries. Ann Intern Med 94:186, 1981
26. Rozanski A, Diamond GA, Forrester JS et al: Alternative referent standards for cardiac normality: implications for diagnostic testing. Ann Intern Med 101:164, 1984
27. Rozanski A, Diamond GA, Berman D, et al: The declining specificity of exercise radionuclide ventriculography. N Engl J Med 309:518, 1983
28. Clements IP, Zinsmeister AR, Gibbons RJ, et al: Exercise radionuclide ventriculography in evaluation of coronary artery disease. Am Heart J 112:582, 1986
29. Okada RD, Boucher CA, Strauss HW, Pohost GM: Exercise radionuclide imaging approaches to coronary artery disease. Am J Cardiol 46:1188, 1980
30. Osbakken MD, Boucher CA, Okada RD, et al: Spectrum of global left ventricular responses to supine exercise: Limitation in the use of ejection fraction in identifying patients with coronary artery disease. Am J Cardiol 51:28, 1983
31. Austin EH, Cobb FR, Coleman RE, Jones RH: Prospective evaluation of radionuclide angiocardiography for the diagnosis of coronary artery disease. Am J Cardiol 50:1212, 1982
32. Jones RH, McEwan P, Newman GE, et al: Accuracy of diagnosis of coronary artery disease by radionuclide measurement of left ventricular function during rest and exercise. Circulation 64:586, 1981
33. Diamond GA, Forrester JS: Analysis of probability as an aid in the clinical diagnosis of coronary-artery disease. N Engl J Med 300:1350, 1979
34. Diamond GA, Forrester JS, Hirsch M, et al: Application of conditional probability analysis to the clinical diagnosis of coronary artery disease. J Clin Invest 65:1210, 1980
35. Epstein SE: Implications of probability analysis on the strategy used for noninvasive detection of coronary artery disease: Role of single or combined use of exercise electrocardiographic testing, radionuclide cineangiography and myocardial perfusion imaging. Am J Cardiol 46:491, 1980
36. Cannon RO III, Bonow RO, Bacharach SL, et al: Left ventricular dysfunction in patients with angina pectoris, normal epicardial coronary arteries, and abnormal vasodilator reserve. Circulation 71:218, 1985
37. Port S, Cobb FR, Jones RH: Effects of propranolol on left ventricular function in normal men. Circulation 61:358, 1980
38. Wasserman AG, Katz RJ, Varghese PJ, et al: Exercise radionuclide ventriculographic responses in hypertensive patients with chest pain. N Engl J Med 311:1276, 1984
39. DePace NL, Hakki A-H, Weinreich DJ, Iskandrian AS: Noninvasive assessment of coronary artery disease. Am J Cardiol 52:714, 1983
40. DePace NL, Iskandrian AS, Hakki A-H, et al: Value of left ventricular ejection fraction during exercise in predicting the extent of coronary artery disease. J Am Coll Cardiol 1:1002, 1983
41. Clements IP, Gibbons RJ, Mankin HT, et al: Guidelines for the interpretation of the exercise radionuclide ventriculogram for diagnosing coronary artery disease. Am J Cardiol 60:1265, 1987
42. Weintraub WS, Schneider RM, Seelaus PA, et al: Prospective evaluation of the severity

of coronary artery disease with exercise radionuclide angiography and electrocardiography. Am Heart J 111:537, 1986

43. Gibbons RJ, Fyke FE III, Clements IP, et al: Noninvasive identification of severe coronary artery disease using exercise radionuclide angiography. J Am Coll Cardiol 11:28, 1988

44. Gibbons RJ, Clements IP, Zinsmeister AR, et al: Left main and 3-vessel disease have similar exercise physiology despite their difference in prognosis. Circulation, 74(suppl 2):221, 1986

45. Vlietstra RE, Assad-Morell JL, Frye RL, et al: Survival predictors in coronary artery disease: Medical and surgical comparisons. Mayo Clin Proc 52:85, 1977

46. The Multicenter Postinfarction Research Group: Risk stratification and survival after myocardial infarction. N Engl J Med 309:331, 1983

47. Jones RH, Floyd RD, Austin EH, Sabiston DC Jr: The role of radionuclide angiocardiography in the preoperative prediction of pain relief and prolonged survival following coronary artery bypass grafting. Ann Surg 197:743, 1983

48. Pryor DB, Harrell Fe Jr, Lee Kl, et al: Prognostic indicators from radionuclide angiography in medically treated patients with coronary artery disease. Am J Cardiol 53:18, 1984

49. Bonow RO, Kent KM, Rosing DR, et al: Exercise-induced ischemia in mildly symptomatic patients with coronary-artery disease and preserved left ventricular function. Identification of subgroups at risk of death during medical therapy. N Engl J Med 311:1339, 1984

50. Taliercio CP, Clements IP, Zinsmeister AR, Gibbons RJ: Prognostic value and limitations of exercise radionuclide angiography in medically treated coronary artery disease. Mayo Clin Proc 63:573, 1988

51. Théroux P, Waters DD, Halphen C, et al: Prognostic value of exercise testing soon after myocardial infarction. N Engl J Med 301:341, 1979

52. Epstein SE, Palmeri ST, Patterson RE: Evaluation of patients after acute myocardial infarction: Indications for cardiac catheterization and surgical intervention. N Engl J Med 307:1487, 1982

53. Borer JS, Rosing DR, Miller RH, et al: Natural history of left ventricular function during 1 year after acute myocardial infarction: comparison with clinical, electrocardiographic and biochemical determinations. Am J Cardiol 46:1, 1980

54. Corbett JR, Dehmer GJ, Lewis SE, et al: The prognostic value of submaximal exercise testing with radionuclide ventriculography before hospital discharge in patients with recent myocardial infarction. Circulation 64:535, 1981

55. Hung J, Goris ML, Nash E, et al: Comparative value of maximal treadmill testing, exercise thallium myocardial perfusion scintigraphy and exercise radionuclide ventriculography for distinguishing high- and low-risk patients soon after acute myocardial infarction. Am J Cardiol 53:1221, 1984

56. Morris KG, Palmeri ST, Califf RM, et al: Value of radionuclide angiography for predicting specific cardiac events after acute myocardial infarction. Am J Cardiol 55:318, 1985

57. Wasserman AG, Katz RJ, Cleary P, et al: Noninvasive detection of multivessel disease after myocardial infarction by exercise radionuclide ventriculography. Am J Cardiol 50:1242, 1982

58. Borer JS, Bacharach SL, Green MV, et al: Exercise-induced left ventricular dysfunction in symptomatic and asymptomatic patients with aortic regurgitation: Assessment with radionuclide cineangiography. Am J Cardiol 42:351, 1978

59. Huxley RL, Gaffney FA, Corbett JR, et al: Early detection of left ventricular dysfunction in chronic aortic regurgitation as assessed by contrast angiography, echocardiography, and rest and exercise scintigraphy. Am J Cardiol 51:1542, 1983

60. Dehmer GJ, Firth BG, Hillis LD, et al: Alterations in left ventricular volumes and ejection fraction at rest and during exercise in patients with aortic regurgitation. Am J Cardiol 48:17, 1981

61. Gerson MC, Engel PJ, Mantil JC, et al: Effects of dynamic and isometric exercise on the radionuclide-determined regurgitant fraction in aortic insufficiency. J Am Coll Cardiol 3:98, 1984

62. Johnson LL, Powers ER, Tzall WR, et al:

Left ventricular volume and ejection fraction response to exercise in aortic regurgitation. Am J Cardiol 51:1379, 1983

63. Bonow RO, Picone AL, McIntosh CL, et al: Survival and functional results after valve replacement for aortic regurgitation from 1976 to 1983: Impact of preoperative left ventricular function. Circulation 72:1244, 1985

64. Massie BM, Kramer BL, Loge D, et al: Ejection fraction response to supine exercise in asymptomatic aortic regurgitation: Relation to simultaneous hemodynamic measurements. J Am Coll Cardiol 5:847, 1985

65. Gee DS, Juni Je, Santinga JT, Buda AJ: Prognostic significance of exercise-induced left ventricular dysfunction in chronic aortic regurgitation. Am J Cardiol 56:605, 1985

66. Boucher CA, Wilson RA, Kanarek DJ, et al: Exercise testing in asymptomatic or minimally symptomatic aortic regurgitation: Relationship of left ventricular ejection fraction to left ventricular filling pressure during exercise. Circulation 67:1091, 1983

67. Borow KM: Surgical outcome in chronic aortic regurgitation: A physiologic framework for assessing preoperative predictors. J Am Coll Cardiol 10:1165, 1987

68. Austin EH, Oldham HN Jr, Sabiston DC Jr, Jones RH: Early assessment of rest and exercise left ventricular function following coronary artery surgery. Ann Thorac Surg 35:159, 1983

69. Kent KM, Borer JS, Green MV, et al: Effects of coronary-artery bypass on global and regional left ventricular function during exercise. N Engl J Med 298:1434, 1978

70. Kent KM, Bonow RO, Rosing DR, et al: Improved myocardial function during exercise after successful percutaneous transluminal coronary angioplasty. N Engl J Med 306:441, 1982

71. O'Keefe JH, Lapeyre AC III, Holmes DR Jr, Gibbons RJ: Usefulness of early radionuclide angiography for identifying low-risk patients for late restenosis after percutaneous transluminal coronary angioplasty. Am J Cardiol 61:51, 1988

7

Dipyridamole Stress-Thallium Imaging: Principles and Applications

E. Edmund Kim
K. Lance Gould

Exercise testing with thallium 201 imaging has been widely used for the noninvasive evaluation of patients suspected of having coronary artery disease (CAD).[1-3] However, many patients referred for stress testing cannot exercise adequately for either physical or psychological reasons, and as a result may have nondiagnostic or suboptimal test results.[4] This problem is seen most often in patients with peripheral vascular disease, in patients with poor physical conditioning, and in patients taking β-blockers. Myocardial ^{201}Tl imaging with pharmacologic coronary vasodilation using dipyridamole has been shown to be a reasonable alternative to exercise ^{201}Tl imaging.[1-3]

There are substantial differences between exercise-induced increased coronary blood flow and that due to pharmacologic vasodilation.

The effectiveness of exercise as a stimulus for coronary flow depends on the level of work achieved. Dipyridamole, a potent coronary arteriolar vasodilator, greatly increases myocardial blood flow with lesser changes in heart rate, blood pressure, myocardial work, and cardiac output than with exercise stress.[5] Intravenous (IV) dipyridamole results in a greater increase in myocardial thallium uptake than does exercise. Since ischemia is not an end point with pharmacologic perfusion imaging, disparate flow in normal compared with stenosed coronary arteries may be achieved with diagnostic perfusion defects without significant ischemia. When ischemia does occur with dipyridamole infusion, it may be immediately reversed by the administration of aminophylline. Dipyridamole may also be used in conjunction with other pharmacologic agents or other forms of stress

119

to achieve maximum coronary flow.[6] Intravenous dipyridamole combined with handgrip stress provides a potent stimulus for purposes of diagnostic myocardial perfusion imaging and has gradually become used in many institutions for screening of coronary arterial disease in asymptomatic or symptomatic patients. The diagnostic sensitivity and specificity of serial ^{201}Tl imaging after dipyridamole infusion are comparable with those reported for ^{201}Tl exercise stress testing.[7] The ^{201}Tl stress test is also used now in guiding many management decisions in patients with established CAD, based on the ability of this test to assess the extent and severity of myocardial ischemia, the functional significance of coronary stenoses, and myocardial viability. Specific uses beyond diagnosis include decisions regarding whom to catheterize, whom to send to coronary bypass surgery, and whom to send to angioplasty; risk stratification following myocardial infarction or before noncardiac surgery; and evaluation of the results of therapy.[8] Intravenous dipyridamole is relatively safe for nonexercise stress testing and has few serious side effects. It is not currently available from commerical sources for widespread routine use. The major disadvantage of dipyridamole imaging is the lack of additional information (i.e., rate-pressure product, exercise capacity) provided by the electrocardiographic (ECG) response to exercise. This chapter reviews the physiologic basis of dipyridamole stress ^{201}Tl imaging and its application to patient care.

EXERCISE STRESS MYOCARDIAL SCINTIGRAPHY

In the presence of clinically significant CAD, exercise frequently causes regional myocardial ischemia associated with angina, ECG abnormalities, and defects on ^{201}Tl perfusion images. Therefore, diagnostic exercise stress has been a practical and useful procedure in evaluating CAD. Upright dynamic (isotonic) muscular exercise is most commonly performed on a treadmill or a bicycle ergometer. The most commonly employed isometric exercise testing is the handgrip test.

During exercise in normal subjects, there is an increase in the heart rate, cardiac output, systolic blood pressure, myocardial blood flow, total oxygen consumption, and a widening of the arteriovenous oxygen difference. Generally, patients with CAD have lower than normal maximal cardiac output during exercise, and lower maximal total body oxygen uptake. The blood pressure response to exercise is variable. The peripheral circulatory regulation during exercise in patients with CAD is similar in many respects to that observed in healthy individuals.[9] Because of the lower cardiac output during exercise in patients with CAD, the oxygen extraction may even be greater than normal, resulting in lower pulmonary artery oxygen saturations.

Current noninvasive diagnostic techniques have limited accuracy for the detection of CAD not only in symptomatic patients, but particularly in asymptomatic patients. The sensitivity and specificity of exercise ECG for asymptomatic patients are so limited as to make it almost useless as a screening procedure.[10] While typical angina is associated with anatomic CAD in more than 90 percent of cases, silent ischemia occurs far more frequently than ischemia accompanied by pain,[11] and may account for more than two-thirds of all ischemic episodes.

The use of ionic ^{201}Tl for evaluation of myocardial ischemia is based on its rapid concentration in the myocardium in proportion to myocardial perfusion. After IV injection of thallium with the patient at rest, approximately 3.5 percent of the injected dose localizes in the myocardium; after injection during large muscle dynamic exercise, approximately 4.4 percent of the injected dose localizes in the myocardium.[12] The thallium in the myocardium is in dynamic equilibrium with that in the blood. In zones of normal perfusion, the intracellular thallium concentration is high compared with the residual amount in the blood, and a net loss of thallium from the myocardium occurs. In zones of ischemia, where the initial concentration of thallium is relatively low, the gradient between the intracellular and extracellular environments is lower, and the rate of loss is much lower.[13] Areas of fibrosis have minimal perfusion, and hence low initial concentration of thallium. The loss of thallium from these areas occurs at about the same rate as the loss from normal myocardium. Abnormal stress images indicate sufficiently severe CAD to limit the regional blood flow increase in response to stress as compared with the normally greater flow increase through coronary arteries without significant disease.

Thallium redistribution (Fig. 7-1) is usually due to a difference in clearance of thallium, with the normally perfused zones clearing more rapidly than the ischemic areas. Although most ischemic lesions exhibit redistribution, in some patients with ischemia, lesions on initial scans do not redistribute.[14] This may be due to a difference in metabolism between acutely and chronically ischemic myocardium. Rarely, an abnormal myocardial perfusion scan can be seen in the absence of large vessel CAD. This has been reported in cardiomyopathy, sarcoidosis, Chagas' disease, aortic stenosis, and left bundle branch block.[15] The cause of these abnormalities is not clear and may involve many factors, such as change in the shape and size of the ventricular cavity, or it may represent disease at the level of either the myocyte or the capillary/sarcolemmal membrane.[16]

Thallium imaging has gained clinical acceptance in detection of coronary disease, prognostication of the likelihood of a major ischemic event, and as a post-therapy follow-

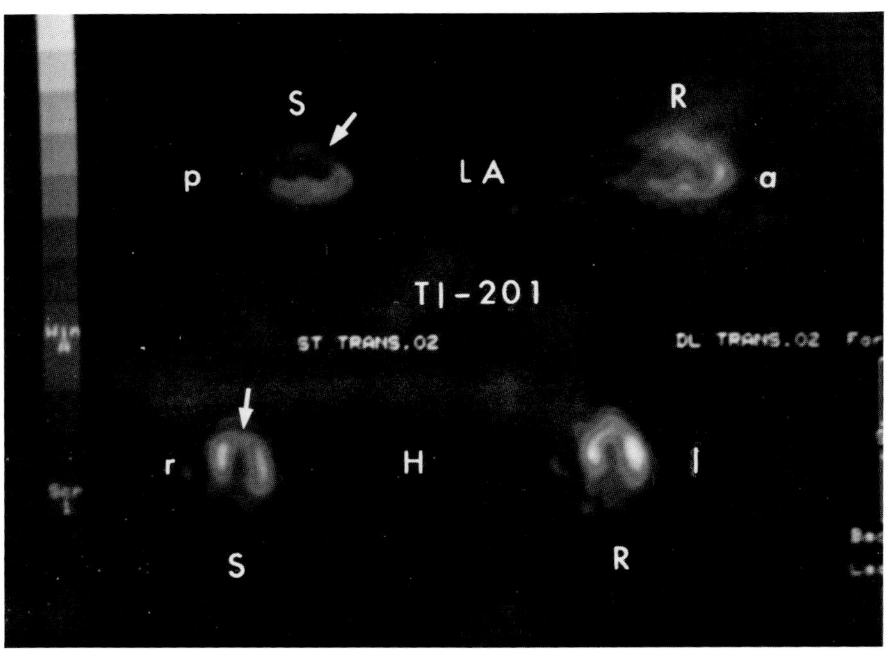

Fig. 7-1 Long axis (LA) and horizontal (H) tomographic views of the heart with ^{201}Tl show anterior perfusion defects on stress (S) images that are partially filled on resting (R) images. A, anterior; P, posterior; L, left; R, right.

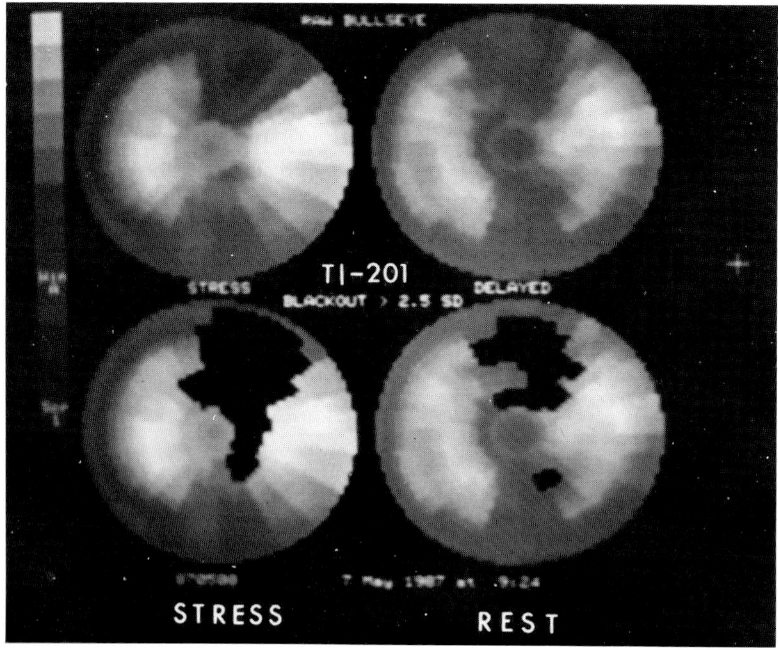

Fig. 7-2 Bull's-eye views of ^{201}Tl myocardial SPECT study show anterior perfusion defects on stress images that were partially filled on resting images.

up study. The average sensitivity of the exercise ECG is about 58 percent, and the average sensitivity of either qualitative or quantitative exercise thallium imaging is about 90 percent.[17] The sensitivity of thallium changes with the number of vessels diseased: 80 percent for single-vessel disease, 83 percent for two-vessel disease, and 96 percent for three-vessel disease.[18] The specificity of exercise thallium imaging for the detection of CAD is about 90 percent, compared with 82 percent for ECG. Thallium-201 imaging is particularly useful in assessing the posterior and inferior regions of the myocardium, where the ECG is relatively insensitive.[19] Most investigators now believe that single-photon emission computed tomography (SPECT) will not enhance the sensitivity for detection of disease but can provide additional data about the location of lesions and thereby help differentiate multivessel from single-vessel disease. One unique approach to the presentation of quantitative data creates a bull's-eye (Fig. 7-2) by portraying the data from each successive section as a concentric ring.[20]

Many studies, in diverse patient populations, confirm that the number and extent of myocardial segments with thallium redistribution are among the best methods of prognostication in a variety of coronary artery disease syndromes.[15] Serial testing with exercise ^{201}Tl imaging is also helpful to document whether any interventional therapy has continued to be successful.

PHARMACOLOGY AND PHARMACOKINETICS OF DIPYRIDAMOLE

Dipyridamole (2,6-bis[diethanolamino]-4,8-dipiperidinopyrimido[5,4-d]pyrimidine) (Persantine) is a non–nitrate coronary vasodilator with few systemic side effects (Fig. 7-3). It is similar to papaverine in many of its pharmacologic properties. Dipyridamole increases coronary blood flow and coronary sinus oxygen saturation. Intravenous dipyridamole has been reported to increase mean coronary flow by up to 3.4 to 4.1 times baseline values in humans in studies using inert gas tracers.[21] Using coronary sinus thermodilution, Brown et al.[6] reported an increase in coronary sinus flow of 1.5 to 1.7 times baseline in patients with CAD and 2.4 times baseline in normal patients after administration of IV dipyridamole. It appears to act predominantly on small resistance vessels of the coronary bed, with little effect on vascular resistance in ischemic coronary areas where small vessels are already maximally dilated. Cardiac work and myocardial oxygen consumption are not markedly affected. Blood pressure and heart rate changes after infusion of dipyridamole have been reported by many investigators.[22] Responses were all similar, with increases of 20 to 40 percent in heart rate and decreases of 4 to 10 percent in systolic blood pressure. Mean and diastolic pressure also decreased significantly.[6] The mean rate-pressure product increased significantly by 11 to 28 percent, but not to the high levels induced by either isometric or dynamic exercise. There was no change in ejection fraction, but cardiac output increased by 33 percent.[6]

The usual therapeutic oral doses (50 mg tid) of dipyridamole generally produce no significant change in blood pressure or in blood flow in peripheral arteries. Gould et al.[5] reported a significant reduction of supine systolic blood pressure compared with the resting supine level following the oral administration of dipyridamole (300 mg). However, a significant decline in systolic blood pressure was not evident on standing. Supine heart rate after high-dose oral dipyridamole increased significantly from 68 ±

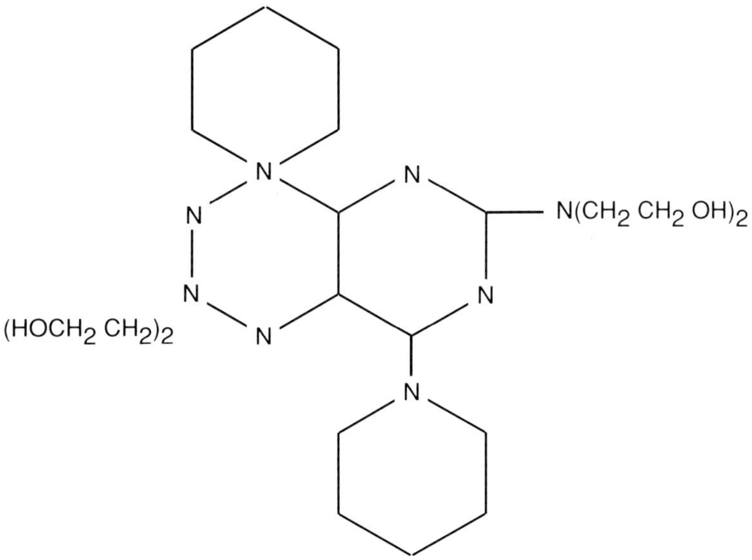

Fig. 7-3 Chemical structure of dipyridamole.

9 to 74 ± 10 bpm. Standing heart rate was also significantly elevated compared with the supine control and supine dipyridamole levels.

The coronary vasodilator effect of dipyridamole probably results from its ability to inhibit adenosine deaminase in the blood, leading to an accumulation of adenosine, a potent vasodilator, which is released from the hypoxic myocardium. Dipyridamole may also cause vasodilation by delaying the hydrolysis of cyclic 3′,5′-adenosine monophosphate (cAMP) by inhibiting the enzyme phosphodiesterase. Dipyridamole inhibits platelet aggregation caused by adenosine diphosphate, by platelet release-inducing agents, by epinephrine, and by norepinephrine. It apparently has no effect on plasma prothrombin levels but may increase platelet count. Dipyridamole prolongs platelet survival time in patients with valvular heart disease in whom platelet survival is shortened. Since dipyridamole may inhibit platelet aggregation, patients receiving heparin and dipyridamole concomitantly should be monitored closely to prevent bleeding. Aspirin and dipyridamole appear to have at least additive inhibitory effects on platelet function. Aspirin and dipyridamole also appear to have a synergistic antithrombotic effect, at least in small blood vessels.

Dipyridamole is widely distributed in body tissues and is metabolized in the liver and excreted in the bile, chiefly as the monoglucuronide and a small amount as the diglucuronide. Dipyridamole and its glucuronides may undergo enterohepatic circulation and are excreted mainly in feces. Small amounts are excreted in urine.

PHYSIOLOGIC BASIS OF DIPYRIDAMOLE-THALLIUM IMAGING

Methods for substantially increasing coronary blood flow are potentially useful within the context of myocardial perfusion imaging.

With isotopes that accumulate in the myocardium in rough proportion to coronary flow, the diagnostic sensitivity improves in concert with the magnitude of increase in coronary blood flow,[23] whereas the scintigraphic image quality generally improves with the ratio of coronary flow to cardiac output. Thus, the ideal isotope for mycocardial imaging would be one whose myocardial accumulation is proportional to coronary blood flow over its entire range and is reduced in association with ischemia. The ideal coronary vasodilator would maximally increase coronary blood flow but not cardiac output.

Thallium 201, although not ideal, is a good agent because 88 percent of the isotope that enters the coronary circulation is taken up in the myocardium in its first coronary transit, when the coronary flow rate is in the normal range. Its long effective half-life limits the administered dose to less than 3 mCi for a radiation burden of 5 rad to the kidneys. The limited photon flux and the poor spatial resolution as well as problems with scatter and attenuation also contribute to a procedure that requires 8 to 10 minutes to record an image.

Dipyridamole is a good agent for vasodilation because its effect is relatively selective for the coronary resistance bed. In the setting of induced maximal coronary dilation, the increased flow goes largely to normally perfused myocardial regions; myocardium supplied through significant coronary stenoses has limited vasodilatory reserve and may have little increase in perfusion.[6] Gould[23] demonstrated that ^{201}Tl imaging defects are detectable during induced hyperemia when flow into the normal coronary vessels exceeds that into a stenotic vessel by a ratio of 2.4 ± 0.3 or greater. Josephson et al.[24] also showed in clinical studies that coronary stenoses as mild as 40 percent frequently cause scintigraphic defects when the ^{201}Tl is given during dipyridamole- or exercise-induced coronary hyperemia. These defects in hyperemic myocardial perfusion imaging occur despite an increase in the absolute flow into the diseased coronary vascular bed. The perfusion in the diseased region is reduced relatively in comparison with that in the maximally dilated normal region. Increased stenotic flow and reduced mean aortic pressure diminish the perfusion pressure distal to the stenosis to the point that the blood supply to the subendocardial vessels it critically compromised. With decreasing distal pressure, the already dilated subendocardial resistance vessels cannot further dilate to increase local perfusion. In effect, a subendocardial steal phenomenon occurs in which a portion of the required subendocardial flow is shunted away through the pharmacologically dilated subepicardial vascular bed. To the extent that thallium behaves like potassium, an additional mechanism may play a role. In areas of myocardial ischemia or injury, the uptake of potassium or thallium is proportionately reduced on a metabolic basis.[25] The relative importance of this metabolic mechanism in producing image defects over and above defects produced by regional flow abnormalities depends on the severity of the stenosis and myocardial oxygen requirements.

The basic physiologic requirement of any method for assessing coronary flow reserve is that the myocardial uptake of the imaging agent be proportional to flow at high coronary flow rates of at least four times resting levels. Gould[23] found that the maximal thallium uptake by tissue counting during peak coronary vasodilation after dipyridamole was only 50 to 60 percent higher than control levels. It has also been reported that myocardial uptake of ^{201}Tl is proportional to flow (or extraction is constant) if the increase in coronary flow is induced by elevating myocardial oxygen demands, as opposed to pharmacologic coronary vasodilation, which does not increase myocardial oxygen requirements.[25] The evidence suggests that thallium uptake in the myocardium is increased as coronary blood flow increases regardless of the stimulus but is not linearly related to flow at flow rates higher than resting control values.[23]

Uptake of an isotope into myocardium is determined by the expression: (coronary blood flow/cardiac output) × (extraction fraction) × (dose of isotope). Because the background counts are, in part, a function of the dose of the isotope, the intensity of the myocardial image relative to background is determined by a product of the extraction fraction and the ratio of coronary to systemic flows. Unlike exercise, dipyridamole increases coronary flow much more than cardiac output. Because handgrip after administration of dipyridamole has little effect on cardiac output, one would predict that the increase in coronary flow during this maneuver would further improve the myocardial to background count ratio. Myocardial uptake of ^{201}Tl is greater with dipyridamole than with exercise stress in cardiac regions in normal volunteers.[7] There is no significant difference in lung uptake, and clearance rates from myocardial segments and lung do not differ. There is significantly greater initial uptake of thallium by the liver, spleen, and splanchnic regions with dipyridamole as compared with exercise. However, there is clearance of this activity with time with dipyridamole, but an increase in activity with time with exercise.[7]

DIPYRIDAMOLE ADMINISTRATION AND SIDE EFFECTS

The standard regimen for the administration of the IV and oral forms of dipyridamole is shown in Figure 7-4.

The optimal IV dose rate of dipyridamole for thallium myocardial imaging is 0.14 mg/kg/min, diluted with 20 ml 5 percent dextrose in water (D_5W) or normal saline, for 4 minutes.[7] Smaller doses given more rapidly failed to produce comparable responses, and significant side effects have been reported with larger doses.[26] Injection in the upright or standing position or with isometric handgrip may increase myocardial uptake.[6] The quality of images and the myocardial-to-

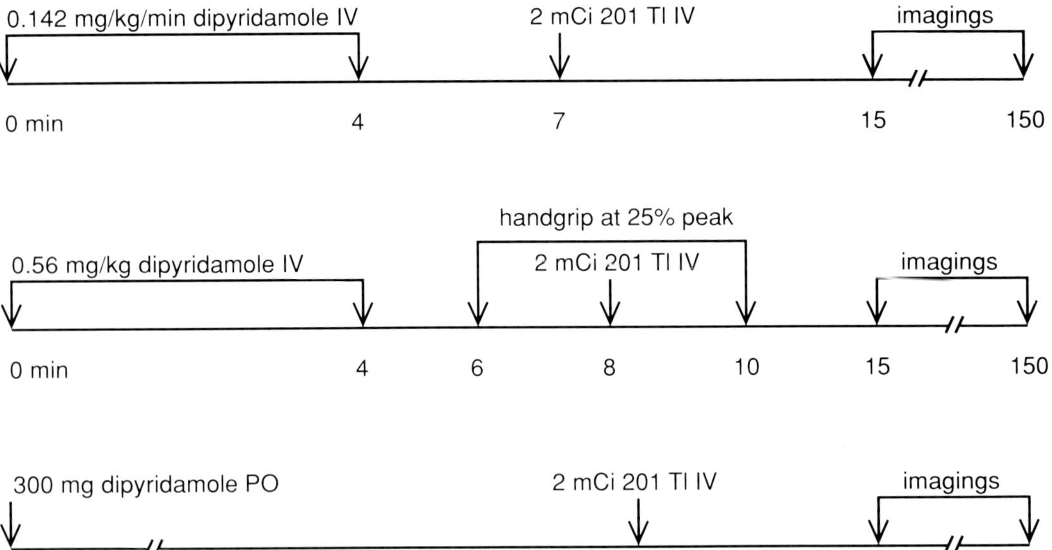

Fig. 7-4 Regimen for dipyridamole administration with corresponding imaging protocol.

background ratios are considerably improved by having the patient walk in place for 1 to 2 minutes before and during and 3 to 5 minutes after the injection of thallium. Either the upright position or exercise, or both, decreases pulmonary blood volume and transit time and would be expected to result in reduced lung uptake of thallium and improved myocardial-to-background ratios.[26] Peak coronary blood flow has been reported to occur 1 to 2 minutes after the 4-minute drug infusion and then to decrease exponentially with a half-life $(t_{1/2})$ of 33 minutes.[6] Wilson et al.[27] found that the mean time from onset of infusion to peak flow velocity was 6.5 minutes. However, it has been stated that the regional coronary blood flow and resistance responses may persist for 15 minutes after an IV bolus dose and that the coronary hemodynamic changes are not apparent after 20 minutes.[28]

Oral dipyridamole has been found to cause sufficient coronary arteriolar vasodilation and increase of coronary flow in nonstenotic arteries to identify perfusion defects comparable to those seen on maximum exercise stress in at least 75 percent of cases.[5] Oral dipyridamole imaging is performed in the fasting state with all dipyridamole antagonists, especially xanthines (theophylline preparations and caffeinated beverages) withheld. Forty-five minutes after dipyridamole ingestion, the patient walks slowly in place for 90 seconds and is injected with 3 mCi [201]Tl. Cardiac imaging follows immediately. Okada et al.[29] demonstrated that the split-dose thallium subtraction imaging technique permits technically adequate imaging before and immediately after dipyridamole infusion within a relatively short time period. Using this technique, 1 mCi ^{201}Tl was injected intravenously while the patient was in the supine position, and imaging was performed in the anterior and the left anterior oblique (LAO) projections for a preset time period. Immediately after acquisition of the images, and without moving the camera, dipyridamole infusion was performed at 0.14 mg/kg/min for 4 minutes, followed by injection of an additional 1 mCi [201]Tl. The LAO and anterior images were again acquired, and redistribution images were repeated in two projections. The intitial images were then subtracted from the realigned dipyridamole images to produce images representing perfusion during dipyridamole-induced hyperemia.

Adverse effects with dipyridamole are generally dose related and reversible. In the doses that are usually employed clinically, dipyridamole is quite nontoxic. Cardiac and noncardiac side effects were studied in 293 consecutive patients referred for nonexercise stress thallium imaging with IV dipyridamole (total dose 20 to 78 mg).[30] Cardiac side effects included chest pain in 76 patients (26 percent), of whom 70 percent were given aminophylline for relief of symptoms. Sixty patients (20 percent) had ischemic ST-segment depression, and 56 (19 percent) had arrhythmias (ventricular in 50 and atrial in 6). There were no deaths, myocardial infarctions, or sustained arrhythmias due to dipyridamole administration. Dipyridamole infusion can cause myocardial ischemia, and the mechanism is probably a coronary steal of blood flow away from the least adequately perfused zone in the myocardium.[6] Therefore, as in exercise stress testing, close monitoring of ECG, heart rate, and blood pressure is suggested. Symptoms of angina pectoris can be alleviated by the IV injection of aminophylline (125 mg over 1 minute), a direct antagonist to the effects of dipyridamole on the coronary vasculature.[31] If a large dose of aminophylline (approximately 200 mg) does not relieve the patient's symptom within several minutes, sublingual nitroglycerin can be administered, relieving angina by its direct effect on coronary stenoses and through its reduction of preload. It has been recommended that aminophylline (50 mg) be given empirically 20 minutes into the study after initial image acquisition to prevent the occurrence of adverse effects.[32] Noncardiac side effects of IV dipyridamole include headache (11 percent), light-headedness or dizziness (5 percent), nausea (4 percent), facial flushing (2 percent), and vomiting (1 percent).[30] One patient with severe asthma whose theophylline preparation was withheld for 2 days had bronchospasm during dipyridamole infusion. Although unproved, dipyridamole may have contributed to the bronchoconstriction by preventing access of prostaglandin E_2 (PGE_2) to its effective site.[33]

APPLICATIONS OF DIPYRIDAMOLE-THALLIUM IMAGING

Many patients in whom a noninvasive assessment of the severity of CAD would be desirable cannot exercise adequately for a stress test. In patients who are not obvious candidates for cardiac catheterization because they do not have unstable or severe symptoms, an alternative form of stress testing such as dipyridamole may be considered. The most common situation for using this approach is in the patient with peripheral vascular disease and claudication, arthritis, neurologic deficit, amputation, myopathy, or poor conditioning. The only group in whom it would be useful, but in whom it cannot be easily used, consists of patients with bronchospasm and chronic lung disease who are receiving theophylline preparations.

Dipyridamole stress-thallium imaging is particularly helpful in the following groups of patients: those with atypical chest pain or nonspecific rest ST-segment abnormalities, those without pain but with ST-segment depression during a stress test, those with chest pain and a negative or nondiagnostic ECG stress test, and those with multiple and severe coronary risk factors to establish the diagnosis of CAD with greater accuracy. It has been found that the use of ^{201}Tl scanning in patients with an intermediate (10 to 90 percent) pretest probability of CAD results in a marked increase in the proportion of patients with a post-test high (more than 90 percent) or low (less than 10 percent) probability of CAD, and that ^{201}Tl imaging can be used to reduce unnecessary catheterization without loss of diagnostic accuracy.[34] Leppo et al.[32] reported 93 percent sensitivity and 80 percent specificity of the ^{201}Tl study after dipyridamole infusion. Test results were not affected by the extent of CAD, the presence of Q waves, or propranolol therapy.

Detection of CAD in patients with aortic value stenosis has been difficult by conventional clinical methods. However, thallium imaging during combined IV dipyridamole and handgrip test demonstrated 85 percent sensitivity and 86 percent specificity in the detection of CAD in 27 patients with aortic valve stenosis.[35] The predictive accuracy of an abnormal ^{201}Tl scan with quantitative tomographic imaging (98 percent) was significantly better with much higher specificity than either qualitative planar or pinhole imaging.[36]

In addition to the application of diagnostic ^{201}Tl stress testing to patients with suspected CAD, the tests have also been used increasingly in patients with established CAD, largely to help in choosing between alternative forms of medical or surgical therapy and to help in assessing the efficacy of a chosen form of therapy. These uses are based on the ability of ^{201}Tl stress tests to assess the extent and severity of CAD, predict prognosis, assess the functional significance of known stenoses, and assess myocardial viability. These tests also have become employed increasingly in the everyday management of patients with known CAD in deciding the need for cardiac catheterization, in determining the need for coronary angiography, in deciding whether to treat patients with borderline stenosis, in deciding the need for coronary bypass surgery, in deciding the need for coronary angioplasty, in risk stratifi-

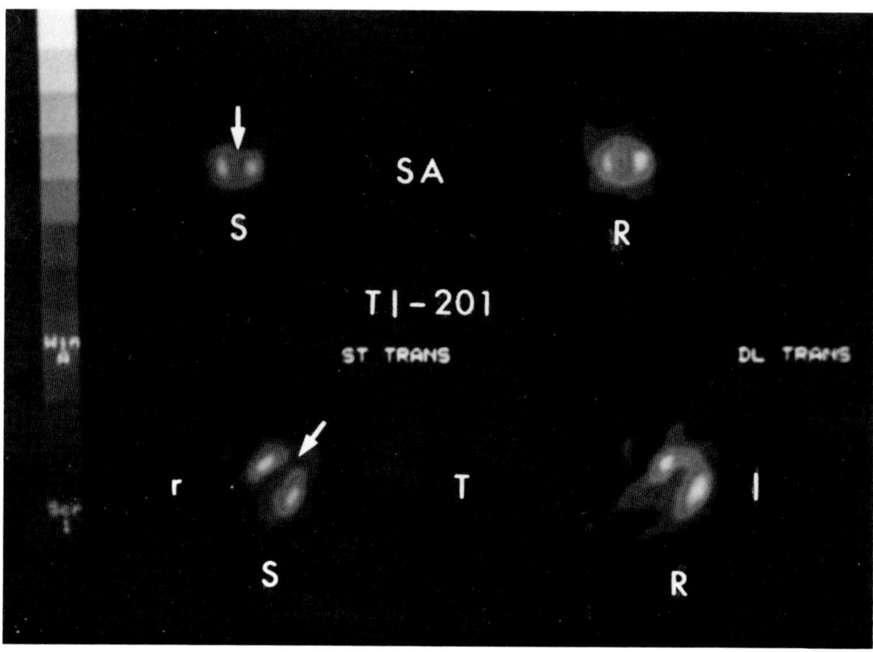

Fig. 7-5 Short axis (SA) and transverse (T) tomographic views of ^{201}Tl myocardial imaging show anterolateral perfusion defects on stress (S) images that were partially filled on resting (R) images.

cation in patients following myocardial infarction, in risk stratification in patients who are candidates for noncoronary surgery, and in evaluating the efficacy of the therapy. In most of these settings, ^{201}Tl dipyridamole stress imaging offers a strong alternative to the thallium exercise stress test.

Finally, it has been reported that the dipyridamole-thallium scan appears to be a more sensitive predictor of subsequent cardiac events than a submaximal exercise stress test after acute myocardial infarction, and that patients with thallium redistribution are at higher risk of future mortality and recurrent infarction.[37] Dipyridamole-thallium imaging also facilitates selection of the subset of truly high-risk patients in whom preoperative coronary angiography may be warranted. There were no cardiac ischemic complications in 32 patients with normal scans or persistent defects (scar), while 7 of 15 patients with thallium redistribution (ischemia) (Fig. 7-5) on preoperative scanning had perioperative ischemic events.[38] Boucher et al.[31] also concluded that dipyridamole-thallium imaging is superior to clinical assessment and is safer and less expensive than coronary angiography for the determination of cardiac risk in patients with severe peripheral vascular disease requiring operation.

ORAL VERSUS INTRAVENOUS DIPYRIDAMOLE

Published reports indicate that comparable diagnostic results may be obtained with dipyridamole imaging using either the PO or IV routes of administration. The sensitivity of the examination in either instance appears to be dose related. Homma et al.[39] found similar serum drug levels with a 300 mg oral dose suspension and IV dipyridamole. Thus the implication is that adequate pharmacologic effects can be achieved with both methods. In addition, oral dipyridamole has the advantages of being readily available with less frequent and less severe side effects with either 200 or 400 mg (except for headache or nausea). Even as the use of the intravenous form of dipyridamole becomes more widespread, the lower incidence and severity of side effects of oral dipyridamole may prove advantageous at least in some patients. On the other hand, oral administration requires longer medical supervision with much more variability in the time of onset and peak of adequate serum blood levels and thus pharmacologic effects. The intravenous route is more efficient and precise in these respects. Whether PO or IV routes of administration are employed, dipyridamole-thallium imaging has been shown to be a reliable alternative in the evaluation of coronary perfusion in patients unable to achieve adequate exercise levels on conventional stress testing.

REFERENCES

1. Botvick EH, Taradash MR, Shames DM, Parmley WW: Thallium-201 myocardial perfusion scintigraphy for the clinical clarification of normal, abnormal and equivocal electrocardiographic tests. Am J Cardiol 41:43, 1978
2. Turner DA, Battle WE, Deshmukh H, et al: The predictive value of myocardial perfusion scintigraphy after stress in patients without previous infarction. J Nucl Med 19:249, 1978
3. Melin JA, Piret LJ, Vanbutsele RJM, et al: Diagnostic value of exercise electrocardiography and thallium myocardial scintigraphy in patients without previous myocardial infarction: A Bayesian approach. Circulation 63:1019, 1981
4. Diamond GA, Forrester JS: Analysis of probablity as an aid in the clinical diagnosis of coronary artery disease. N Engl J Med 300:1350, 1979
5. Gould KL, Sorenson SG, Albro P, et al: Thallium-201 myocardial imaging during coronary vasodilation induced by oral dipyridamole. J Nucl Med 27:31, 1986
6. Brown BG, Josephson MA, Petersen RB, et al: Intravenous dipyridamole combined with

isometric handgrip for near maximal acute increase in coronary flow in patients with coronary artery disease. Am J Cardiol 48:1077, 1981

7. Gill JB, Miller D, Boucher CA, Strauss HW: Clinical decision making: Dipyridamole thallium imaging. J Nucl Med 27:132, 1986

8. Rozanski A, Berman DS: The efficacy of cardiovascular nuclear medicine exercise studies. Semin Nucl Med 17:104, 1987

9. Clausen JP: Circulatory adjustments to dynamic exercise and effect of physical training in normal subjects and in patients with coronary artery disease. Prog Cardiovasc Dis 18:459, 1976

10. Hamilton GW: Myocardial imaging with thallium-201: The controversy over its clinical usefulness in ischemic heart disease. J Nucl Med 20:1201, 1979

11. Gottlieb SO, Weisfeldt ML, Ouyang P, et al: Silent ischemia as a marker for early unfavorable outcomes in patients with unstable angina. N Engl J Med 314:1214, 1986

12. Svensson SE, Lomsky M, Olsson L, et al: Non-invasive determination of the distribution of cardiac output in man at rest and during exercise. Clin Physiol 2:467, 1982

13. Pohost GM, Alpert NM, Ingwall JS, Strauss HW: Thallium redistribution: mechanism and clinical utility. Semin Nucl Med 10:70, 1980

14. Liu P, Kiess MC, Okada RD, et al: The persistent defect on exercise thallium imaging and its fate after myocardial revascularization: Does it represent scar or ischemia? Am Heart J 110:996, 1985

15. Strauss HW, Boucher CA: Myocardial perfusion studies: lessons from a decade of clinical use. Radiology 160:577, 1986

16. Gewirtz H, Grotte GJ, Strauss HW, et al: The influence of left ventricular volume and wall motion on myocardial images. Circulation 59:1172, 1979

17. Beller GA, Watson DD, Gibson RS: Assessment of myocardial perfusion. p. 125. In Come PC (ed): Diagnostic Cardiology: noninvasive imaging techniques. JB Lippincott, Philadelphia, 1985

18. Gibson RS, Beller GA: Should exercise electrocardiography be replaced by radionuclide methods? p. 1. In Rahimtolla SH, Brest AM (eds): Controversies in Coronary Artery Disease. FA Davis, Philadelphia, 1982

19. Kaul S, Kiess M, Liu P, et al: Comparison of exercise electrocardiography and quantitative thallium imaging for one-vessel coronary artery disease. Am J Cardiol 56:257, 1985

20. Garcia EV, Van Train K, Maddahi J, et al: Quantification of rotational thallium-201 myocardial tomography. J Nucl Med 26:17, 1985

21. Tauchert M: Koronarreserve und maximaler saverstoffverbrauch des menschlichen herzen. Basic Res Cardiol 68:183, 1973

22. Gould KL: Pharmacologic intervention as an alternative to exercise stress. Semin Nucl Med 17:121, 1987

23. Gould KL: Noninvasive assessment of coronary stenoses by myocardial perfusion imaging during pharmacologic coronary vasodilation. I. Physiological basis and experimental validation. Am J Cardiol 41:267, 1978

24. Josephson MA, Brown BG, Hecht HS, et al: Detection and localization of $\geq$ 40% coronary stenosis in patients: Comparison of exercise and dypyridamole thallium-201 myocardial imaging. Am J Cardiol 45:399, 1980 (abst.)

25. Weich HF, Strauss HW, Pitt B: The extraction of thallium-201 by the myocardium. Circulation 56:188, 1977

26. Gould KL, Westcott RJ, Albro PC, Hamilton GW: Noninvasive assessment of coronary stenoses by myocardial imaging during pharmacologic coronary vasodilation. II. Clinical methodology and feasibility. Am J Cardiol 4:279, 1978

27. Wilson RF, Laughlin DE, Ackell PH, et al: Transluminal, subselective measurement of coronary artery blood flow velocity and vasodilator reserve in man. Circulation 72:82, 1985

28. Feldman RL, Wilmer MD, Nilchols WW, et al: Acute effect of intravenous dipyridamole on regional coronary hemodynamics and metabolism. Circulation 64:333, 1981

29. Okada RD, Lim YL, Rothendler J, et al: Split dose thallium-201 dipyridamole imaging: A new technique for obtaining thallium images before and immediately after an intervention. J Am Coll Cardiol 1:1302, 1983

30. Homma S, Gilliland Y, Guiney TE, et al: Safety of intravenous dipyridamole for stress testing with thallium imaging. Am J Cardiol 59:152, 1987

31. Boucher CA, Brewster DC, Darling RC, et

al: Determination of cardiac risk by dipyridamole-thallium imaging before peripheral vascular surgery. N Engl J Med 312:389, 1985

32. Leppo J, Boucher CA, Okada RD, et al: Serial thallium-201 myocardial imaging after dipyridamole infusion: diagnostic utility in detecting coronary stenoses and relationship to regional wall motion. Circulation 66:649, 1982

33. Heikela A, Haavisto M, Grannas R: Pulmonary uptake of PGE_2 is inhibited by dipyridamole in rat isolated lungs. Prostaglandins 23:147, 1982

34. Melin JA, Wijns W, Vanbutsele RJ, et al: Alternative diagnostic strategies of coronary artery disease in women: Demonstration of the usefulness and efficiency of probability analysis. Circulation 71:535, 1985

35. Huikuri HV, Korhonen UR, Ikaheimo MJ, et al: Detection of coronary artery disease by thallium imaging using a combined initravenous dipyridamole and isometric handgrip test in patients with aortic valve stenosis. Am J Cardiol 59:336, 1987

36. Francisco DA, Collins SM, Go RT, et al: Tomographic thallium-201 myocardial perfusion scintigrams after maximal coronary artery vasodilation with intravenous dipyridamole. Comparison of qualitative and quantitative approaches. Circulation 66:370, 1982

37. Leppo JA, O'Brien J, Rothendler JA, et al: Dipyridamole-thallium-201 scintigraphy in the prediction of future cardiac events after acute myocardial infarction. N Engl J Med 310:1014, 1984

38. Brewster DC, Okada RD, Strauss HW, et al: Selection of patients for preoperative coronary angiography: Use of dipyridamole-stress-thallium myocardial imaging. J Vasc Surg 2:504, 1985

39. Homma S, Callahan RJ, Ameer B, et al: Usefulness of oral dipyridamole suspension for stress thallium imaging without exercise in detection of coronary artery disease. Am J Cardiol 57:503, 1986

8

Qualitative SPECT Thallium Imaging: Technical Considerations and Clinical Applications

Keith C. Fischer

Single photon emission computed tomography (SPECT) has become the preferred imaging technique for ^{201}Tl myocardial perfusion studies.[1-4] Nevertheless, although providing clear advantages for cardiac imaging, this technique poses new challenges for the technologists who perform the examination and the physicians who interpret it. Both must be involved as never before in a rigorous quality-assurance program to maintain the equipment at peak performance and to detect faults in the system that would degrade the clinical images. With a solid basis in knowledge, however, personnel with the equipment and commitment can perform SPECT thallium imaging routinely.

This chapter focuses on qualitative techniques of thallium imaging, while Chapter 9 presents the substantial progress made in developing quantitative algorithms for the processing, display, and interpretation of these examinations.

Tomographic imaging, which produces thin sections of the organ of interest, offers distinct advantages over planar imaging. By focusing on a thin slice of an organ, overlying and underlying activity is minimized. This results in marked improvement of image contrast.[5] Although tomography is not immune to partial volume effects, SPECT clearly increases target-to-background ratios above those obtainable in planar imaging.[6,7]

Just as important is the three-dimensional nature of SPECT. Images are obtained from multiple projections around the organ and, when reviewed in a cine format, give an image of the organ rotating in space that can be useful in interpretation. Furthermore, after initial reconstruction in the transaxial plane, the image set has the potential to be reoriented to display the organ from other perspectives.[8] As will be seen, this is of particular advantage in an anatomically complex organ such as the heart, in which the ability to reorient images leads to superior localization of perfusion defects in the myocardium.[4,9] In addition, although many problems remain to be solved, true quantification of this three-dimensional tomographic image data is a valid hope.[10–12] Two-dimensional planar images suffer greatly from overlapping structures and higher background levels, making true quantification impractical.

PRINCIPLES OF SPECT

The discussion in this chapter refers exclusively to transaxial tomography rather than to longitudinal tomography. Seven-pinhole[13,14] and rotating slant-hole collimator tomography[15,16] are examples of longitudinal techniques that have been applied to thallium cardiac imaging. Clinical and phantom studies, however, have demonstrated that the transaxial technique is superior to these longitudinal techniques for thallium myocardial perfusion studies.[7,17,18] Both these methods suffer from the artifactual propagation of defects into tomographic slices proximal and distal to the actual defect,[18,19] a problem thought to be related to the limited angle of data acquisition of these techniques. Transaxial tomography, which accumulates data from a wider angle of coverage, gives a truer representation of the isotope distribution.

Acquisition

The initial step in the production of the transaxial SPECT images is the acquisition of multiple planar images from around the patient. Elliptical and body contour imaging, while possible, are not widely used in clinical thallium imaging; for this discussion of principles, only a circular orbit about the patient is considered. Figure 8-1 diagrams that motion and establishes the coordinate system used in this discussion. The camera moves in a circular orbit around the central axis of rotation (AOR). The distance from this axis to the camera face is termed the radius of rotation (ROR). The camera is essentially a standard Anger (gamma) camera head placed on a gantry that allows 360-degree motion around the patient resulting in acquisitions from a preset number of angles. Thus, if a 360-degree orbit is accomplished at angular increments of 6 degrees, 60 images are obtained. Even if, as some cameras permit, motion of the camera head is continuous rather than "step-and-shoot," the planar images are discrete and are of a preprogrammed number.

The separate images obtained by the analog camera are converted to digitized matrices of appropriate size by the analog-to-digital converters (ADC) of the computer. The matrix size (64 × 64 or 128 × 128 are the two practical choices) is assigned by the operator based on the resolution obtainable in the study. Among the factors that influence resolution are the intrinsic resolving characteristics of the camera, the collimator being used, the object distance from the collimator face, intervening scattering material, and the total counts obtained. The size and particularly the motion of the patient and target organ also affect resolution. In clinical thallium imaging, the distance from the heart, the heart motion, the scatter in the thorax, and the collimator used all conspire to make the FWHM in the range of 12 to 18 mm.[2,20,21]

Backprojection

In the digitized images, each pixel contains a numerical value of counts for a discrete square of the image matrix. Each row and

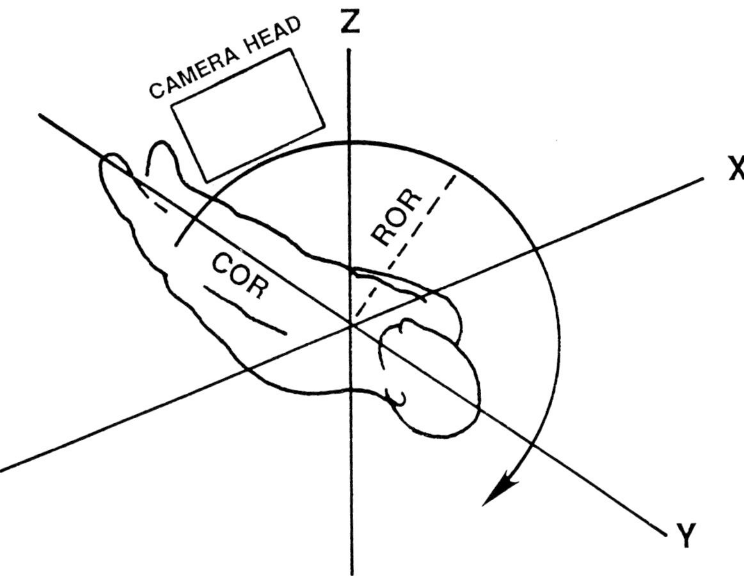

Fig. 8-1 As viewed from the patient's head, the camera travels in a clockwise arc about the center of rotation (COR). The distance from the COR to the camera face is the radius of rotation (ROR). In this coordinate system, the transaxial images are in the x, z plane. The y axis is parallel to the COR.

column of pixels·is thus a projection of count intensity across the field of view at each of the camera stops (Fig. 8-2A). The SPECT algorithm reconstructs a three-dimensional image of the original object combining these multiple-count intensity profiles. The method routinely used in clinical computer systems for this reconstruction is backprojection.[22] By this method, the intensity of each pixel in the reconstructed image is the sum of all count profiles that pass through it (Fig. 8-2B).

The mathematical processes used to achieve this are outlined elsewhere,[22] but what is important is that the simple backprojection method does not produce clinically useful images. In fact, the reconstructed images are dominated by star-burst artifacts, which consist of a central density with radiating arms of lesser intensity (Fig. 8-2B). These "arms" represent the backprojection through the en-

tire matrix of the counts in each profile. Back-projection of these profiles causes extraneous counts to be spread over surrounding pixels. This slurring of counts over the matrix causes a reduction of contrast and a loss of detail.

Filters

To project a truer distribution of activity in the object being imaged, the count profiles must be filtered before reconstruction; alternatively, the resulting unacceptable transaxial images must be filtered after reconstruction. These are mathematically analogous processes, but most commercial algorithms perform digital filtering before proceeding with the backprojection in a process termed filtered backprojection. The filter introduces negative values for counts in the tails of the point-spread functions to cancel out the positive values that constitute the arms of the

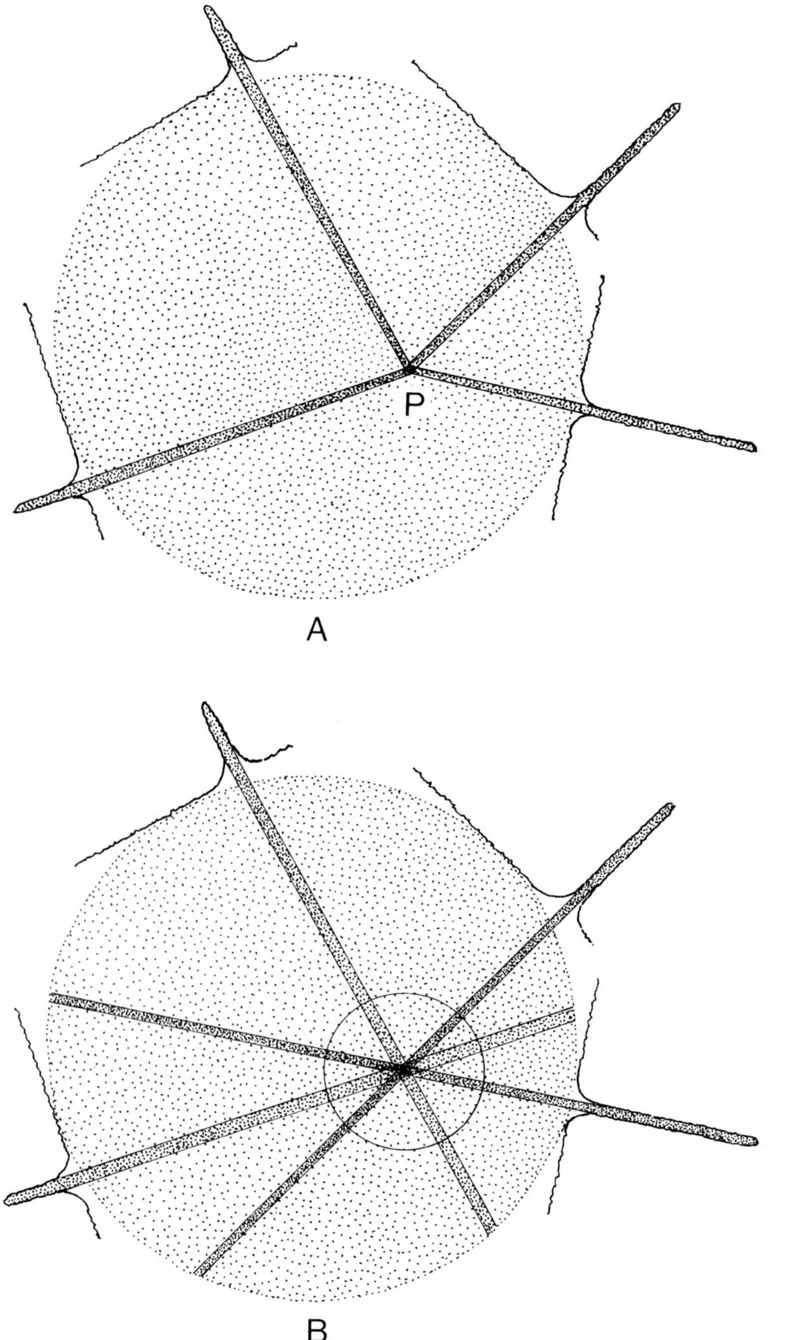

Fig. 8-2 (A) The first step in the production of SPECT images is the creation of count-intensity profiles at each camera stop around the patient. Here four such profiles of a point source (P) are represented. The height and FWHM of the profiles vary with distance and intervening scatter. **(B)** During backprojection, each count profile is projected onto the matrix so that the intensity of each resulting pixel represents the sum of all profiles passing through it. This process results in the creation of star-burst artifacts (circle).

star burst (Fig. 8-3). This preserves the contrast of the image.

Expansion on the subject of digital filters is warranted here because although they are stated in complex mathematical terms that make a thorough understanding of them beyond the confines of this discussion, they are essential for the production of interpretable images. Besides making the backprojection process clinically usable, filters can also be used in either pre- or postbackprojection processing of data, or both, to enhance the images. A further practical reason to gain a basic understanding of filters is that commercial SPECT software packages provide multiple predefined and operator–definable filters from which to choose. Although there may be more art than science in picking filters to produce the final thallium reconstructions, a basic intuitive understanding of filters makes these choices more rational.

The digital filters used in the backprojection process are complex integral functions that, when multipled or convolved with each count profile, alter the distribution of counts in the profiles. Using the description of filters in frequency space that Galt et al.[23] reported as a model, one can gain a better understanding of the effect of filtering and convolution. Count profiles obtained by the angular sampling around the patient can be thought of as made of various distributions of count frequencies. Frequency refers to the rate of change in counts over a distance and can be measured in cycles per pixel. A complete cycle (from peak to peak) can be accomplished in two pixels, so the highest frequency that can be demonstrated is 0.5 cycles/pixel. This is called the Nyquist frequency (F_N). Higher frequencies are cut off and cannot be displayed by the computer. Because pixel size is smaller for larger matrices, 128 × 128 matrices can potentially display higher frequencies than 64 × 64 matrices. In an image, the higher frequencies define the rapidly changing count-rate areas, such as edges. Unfortunately, the statistical

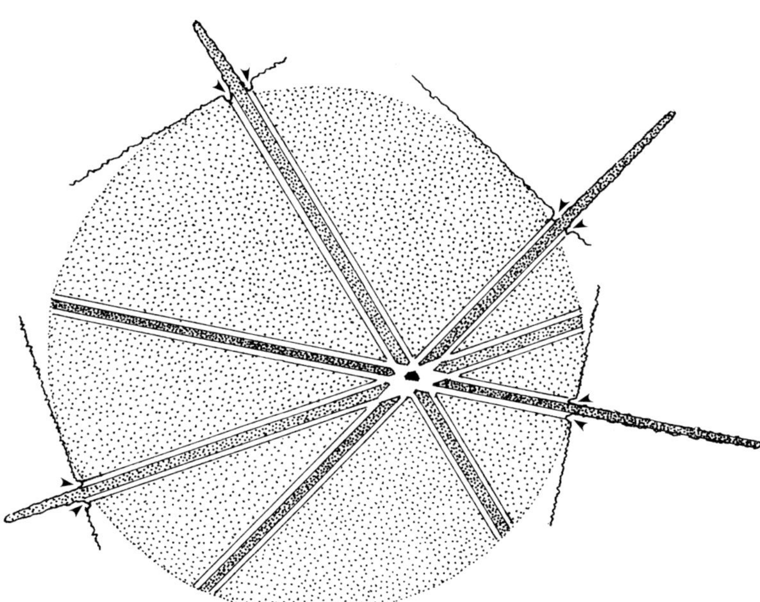

Fig. 8-3 Filtered backprojection introduces negative values into the projections (arrowheads) canceling out the long arms of the star-burst artifacts.

uncertainty or *noise* in the data is also in the higher frequency ranges. Lower frequencies define the more gradual shifts of count rate that might be found in the middle of organs.

Filters can thus be described by the frequencies they allow to pass through so that filters that pass relatively more high frequencies (high pass) result in sharper (but noisier) images with better edge definition, and filters that pass relatively fewer high frequencies (lower pass) produce smoother images where edges are less distinct.

The prototype Ramp filter is diagrammed in Figure 8-4A. It allows all frequencies to pass up to the Nyquist frequency ($F/F_N = 1$). In fact, it enhances the higher frequencies linearly, at the expense of the lower frequencies. This enhancement of the higher edge-forming frequencies maximizes contrast and resolution in the reconstructed image. In clinical thallium studies, however, the images formed with this filter are unacceptably coarse because in these low-count studies, noise is also amplified and can overpower the useful clinical data (Fig. 8-4B).

Image noise follows Poisson statistics. Thus, if a pixel in one of the planar projections contains 100 counts, as it might in a thallium image, the standard deviation is the square root of 100 or 10 counts. This standard deviation represents 10 percent (10/100) of the counts in the pixel. Thus, it is clear why low-count planar data with such a large noise component results in unacceptably noisy transaxial images after filtered backprojection with a Ramp filter that enhances higher frequencies.

Filters can be described by their characteristic shape and, within a family of filters, by their different cutoff frequencies. The lower the cutoff, the fewer high frequencies passed, and in general the smoother the image. Many filters with such names as Hanning, Parzan,

Hamming, Hann, Shepp-Hanning-Logan, and Butterworth have been described. However, the filters used in a particular laboratory often depend on which filters are available on the computer system employed. Some of these filters are shown in Figure 8-4C to J, and the resulting transaxial images of the heart can be compared with those produced by the Ramp filter (Fig. 8-4B). The most clinically useful filters for thallium imaging will have the characteristics of not overamplifying the high-frequency noise and of rolling off gradually at the cutoff frequency, to avoid artifacts. It should be re-emphasized here that filters used in SPECT processing and display algorithms are not confined to the backprojection process alone. Prefiltration of image data before filtered backprojection can be performed with a low-pass filter, permitting the use of a coarser (more Ramp-like) filter in the backprojection process, potentially preserving more contrast in the reconstructed images.[24]

The images produced by the filtered backprojection process are a series of transaxial tomographs reconstructed perpendicular to the axis of rotation. If a 64×64 matrix was used, these transaxial images are 1 pixel thick in the y direction and 64 pixels along the x and z coordinates. At this point, additional postprocessing filtration to reduce noise in the data can be performed if needed. This is often in the form of spatial smoothing in which adjacent transverse images are either simply added together in the y axis or a more complex volume smooth performed on these three-dimensional images. For reasons to be discussed, transverse images of the heart are not ideal for visualizing all myocardial segments and are generally reoriented before final display and interpretation.[8]

System Uniformity

The tomographic reconstruction process amplifies statistical noise and other system nonuniformities[25] despite the use of digital

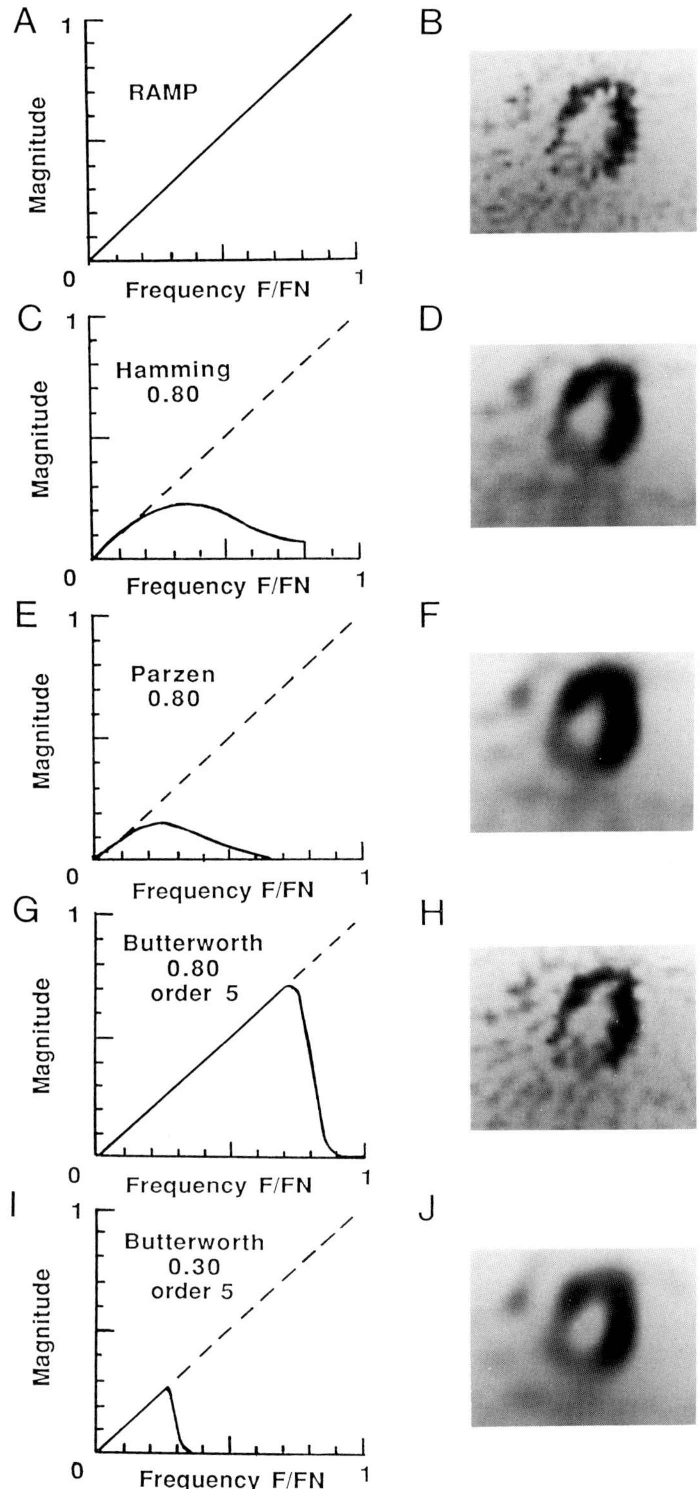

Fig. 8-4 Examples of different filters and the resultant transverse reconstructions of a normal heart. The Ramp filter **(A)** allows all frequencies to pass, **(B)** amplifying the higher frequencies and producing coarse noisy images. **(C,E,G)** Filters with a cutoff at 0.8 of the Nyquist frequency ($F/F_N = 0.8$) that vary as to the pattern of frequencies passed below this cutoff. **(G,I)** The two Butterworth filters differ in their cutoffs. Generally, the fewer high-frequency data passed and the lower the cutoff frequency, the smoother the image.

filters, which can only partially eliminate this effect. Thus, if not minimized, these nonuniformities are propagated in the reconstructed images, resulting in the creation of artifacts in the transaxial slice data. These take the form of bull's-eyes (hot or cold spots) in the center of the field or ring artifacts off center.[26] In actuality, very high-count images must be obtained to see the complete geometry of the artifacts. At the level of total counts in thallium images, the Poisson noise almost completely masks the definition of these artifacts. Although not clearly defined by the low-count statistics of thallium images, their effect is a loss of precision in the images. This is experienced by the observer as a blurring of the image with potential loss of resolution.

Because the backprojection process amplifies nonuniformities causing artifacts, excellent system uniformity is demanded for SPECT imaging. To obtain this, all causes of inhomogeneous response in the total system (camera, collimator, computer interface, and software) must be minimized. Realization of this goal requires close attention to many of the acceptance testing and quality-control procedures that must be performed to produce the highest-quality SPECT images.

Since the production of SPECT images begins with the accumulation of multiple planar projections, high-quality SPECT images require optimization of the intrinsic performance specifications of the gamma camera used to acquire the images. Excellent linearity of the camera is fundamental because multiple count profiles are used to reconstruct the images. These must be projected in parallel arrays across the matrix to maintain resolution in the x and z directions. Furthermore, slice thickness would vary in a nonlinear camera; thus, resolution in the y axis would be degraded.[27] The camera manufacturers have responded to this need for superior linearity; in most instruments, a linearity correction to less than 1 percent is achieved.

The variation in response across the detector face is another important consideration in determining system uniformity. Despite matched photomultiplier tubes and digital correction circuitry, the variation of response is approximately 3 to 5 percent. This degree of nonuniformity of response is in general an unacceptable level for SPECT imaging. If the counting statistics are adequate, artifacts will be seen in the reconstructed transaxial images with this level of nonuniformity.[28] Even in lower count studies, such a level of nonuniformity results in noise in the back-projected images and in all images derived from them.

In addition to these intrinsic camera factors, the collimators must be considered for their effect on system uniformity. Variations in septal diameter, length, or angulation will result in a nonuniform distribution of counts.

Finally, due to differential nonlinearities in the ADC, nonuniformities are introduced at the camera-computer interface as well. The ADCs are responsible for turning the analog positioning signals into digital information and must faithfully digitize all pulses presented to them by the camera.

Uniformity Correction

It is a general goal in SPECT imaging to reduce system inhomogeneity to 1 percent or below.[28] For low-count studies such as thallium studies, however, where counts per pixel in our experience may range from 35 to 200, it is problematic whether such a high degree of uniformity is required. Since the camera, collimator, and interface problems discussed above produce inhomogeneity of 3 to 5 percent, to reduce this to 1 percent, a uniformity correction is needed in SPECT cameras that is not employed for planar imaging. This correction is provided by the acquisition of a high count flood. Coming as it does at the end of the imaging chain, it has the potential to alter the nonuniformities introduced by the camera, collimator, and

ADC. Since this technique is meant to correct for both intrinsic and extrinsic nonuniformities, as well as the ADC, the flood is accumulated with the collimator in place and is digitized and stored on the computer to be applied to each planar slice for correction of count inhomogeneity before reconstruction takes place. Thus, each pixel value in a projection is altered by a correction factor specific for that pixel, taking into account the mean flood counts for that pixel divided by the counts in the planar images to be reconstructed.[25]

Obviously, the uniformity of this flood must exceed the uniformity one is trying to obtain in the system. The number of counts needed to obtain field uniformity of ± 1 percent has to be 10,000 counts per pixel ($\sqrt{10,000} = 100$; $\pm 100/10,000$ counts per pixel is ± 1 percent variation). About 3,000 pixels of the 64×64 matrix are actually used in images from a circular camera face, so for this matrix size, $3,000 \times 10,000$ or 30 million counts are needed. For a 128×128 matrix, four times this number of counts (approx. 120,000,000) would be needed for a 1 percent flood field correction. It is important to point out that these floods are specific for the acquision parameters used in a study. Thus, separate floods have to be accumulated for each different collimator and for each zoom factor used in the acquisitions. The computers should permit the storing of several such floods, which can be applied to the appropriate acquisition data sets. It is simplest to acquire a flood with a solid ^{57}Co sheet source because, with current production methods, a 1 percent uniformity can be achieved in these sources. The floods collected on the photopeak of ^{57}Co can be applied to thallium acquisitions.

Rotation Effects

Although the flood field correction is meant to neutralize many sources of nonuniformity in the imaging chain, some sources of nonuniformity cannot be corrected by this strata-

gem. The rotation of the gantry itself subjects the camera head and its components to thermal, magnetic, and gravitational forces not experienced during planar imaging. The collimator may shift as a function of position with rotation around the patient. This problem may be greater with insert-type collimators. The photomultipler tubes themselves may shift slightly in position, altering the gains on the dynodes, which would alter uniformity. More predictably, as the head orientation changes with relationship to the earth's gravitational field, the magnetic fluxes to which the tubes are subjected change. The tubes are shielded with μ metal in the cameras to protect against the changing magnetic fields during rotation, but this protection is only effective to near-field strengths of 0.5 gauss—approximately the strength of the earth's gravitational field. If strong electrical fields exist around the camera as its head moves, the magnetic effects created could alter the electron paths in the photomultipler tubes and distort the images. Electrical motors if not appropriately shielded are the most common cause of these effects.

Electronic Alignment

One major problem arising at the interface between the camera and computer that cannot be altered by the flood correction is malalignment of the center of the computer matrix with the COR of the camera. The projected center of rotation of the camera and the center of the computer matrix must be shifted to be within 0.3 pixels of each other.[29] To facilitate this, the manufacturers have developed software that allows the customer to use either a point or line source around which to acquire several stops, so that the computer can calculate an offset from the center of the matrix. This offset is stored in the computer; subsequent image sets are shifted according to this figure to align them before filtered backprojection is performed. If the images are not shifted to bring them into alignment before the filtered backprojec-

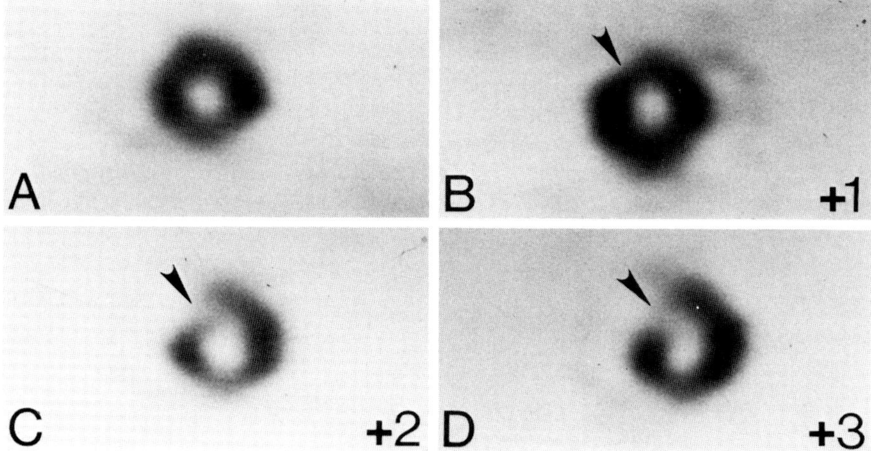

Fig. 8-5 Effect of malalignment of the center of rotation and the center of the computer matrix is demonstrated. A defect (arrowhead) becomes increasingly apparent in these axial reconstructions as the malalignment is increased by 1-pixel increments from an aligned configuration **(A)** to an offset of 3.0 pixels **(D)**.

tion, the resulting imprecision can cause blurring or more gross artifacts in the images (Fig. 8-5).

QUALITY CONTROL

Extrinsic Camera Parameters

The preceding discussion briefly points up some of the more important factors that affect image quality in a SPECT system. Superior SPECT images will result only if these and other potential problems in the equipment are minimized. To ensure this, both adequate acceptance testing and, more importantly, an ongoing program of quality control must be in place in the laboratory that expects to use this technique with consistent results. Those laboratories with the equipment, personnel, knowledge, and time may be able to maintain a very sophisticated ongoing testing routine, but for the smaller clinical center that lacks physics support, simplified procedures that leave no essential task undone are more practical. Table 10-1 summarizes an acceptable frequency of performance of these various tests and procedures.

The complete SPECT system consists of a special imaging table on which the patient lies, the gamma camera with gantry allowing 360-degree rotation of its head, collimators, computer and interface, software, and some sort of imager for making hard copy. Acceptance testing of the components of the system should be performed by the user and/or the vendor at installation. An ongoing testing program should then be instituted.

The table with its cantilevered pallet around which the camera must rotate should support approximately 250 pounds without significant bending of the unsupported head end. At installation, a reproducible, fixed method of securing the table in position for patient studies should be provided. If the table is secured to the floor permanently, however, the flexibility of using the camera as a planar imaging device will be compromised. The user should ascertain by simple measurement that the table position is in the center of rotation of the camera by measurement of the distance from the vertical camera head to the table edge on both sides of the table.

TABLE 8-1 Quality-Control Schedule

Test Frequency	Quality-Control Test
Daily	Low-count intrinsic flood (2–5 Mct)
	Careful peaking on ^{201}Tl with documentation of photopeaks and windows
	Leveling camera head before each patient acquisition
Semiweekly	Center of rotation correction
Weekly	Uniformity correction flood
	Extrinsic uniformity evaluation (5–10 Mcts)
	Check of gantry leveling
	Pixel width calibration (if needed for attenuation correction and/or lesion sizing)
Quarterly	Evaluation of uniformity of camera at several stops
	Phantom studies of 50–100 Mct for resolution, uniformity, and contrast evaluation

More critically, the collimator face must be parallel to the axis of rotation as the camera rotates around the patient. Manufacturers usually supply both a digital readout of pitch or angle of the camera head and a bubble on the side of the head to confirm the level. Nevertheless, as part of acceptance testing, the collimator surface should be confirmed to be parallel to the horizon when the readout says 0. Testing to confirm that the camera stays parallel to the axis of rotation should be done at multiple stops around the table. If the collimator is not level and the septa are not perpendicular to the AOR, there will be a variation of sensitivity and resolution across the face of the collimator, since profiles will actually be collected with different ROR.[25] It appears that as little as ½ to 1 degree variance from true parallel can degrade high-count phantom images.[30,31] However, angulation on the order of 5 degrees is needed to alter thallium images detectably[32] (Fig. 8-6). This artifact is not corrected by the uniformity flood.

Also as part of acceptance testing, the gamma camera head support should be observed for excessive flexing during its circular motion. This could potentially cause misregistration during the backprojection process.[32] All

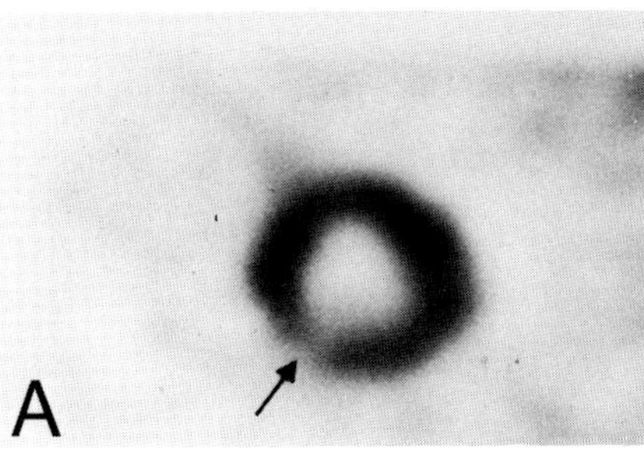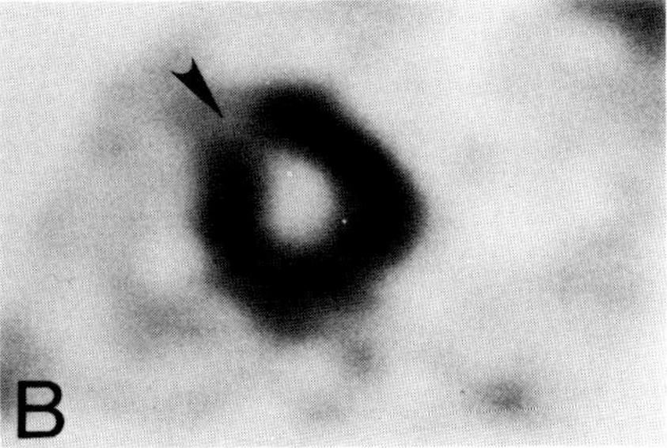

Fig. 8-6 (A) Axial reconstruction at mid-ventricle of a normal patient. The heart is round in this projection with only the normal reduction of counts at the base of the septum (arrow). **(B)** Axial reconstruction of the same heart with image data acquired with a 6-degree angulation toward the feet. The heart is distorted from its normal round shape, and a superior defect can be seen (arrowhead).

safety mechanisms designed to stop the gantry when it hits a patient should be tested at purchase and frequently thereafter.

Intrinsic Camera Parameters

Intrinsic camera parameters should next be evaluated. The camera should be confirmed to be imaging at the manufacturer's specifications for linearity, uniformity, and resolution with various isotopes used in SPECT images. Bar phantom and high count uniformity floods obtained after installation must be critically compared with those provided by the manufacturer as standards for their systems. Count rate performance should be known and not exceeded in phantom acquisitions. Automatic correction circuitry should be understood. The potential gravitational and magnetic effects on count uniformity should be studied during acceptance testing and periodically thereafter. To do this, a flood source is secured to the collimator and 3 to 5 million count floods obtained over eight positions (every 45 degrees in a 360-degree collection). Correction by the uniformity flood should then be performed and the resulting floods inspected visually. If software permits, each of the subsequently collected floods may be subtracted from the flood collected at 0 degrees to see whether any residual counts or reproducible structure is seen.[33]

If all is well, the intrinsic resolution of the camera should be approximately the same for planar acquisitions and reconstructed SPECT images of the same counts. This can be determined by imaging a line source placed parallel with the AOR at a known ROR.[29] After reconstructing the image with a Ramp filter to preserve maximum resolution, it is compared with a planar image of similar counts taken from the same distance as the ROR of the SPECT acquisition. Images should be quite similar. If FWHM values can be calculated, they should be no more than 1 to 2 mm better for the planar than the SPECT study.[29]

The collimators, a very important component of the system, should be carefully inspected at installation and at intervals thereafter. Initially, they should be radiographed to find any significant variation in septal thickness or physical damage that might have occurred during shipping. This radiograph can be preserved and compared with radiographs obtained subsequently. It should be checked that the collimator has not shifted during collection at all angles to the horizon. Extrinsic uniformity and resolution should be evaluated initially and at no less than weekly intervals afterward.

In evaluating the computer and software, some basic observations can be made. The camera field should fill up the computer matrix as closely as possible. The zoom factors should be tested. It should be confirmed that counts registered by the computer are equal to those registered by the camera for the same time. A flood fixed to the collimator should be imaged for 64 stops. The counts should be equal at each stop. The stops should be timed with a stop watch, to confirm that they are equal at multiple positions around the table. The number of stops should correspond to the figure designated for the acquisition.

Before final acceptance, phantom studies should be performed. These can simultaneously evaluate the total system resolution, contrast, and uniformity. Relatively low-count clinical images do not give as good an indication of degradation of the system because changes are masked by the statistical noise in the studies. Keeping a comparison file of high-count phantom reconstructions will allow these comparisons to be made over time.

In most commercial phantoms designed for use with SPECT cameras, different sections evaluate different parameters of SPECT imaging. One section should permit uniform distribution of isotope to look for bull's-eye and ring artifacts in high-count acquisitions. Ten to 20 million counts per slice will have to be collected. To obtain this, multiple slices may have to be summed. A measure of contrast and resolution of the system can be obtained by imaging cold spheres and rods in the phantom. These should be studied at high count densities to compare with vendor-supplied specifications or images. Some phantoms have specific cardiac inserts that permit simulation of myocardial imaging; these may provide further clinical comparisons. The articles by Greer et al.[29] and Areeda et al.[34] provide further information on the acquisition and evaluation of these phantom images.

CLINICAL SPECT MYOCARDIAL IMAGING

Having established a foundation in knowledge of SPECT imaging and equipment quality-control procedures, the imaging physician can then proceed to concentrate on the practical aspects of acquiring, processing, displaying, and archiving a SPECT thallium study. Consistency and accuracy in the performance of these various tasks should be the goals. To produce clinically valid thallium SPECT studies, routines for these tasks should be established that can be followed by all technologists and physicians performing, processing, and interpreting the examinations.

Acquisition

CAMERA PREPARATION

The routine in a SPECT thallium study should begin with daily preparation of the camera. A camera flood should be obtained and carefully inspected for uniformity. If photomultiplier tube voltages and/or tune status readouts are available, these should be studied for photomultiplier tubes that have drifted out of tune.

The camera should be carefully peaked for thallium at the beginning of the day. We use both the mercury daughter x-rays from 68.8 to 81 keV and the higher photopeak of 167.5 keV, which provides a 10 percent abundance of γ-rays. Currently, although our camera is capable of asymmetric peaking, we are using a symmetric window of 20 percent centered over the x-ray spectrum and a 30 percent window on the higher γ-peak. An asymmetric high window would exclude scattered radiation better, improving lesion contrast and resolution. However, there is a trade-off with uniformity, since there is a loss of flood field uniformity as a function of asymmetry of the window. In experiments with planar images, LaFontaine et al.[35] found a small improvement in resolution with asymmetry of the window. However, because of the loss of counts and loss of uniformity demonstrated by these workers, both critical factors to be maximized in SPECT imaging, symmetric windows may be the better alternative despite less scatter rejection. Our use of a 30 percent window on the higher peak increases our counts in clinical studies by 15 to 20 percent over imaging the mercury x-ray spectrum alone. Phantom studies confirm the improvement in resolution of images accumulated at this higher energy and confirm that no detectable degradation of images occurs by simultaneous acquisition of counts from two different energy spectra.

180-DEGREE ACQUISITIONS

In our laboratory, we acquire images in a 180-degree arc around the patient beginning in a 45-degree RAO position and finishing in a 45-degree LPO position (Fig. 8-7). This is the more common method. However, a controversy has developed, with some defending the position that a 360-degree acquisition should be used for cardiac thallium imaging, as it is for other SPECT organ imaging.[36,37] The supporters of 360-degree collections point to the advantages of more uniform spatial resolution and fewer imag-

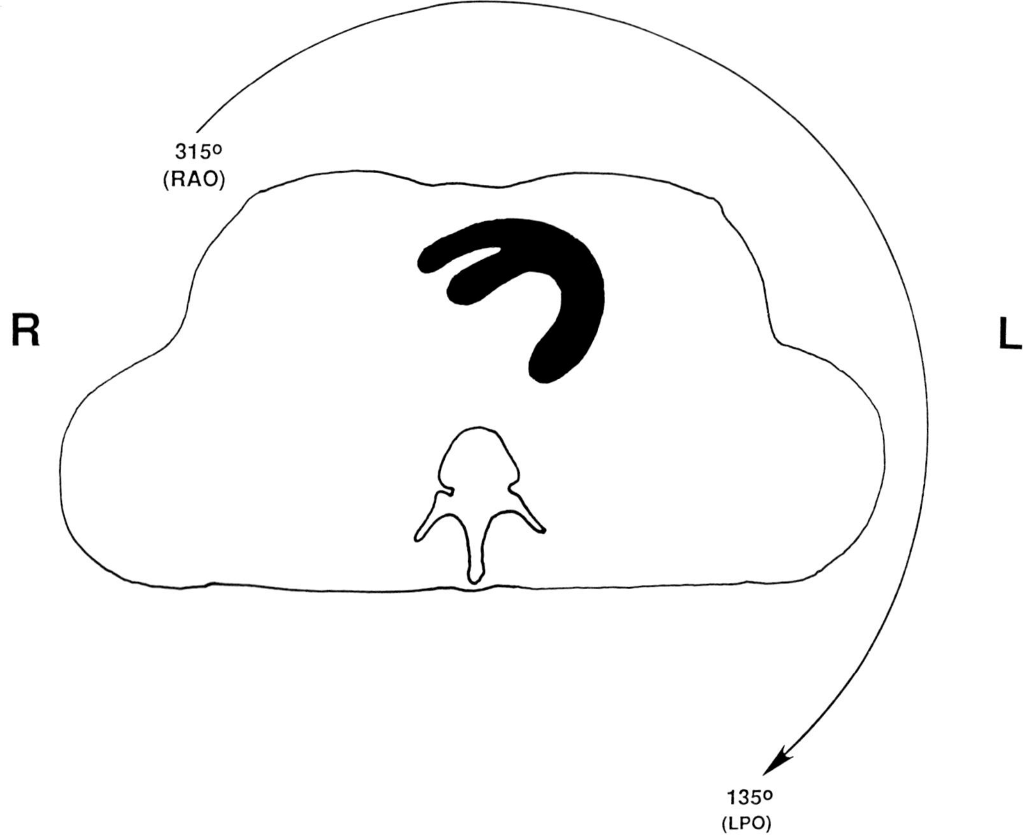

Fig. 8-7 Schematic cross section of the thorax at heart level as viewed from the feet. The 180-degree arc defines the path of the gamma camera during acquisitions.

ing artifacts present in these collections versus 180-degree acquisitions. Furthermore, better attenuation correction is possible for the 360-degree acquisitions.[36,37] However, Hoffman[38] points out that the anterior position of the heart in the left chest makes imaging with thallium, with its low-energy spectrum, a special case; he favors 180-degree acquisitions. Most of the thallium photons detected by the camera as it rotates behind the body in the 360-degree acquisition are scatter. Furthermore, resolution is degraded by the distance from the heart when imaging posteriorly. Absorption of thallium photons by the pallet on which the patient lies also degrades the clinical images. We have documented up to 20 percent absorption of counts

by the pallet in phantom studies. Thus, for the same acquisition times, many more unscattered counts are collected from the anteriorly placed heart in the 180-degree acquisition than in a 360-degree acquisition. Comparing images accumulated in an anterior 180-degree arc versus the posterior 180-degree arc dramatically shows these effects of scatter and attenuation (Fig. 8-8). Eisner et al.[39] pointed out, however, that which particular 180-degree arc is used for acquisition is important; these workers demonstrated marked differences in counts in the different walls of the heart, depending on the angle at which the 180-degree arc is initiated.[39] To minimize these acquisition-dependent effects, Eisner and co-workers sug-

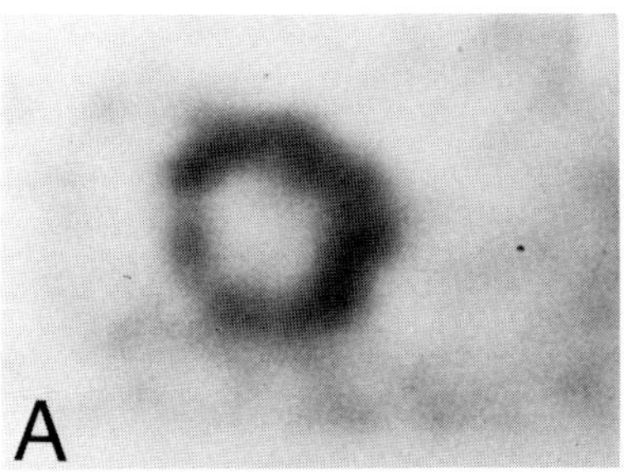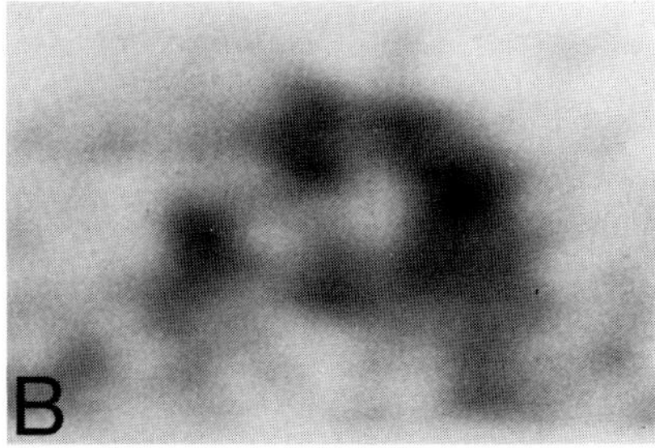

Fig. 8-8 (A) Axial reconstruction from 80-stop data collected in the anterior arc defined in Figure 8-7. **(B)** Axial reconstruction of the same heart from 80-stop data acquired in a 180-degree arc behind the patient from 135 degrees (LPO) to 315 degrees (RAO). The same filter was used for both reconstructions without additional smoothing. Marked distortion of the reconstructed posterior data is apparent; it arises from distance from the anteriorly placed heart, scatter, and attenuation by bony structures and the scanning table.

gest starting with an angle of 270 degrees (right lateral) to 315 degrees (45 degrees RAO).

Clinical studies bear out the increased lesion contrast and confirm the improvement in resolution with 180-degree versus 360-degree acquisitions.[40] It would seem that, at this time, for the reasons mentioned, 180-degree acquisitions would be favored. In the special situations of a dual-headed camera[36] or the need for accurate quantification of myocardial activity when attenuation correction is necessary,[38] 360-degree collections would be the method of choice.

THE PATIENT

There is also some controversy about the dose of ^{201}Tl to be administered. We have had clinically validated success with 2.5-mCi injections, but doses of up to 3.5 mCi have been advocated (Dupuey EG: personal communication). The 2.5-mCi dose of thallium gives us approximately 3 to 4 million counts per acquisition. For the heavier male patients (above 220 pounds), 3.0 mCi may be appropriate to increase the counts obtained, but otherwise we have not found a clinical reason to use a higher dose.

After injection, the patients should be brought to the camera room and imaged as rapidly as possible. In general, SPECT imaging takes longer than planar imaging, with our imaging times being approximately 22 to 26 minutes. The data show that sensitivity for lesions with SPECT is very high, but as a time dependency in seeing lesions has been demonstrated with thallium imaging,[41,42] the less time taken after injection of isotope the better.

Positioning of the patient for SPECT imaging is time consuming for the unskilled. This step has to be well rehearsed by the technologist, to make it as efficient as possible. In positioning the patient, the goal is first and most importantly to place the face of the camera as close to the patient during its arc as possible. This maximizes the counts from the heart. As there is an increase in FWHM with distance from the object being imaged with gamma cameras, the resolution is also improved. Second, positioning for the two acquisitions should be nearly the same as possible so that slice-by-slice comparisons of the postexercise and reperfusion images will be valid.

The parameters that can be varied are the position of the patient on the pallet, table height, and the ROR of the camera head. With semicircular arcs, to come closest to the large patient may require moving him to the right of the pallet. This places the heart closer to the collimator in the RAO position and permits the use of a smaller ROR because the camera head can clear the left side of the body. We have a foam wedge with a depression cut out of it for the head and mark its position for each acquisition to help ensure proper repositioning on the delayed images. The parameters of table height and ROR used on the immediate post-exercise images must be reproduced on the delayed acquisition. We use tape to mark table height and reproduce this position on the delayed images. The vendors have not all been sensitive to the needs of displaying ROR values, and a relative scale may have to be improvised for the camera (Fig. 8-9).

Keeping the patient stationary during the examination is very important. The patient should be comfortable during the examination in order to remain still in the supine position with arms above the head. Additional foam padding of the table should be used, and something for the patients to hold above their heads is useful. Of primary importance is a vigilant but compassionate technologist who watches the patients to ensure that they do not move in such a way as to interfere with the study but who does allow supervised motion such as some relaxation of the right arm after the camera has passed by. It is important to remember that no amount of filtering or postprocessing can save a study that has been corrupted by significant patient motion.

Over the 6 years we have performed SPECT, approximately 1 of 10 patients could not be imaged with this technique. The main reasons were the patient's inability to raise the arms above the shoulders and maintain this position for 20 to 25 minutes, claustrophobia,

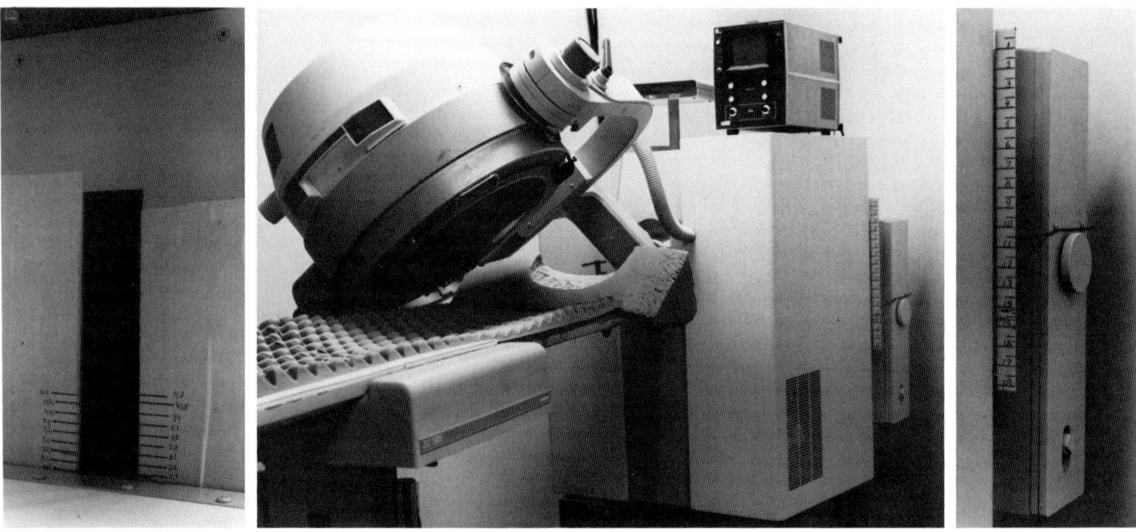

Fig. 8-9 (*Center*) SPECT camera and table prepared for a patient. Foam rubber provides additional comfort. Head rest also provides comfort and permits repositioning of the patient for reperfusion images. Low-budget handgrip (a c-clamp vice) is seen at the head of the table. (*Left*) Tape markings for table height and (*right*) jury-rigged radius of rotation indicator. These simple devices aid the accurate repositioning of the patient for reperfusion images.

or a weight greater than 250 pounds that exceeds the specifications of the pallet on the imaging table. Although we tested a pallet that was rated for weights above 250 pounds, its wide design and the patient's large girth made the ROR excessive. Reconstructed images were not of good quality.

MATRIX SIZE

The matrix size used for our acquisitions is 64 × 64. Although resolution is potentially improved by the smaller pixel size of a 128 × 128 matrix, the count density (if other acquisition parameters remain constant) is reduced, increasing the statistical uncertainty and noise in the data. In addition, with the 128 × 128 matrix, processing times increase, and storage requirements are four times greater. Since some increase in resolution can be obtained by zooming 64 × 64 acquisitions without the marked increase in space requirements of 128 × 128 matrices, this appears to be a reasonable compromise. We routinely use a 1.25 zoom. Keeping the heart in the field during the entire arc becomes more difficult when zoom factors are used, and extra care has to be taken not to exclude the apex of the heart from the image.

NUMBER OF STOPS

Acquisition of the images by our cameras occurs in a step-and-shoot mode. The time per stop and movement time between stops multiplied by the number of stops determines the total imaging time. In deciding on how many stops to make, it is clear that one can make either a relatively few stops (32 would be a minimum) for a longer time or more stops for a shorter time per stop. Theory suggests that for a 64 × 64 matrix, approximately 100 angular samples are necessary to maintain an angular resolution similar to the spatial resolution.[43] We have found this increased number of stops improves our images qualitatively but we have compromised on time and performed 80 or 90 stops in our

acquisitions. To keep the imaging times reasonable when using 90 stops, 10-second acquisitions are used during the postexercise study and 15-second images for the redistribution study (18 and 23 seconds are used for 80 stops). With movement of the camera head between stops, the total imaging times are 24 and 22 minutes, respectively, for the 90-stop and 80-stop studies. As stated, these acquisition parameters, with a low-energy all-purpose collimator, obtain approximately 3 to 4 million counts for the entire acquisition.

Processing

FILTERING

Processing of data that includes possible prefiltering, filtered backprojection, reorientation of images, and possible postprocessing smoothing can be performed with a number of clinically valid protocols. The protocols that are ultimately used should be applicable to most thallium studies performed by a nuclear medicine laboratory and should be validated in comparison with cardiac catheterization data.

Making a selection of filters for SPECT reconstructions means balancing the parameters of image contrast, smoothness, resolution, and noise texture. While some groups favor prefiltering of images with some type of low-pass or medium-pass filter,[24,44] we generally have not performed any preliminary steps but have gone straight to filtered backprojection with a 0.75 Nyquist Shepp-Hanning-Logan filter. On computer systems without this filter, experimentation with the multiple possibilites of the Butterworth filter will yield similar images. Prefiltering with initial removal of some higher frequencies permits use of a coarser, more Ramp-like, filter during backprojection. Because smoothing of images by eliminating higher frequencies lowers contrast and resolution, this would potentially preserve more contrast and resolution than would applying a more smoothing filter with a cutoff further below the Nyquist frequency. However, the order of filtering may not be significant, as filtering the planar images initially and then using a sharper filter for backprojection, or not filtering initially and using a smoother filter for backprojection, are essentially equivalent. We prefer not to apply a prefilter; we use a fairly smooth backprojection filter and then postfilter the images. Postfiltering of the images is routinely performed in our laboratory by a weighted volume smooth. We have used the three-point weighted volume smooth for most of our data, resorting to a five-point weighted smooth only with data of very poor statistical quality (e.g., a large patient who exercises poorly). We recognize that this also reduces contrast and resolution, but the noise reduction in the low-count thallium images is significant. If other options are not available, simply adding two or three adjacent slices together also reduces noise.

REORIENTATION OF IMAGES

Because of partial volume effect, the inferior wall of the heart, which is oblique to the AOR of the SPECT camera, is seen poorly on the transverse images. To overcome this effect, the transverse images containing data from multiple projections are realigned in a process called coordinate transformation into multiple image sets parallel or perpendicular to the long axis of the heart (Fig. 8-10). The computer equipped with an array processor performs this algorithm with its multiple interpolations rapidly. The only input required by the operator is to identify the long axis of the heart. The resultant images are the vertical and horizontal long-axis views parallel to the long axis of the heart and the short-axis or axial image set perpendicular to the long axis of the heart. Some computers do not produce the horizontal long-axis images, and the interpreter has only the transverse images, which are quite similar in appearance.

Croft[45] states that transaxial images that are 1 pixel thick in the y axis should be used to create the reoriented images rather than volume smoothing these images initially. The problem is that the rotational maneuvers used in the reorientation of the images call for many interpolations of the pixels. If the transaxial images are several pixels thick, distortions could arise in the reoriented data during these interpolations.

Display and Archiving

Each computer system has a display algorithm for the tomographic images. Since there are a total of 30 to 40 images of the heart in the three projections of the two image sets, the handling of these images can present a logistical problem.

It is most useful to see the images on the computer screen with the immediate postexercise and delayed images side by side. Thus, the technologist has to match the images to compare similar levels in the heart. This must be carefully done, and experience is the best teacher. The short-axis images should begin with the first image of the cavity and continue through the base of the heart. Although more difficult, proper alignment of the horizontal and vertical long-axis views can be performed with experience.

Permanent storage of images is a necessity. Unfortunately, the raw data and processed images take up a large amount of room on digital storage media. Using dual-density floppy disks with 1.2 megabytes of storage, the raw data, and at least the transverse reconstructions, can be stored if 90 stops are used. More images can be stored if fewer stops are employed in the acquisition. It is important to store the raw data so that, if processing algorithms change over time, data will be available to reprocess for comparison with a more recent study.

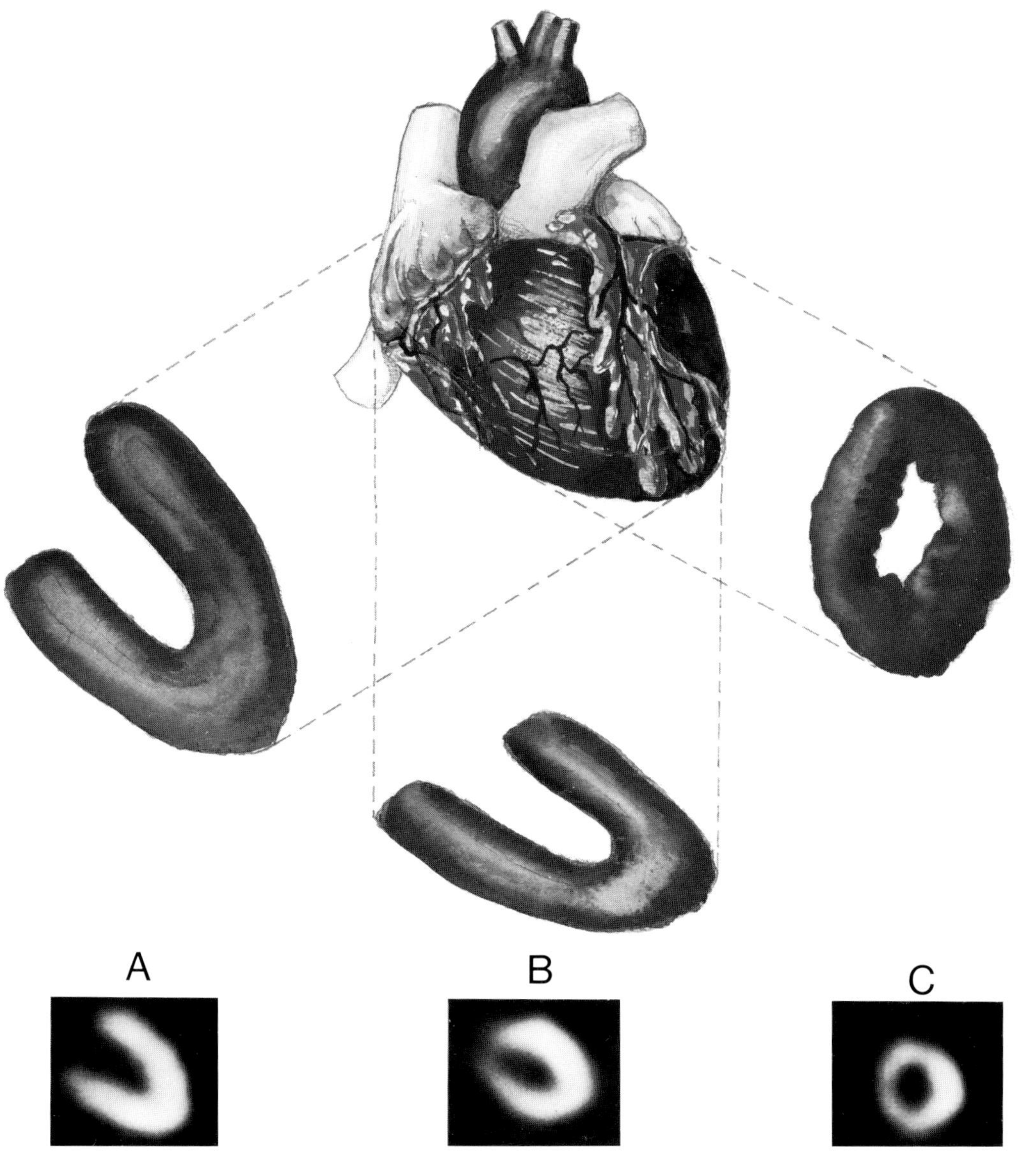

Fig. 8-10 Illustration representing the heart as it is oriented within the chest. From the three-dimensional data collected in the acquisitions, multiple projections of the heart can be reconstructed. The three most commonly produced are shown, with examples of actual mid-ventricular images of each projection. **(A)** Vertical long-axis view. **(B)** Horizontal long-axis view. **(C)** Short-axis, or axial, view.

Filming (hard copy) of the images becomes a noticeable expense in a busy department. It is also a labor-intensive, time-consuming step. We have found it adequate to film selected slices from the short-axis views so that the apical, midportion, and basilar portions of the ventricle are represented. This permits filming of the short-axis images on two sheets of cut film (6 on 1 display) and other image sets (horizontal long axis and vertical

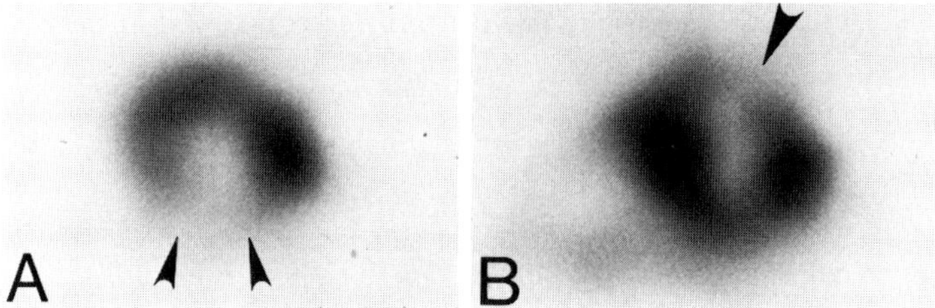

Fig. 8-11 Axial images of a patient with normal coronary arteries who moved during acquisition of both phases of her thallium examination. **(A)** In the postexercise views, an inferior wall defect is present. Cine of raw data showed that the patient moved up in the field during the acquisition. **(B)** Reperfusion images were compromised because the patient moved her left arm over her chest, as clearly seen on the raw data cine. The result was to create a defect in the anterior wall. This set of images might be misinterpreted as inferior wall ischemia. The appearance of an anterior wall defect is unexpected on the reperfusion views, and an artifact should be suspected.

long axis) on one piece of cut film each. For photographic purposes, the gray scale should be as broad as possible. Negative or positive images of the heart are equally satisfactory.

Image Interpretation

The tomographic images are highly processed data that are several steps away from the raw data. This makes it more difficult for the interpreter to detect errors in acquisition and processing that may manifest themselves as myocardial defects and be misinterpreted as ischemia or infarct. Therefore, the initial responsibility of the physician interpreting the thallium tomographic images is to ascertain that the images are valid and that their acquisition and processing have been properly performed. Careful rapid examination of the raw data files in a cine format demonstrates gross movement during the examination or any acquisition error made by

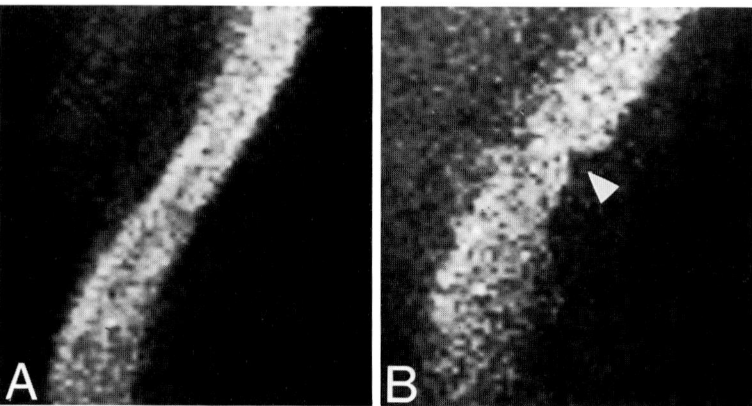

Fig. 8-12 (A) Sinogram of a normal 80-stop collection. Note the smooth sinusoidal curve. **(B)** Sinogram of patient depicted in Figure 8-11 who moved during the acquisition. A disruption (arrowhead) in the curve of the sinogram is apparent where the patient shifted position.

the camera or computer. Gross patient movement can cause defects to appear in the thallium images that are misinterpreted as ischemia (Fig. 8-11). It should be stressed again that little can be done about these acquisition errors once acquired, and they must be prevented or the study re-acquired when marked patient movement is detected by the technologist in attendance.

Some systems provide a display called a sinogram that can be useful in spotting patient motion or other acquisition problems. The sinogram permits the display of the position of a particular pixel or row of pixels from each of the raw data files. If the position of 1 pixel in the planar images is plotted for each angle of the detector during the multiple acquisitions, the plot should resemble a portion of a sine wave for a 180-degree acquisition. Patient motion or other discontinuities in data acquisition disrupt this wave pattern.[46] Studying this image gives a rapid appraisal of possible patient motion (Fig. 8-12).

After determining that the acquisition is artifact free, the interpreter should assess the processing of the data rapidly by checking the short-axis views to make sure they are aligned. If the long axis of the heart is not designated properly by the technologist, distortions can be created (Fig. 8-13). To check for this problem, the short-axis views can be rapidly displayed from the apex to the base to confirm that their centers are superimposed.

THE NORMAL SPECT STUDY

After ascertaining that the images are acquired and processed appropriately according to the protocol in the laboratory, the interpreter can judge the images with respect to myocardial perfusion. Although more sophisticated approaches to correlating coronary artery anatomy with the various re-oriented SPECT image sets exist,[49] a relatively straightforward approach has proved functional in our laboratory. Each cardiac projection can be divided into seg-

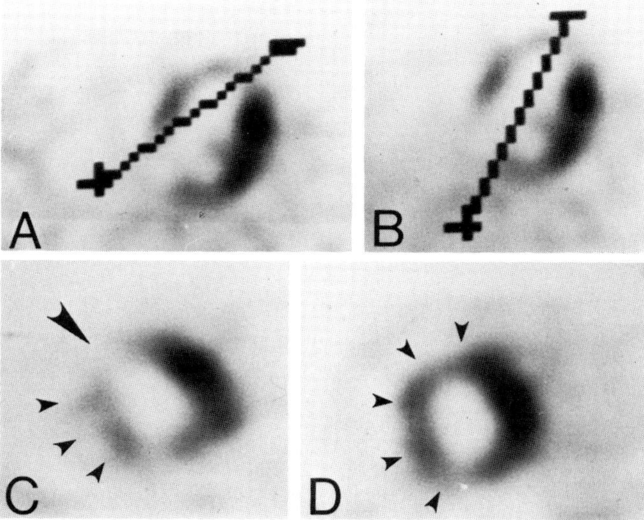

Fig. 8-13 (A) Incorrectly positioned and **(B)** correctly positioned long axis of the heart. **(C)** The axial view resulting from the incorrectly positioned axis shows markedly reduced septal and anterior perfusion (arrowheads). **(D)** The axial view resulting from the correctly positioned axis demonstrates somewhat reduced anterior and septal perfusion (arrowheads). The two studies taken together suggest some reperfusible ischemia of the septum and anterior wall. Actually, when both were correctly processed, only a nonreperfusing anterior septal infarct was found.

ments perfused by individual coronary arteries. The left anterior descending coronary artery (LAD) perfuses the septal, anteroseptal, and anterior segments. The apex is supplied by the LAD but is frequently an overlap area. The left circumflex coronary artery (LCX) supplies the lateral wall and in approximately 10 percent of hearts perfuses the inferior wall to some degree by providing the posterior descending artery.[48] The posterior descending artery is a branch of the right coronary artery (RCA) in approximately 90 percent of hearts.[48] The RCA also supplies the right ventricular (RV) myocardium. Figure 8-14 demonstrates examples of the three projections with diagrams of the vascular territories.

NORMAL VARIANTS

The interpreter of the images must be aware of those regions in the myocardium that, on tomography, normally have relatively fewer counts. When displayed on a high-contrast cathode-ray tube (CRT) screen, perfusion defects can be simulated in these regions. The membranous septum is the lowest count area in the normal heart. This is seen in the more basilar short-axis views. Frequently, an area of relatively decreased count rate is seen in the region of the inferior wall, where it abuts the septum[1,49] (Fig. 8-15A). This defect, which is more prominent in males, is secondary to absorption of counts from those myocardial structures furthest from the

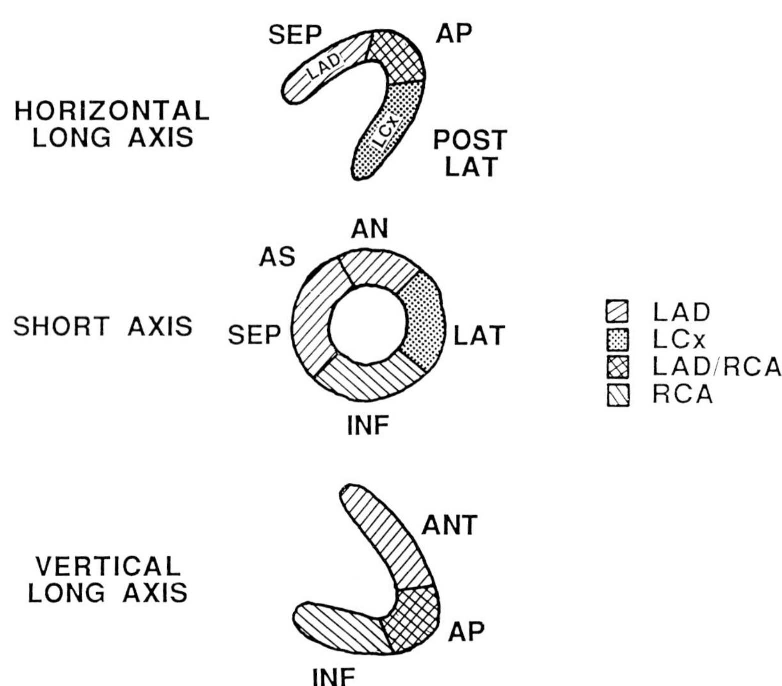

Fig. 8-14 Representative mid-ventricular slices of the three projections most frequently used for SPECT thallium display. The vascular supply is diagrammed. The apex is a segment in which vascular territories may overlap. LAD, left anterior descending; LCx, left circumflex; RCA, right coronary artery; SEP, septum; AP, apical; LAT, lateral; POST LAT, posterior lateral; INF, inferior.

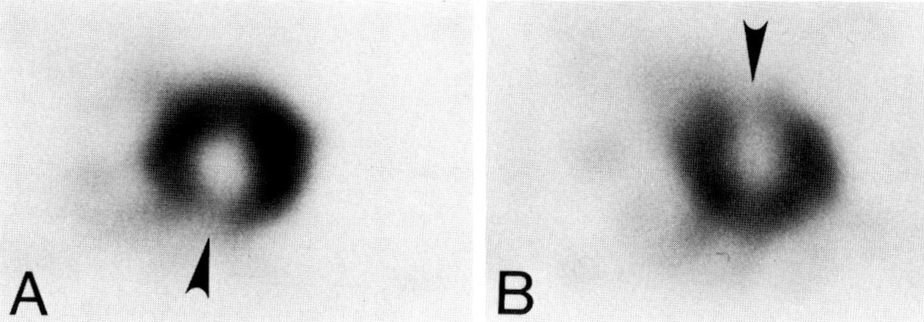

Fig. 8-15 Defects that do not represent coronary artery disease. **(A)** Normal muscular male shows a focal defect in the inferior wall abutting the septum (arrowhead). This defect persisted at rest and is a typical (but somewhat more striking) example of the attenuation defect apparent in males in this location. **(B)** Typical breast-attenuation defect (arrowhead) simulating an anterior wall infarction in a female with large breasts.

rotating camera. This defect is seen both on the postexercise and reperfusion images, but image brightness may have to be manipulated to match the two images, which may not be normalized by the display software. This defect is less obvious in females because absorption from breast tissue evens out the count distribution. However, absorption of counts by large breasts or breast prostheses can create defects as well, and these can become so pronounced that an anterior wall perfusion deficit is simulated[50,51] (Fig. 8-15B). This can be ameliorated in some patients with large breasts by elevation of the breast,[50] but a method must be devised to achieve this consistently on both the postexercise and delayed images.

Friedman and associates[52] reported another cause of apparent perfusion deficit that is unrelated to actual myocardial ischemia, which is seen only on the immediate postexercise images.[53] This apparent reperfusible defect occurs in the inferior wall in patients who exercise to a high heart rate. Friedman et al. termed this "upward creep" of the heart, since the heart can be shown to move cephalad during the acquisition of the immediate postexercise images. One way to prevent this problem is to delay imaging for 10 minutes after exercise in those patients achieving a high heart rate so that the heart rate and respiratory rate can decrease.

Some segments of the myocardium have relatively increased activity compared with other regions; these patterns should also be kept in mind when analyzing the image sets. The lateral myocardium (circumflex territory) closest to the camera during much of its 180-degree arc generally has more counts than do other regions. When this is not observed, it can be a clue to ischemia in this distribution. More focally, the anterior and posterior papillary muscles located in the mid- to apical portion of the axial slices at about 2 o'clock and 7 o'clock can be visualized as areas of more intense activity. Because of the relatively low resolution of the tomographic images, these structures usually appear as part of the myocardial walls[51] (Fig. 8-16A). Rarely, they can be visualized extending into the ventricular chamber (Fig. 8-16B).

THE ABNORMAL SPECT STUDY

Figure 8-17A to K demonstrates multiple views of perfusion defects in the three major coronary artery territories. Smaller defects may represent ischemia or infarct in a portion of a coronary artery distribution. For instance, segmental disease of the LAD can

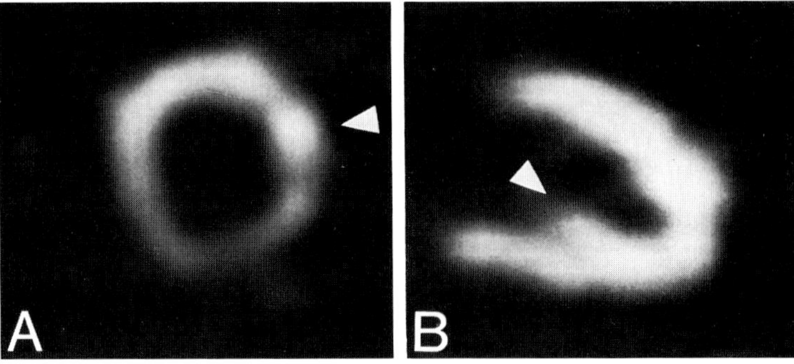

Fig. 8-16 Images of a young male who reached a high heart rate on a stress test. **(A)** Axial view. Arrowhead points to an area of increased activity secondary to a papillary muscle. This cannot be clearly separated from the myocardium (the usual pattern). **(B)** Vertical long-axis view demonstrates the posterior papillary muscle seen as a separate structure (an uncommon pattern).

be demonstrated by isolated defects in the anterior wall when only diagonal branches are involved.

Morton et al.[53] reported their experience in identifying left ventricular aneurysms. These investigators found that the presence of a left ventricular anterior apical aneurysm correlates with the finding on SPECT images of failure of the ventricular walls to converge (Fig. 8-18). SPECT imaging identified 14 of 16 aneurysms with this finding of nonconvergence of walls toward the apex. The overall sensitivity for aneurysm in the series was 94 percent with a specificity of 97 percent.[53]

The perfusion status of the right ventricle can be evaluated on the transverse (or horizontal long-axis views) as well as on the axial images. Right ventricular infarctions have been reported on SPECT thallium studies,[54] and we have identified right ventricular ischemia in a case of subtotal proximal RCA occlusion.[55] However, while the specificity of this finding of RV ischemia is relatively high (86 percent) for detection of a significant RCA lesion, the sensitivity is low (46 percent).[56]

Clinical Applications

MYOCARDIAL INFARCTION: SPECT VERSUS PLANAR IMAGING

The imaging of perfusion defects created by myocardial infarction provides the most direct comparison of planar and SPECT techniques. Unlike the identification of ischemic defects, the order of the tests does not bias the results in favor of the examination performed first, and the comparison can be made with a single injection of the isotope. Several investigators have published results substantiating the superiority of SPECT in imaging infarcts.

In one early series, N. Tamaki et al.[17] demonstrated a sensitivity of 96 percent for SPECT imaging of transmural infarction compared with 75 percent for planar imaging. Specificity of both techniques was 89 percent. Maublant et al.[3] also showed a very high sensitivity of 98 percent with a specificity of 93 percent with SPECT thallium imaging for the identification of infarction. Planar imaging identified 89 percent of infarctions with 93 percent specificity.

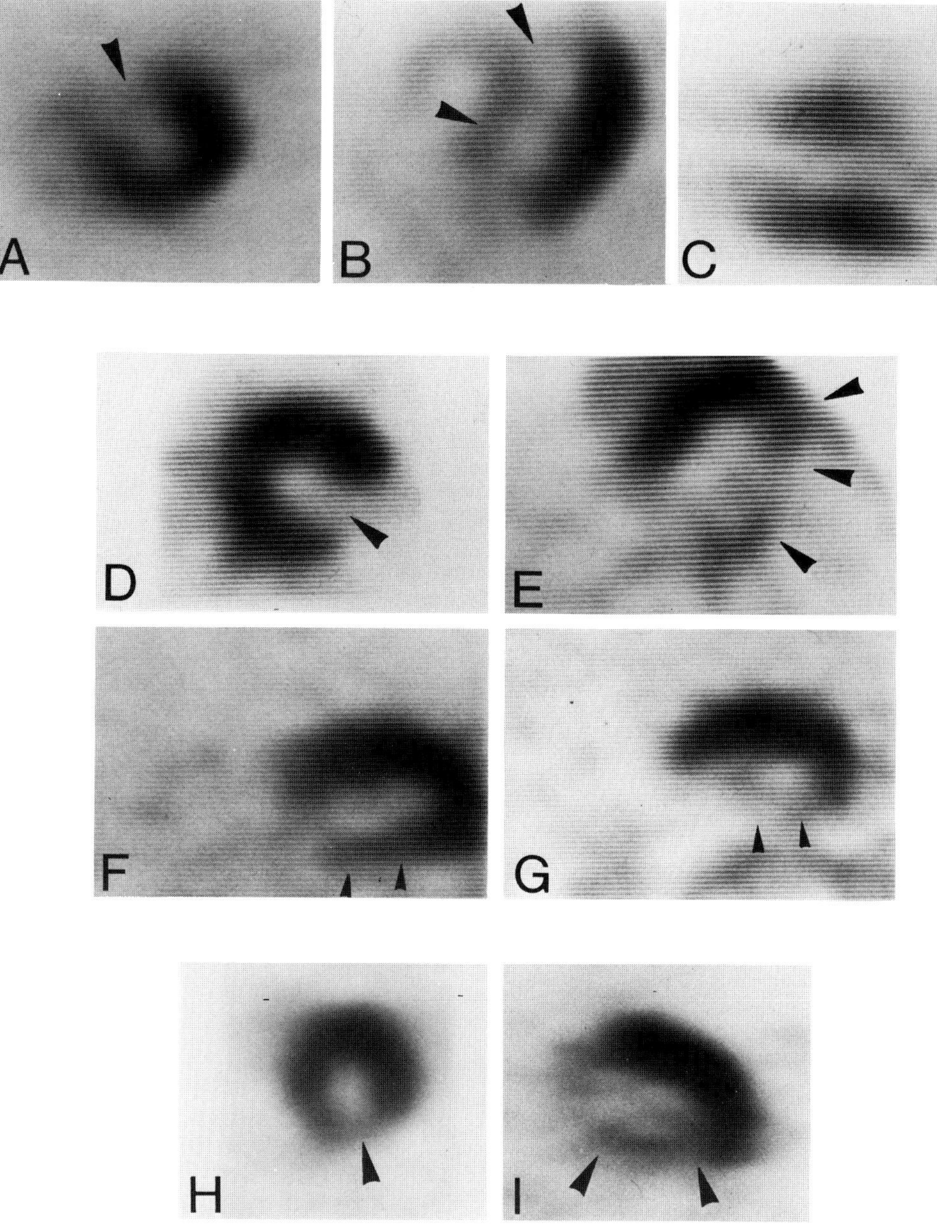

Fig. 8-17 (A–C) Perfusion pattern seen with a proximal lesion in the LAD. **(A)** Axial view shows an anterior septal defect (arrowhead). **(B)** Horizontal long axis shows an anterior and septal defect (arrowheads. **(C)** Vertical long-axis image demonstrates an anterior and apical defect (arrowheads). **(D–G)** Pattern of perfusion with a significant LCX lesion. **(D)** Axial view shows a posterior lateral defect. **(E)** Horizontal long axis shows the entire lateral wall underperfused. **(F)** Mid-ventricular vertical long-axis view shows preserved perfusion to the inferior wall. **(G)** More laterally, perfusion is absent in the LCX territory. **(H,I)** RCA lesion. **(H)** Axial view shows the expected inferior wall defect. **(I)** Vertical long-axis view confirms this inferior defect.

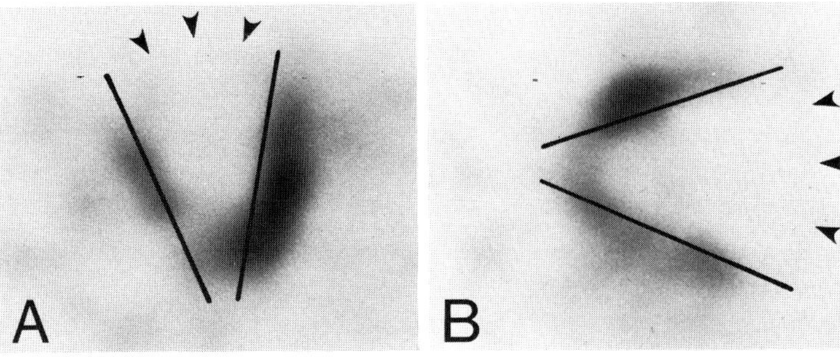

Fig. 8-18 Myocardial walls diverging. **(A)** Horizontal long-axis view. **(B)** Vertical long axis view. Large defect (arrowheads) is a large anterior apical aneurysm. This divergence of walls is highly sensitive and specific for an aneurysm in this location. (From Morton et al.,[53] with permission.)

The work of Ritchie et al.,[9] N. Tamaki et al.,[17] and S. Tamaki et al.[58] confirms the increased sensitivity of SPECT imaging compared with planar techniques for the detection of infarctions and clearly points out its ability to see smaller and lower contrast defects. Ritchie et al.[9] detected infarcts with a sensitivity of 87 percent by SPECT and 63 percent with planar imaging. Their analysis showed that this improved sensitivity derived from the identification by SPECT of subendocardial and inferior wall infarcts not detected by planar imaging. This reinforces the concept that the tomographic method improves detection of perfusion defects by its increased image contrast and by permitting better definition of deep structures obscured by overlying activity on planar images. Ritchie and co-workers also stressed the importance of the three-dimensional nature of the SPECT data, which permits reorientation of the transverse myocardial images to display the myocardial slices from many aspects. In six of nine patients in their series, in which the infarction was detected only by SPECT, realignment of the images along the short and long axes of the heart was essential.[9] This permits viewing of the different vascular territories without the overlap of other distributions. It is especially useful for the inferior wall which is poorly seen on the transverse view.

While noting an increased sensitivity for SPECT imaging of infarcts of both the anterior (96 percent versus 87 percent) and inferior walls (97 percent versus 73 percent), S. Tamaki et al.[57] state that the increased sensitivity arose from detecting smaller infarcts as measured by peak CPK elevation. The sensitivity for nontransmural infarctions in this series was 87 percent versus 47 percent for planar imaging.[57]

N. Tamaki et al.[58] derived a semiquantitative expression for the contrast of nontransmural infarcts by measuring an average of 75.4 ± 7.8 percent of maximum myocardial activity in these infarcts as compared with 47.6 ± 12.1 percent for transmural infarcts. SPECT succeeded in localizing 85 percent of such infarcts, while planar imaging only defined 54 percent.[58]

CORONARY ARTERY DISEASE: SPECT VERSUS PLANAR IMAGING

The qualitative visual interpretation of three-view planar thallium images, despite its acceptable level of sensitivity and specificity for the detection of coronary artery disease (CAD), is suboptimal in several respects. Accurate identification of the specific coronary arteries involved and thus the determination of the presence of multivessel disease is not optimal.[59–61] Sensitivity for moderate CAD, defined as 50 to 70 percent stenosis, is low.[59,60,62] Finally, interobserver variability is high.[63] Quantitative planar imaging with evaluation of relative thallium uptake and washout has improved on these parameters,[62] but early reports suggest that SPECT may be a further improvement.

An initial report by Go et al.[64] demonstrated improved sensitivity for CAD over visual planar interpretation; this has since been substantiated by several investigators.[2,4,65–67] Links et al.[65] made the specific observation that the improved sensitivity and specificity of SPECT imaging, as compared with planar imaging, applies to female as well as male patients.

Nohara et al.[66] studied a CAD population, some of whom had had myocardial infarctions. In comparing planar and SPECT images, these workers found a higher sensitivity and specificity of SPECT for the detection of specific vessel disease: LAD (sens/spec) 88 percent/89 percent versus 73 percent/89 percent; RCA (sens/spec) 96 percent/87 percent versus 85 percent/87 percent; and for the LCX (sens/spec) 78 percent/100 percent versus 39 percent/100 percent. Although these investigators report the sensitivity and specificity for the identification of no-vessel, one-vessel, and two-vessel disease to be statistically similar between the two techniques, SPECT was clearly superior in identifying three-vessel disease with a sensitivity of 63 percent versus 19 percent for planar imaging.[66]

N. Tamaki et al.[4] also showed this to be true. Although the overall sensitivity for CAD with SPECT and planar imaging was similar in their hands (95 percent as compared with 90 percent), the identification of individual-vessel stenoses was improved by SPECT; 83 percent of stenotic vessels were detected by SPECT, but only 57 percent of total lesions by planar imaging. SPECT identified 89 percent of RCA lesions compared with 55 percent for planar and 70 percent of LCX lesions compared with 36 percent for the planar technique. Two-vessel (85 percent versus 50 percent) and three-vessel disease (78 percent versus 44 percent) were detected with more sensitivity with SPECT.[4]

Although these papers confirm the improved sensitivity and specificity of SPECT over planar imaging for defining the extent and severity of CAD, the ability to detect moderate (50 to 75 percent) stenoses of the coronary arteries with qualitative SPECT imaging is limited. In our review of 118 consecutive cases with catheterization correlation, we detected only 53 percent of such lesions. N. Tamaki et al.[49] found only a 56 percent rate of detection of moderate lesions. Even though the detection rate with qualitative SPECT imaging is suboptimal, sensitivity is greater than the 35 percent rate of detection of such lesions by planar imaging.[62] Quantification of SPECT images with washout analysis has yielded an 81 percent sensitivity for moderate lesions,[49] and this methodology may ultimately be the most sensitive test. Nevertheless, initial comparisons of qualitative interpretation of SPECT thallium images to quantitative planar evaluation found SPECT more specific, and for the circumflex coronary artery, more sensitive. Hung et al.[68] found this to be true in their comparison of SPECT to circumferential quantitative analysis of planar thallium images. For the RCA, SPECT demonstrated a sensitivity and specificity of 82 percent and 80 percent respectively, versus 82 percent and 60 percent for the quantitative planar technique. For the LAD, the values were 80 percent and 100 percent versus 88 percent and 80 percent and for the LCX, 80 percent and 100 percent versus 40 percent and 94 percent. For detecting single-vessel disease, SPECT was equal to circumferential analysis, but for two-vessel disease, better than circumferential analysis (80 percent versus 40 percent). For detecting three-vessel disease, SPECT and the quantitative planar had equal sensitivity in their hands.[68] Mahmarian et al.[69] found a higher specificity (89 percent versus 41 percent) and predictive accuracy (85 percent versus 48 percent) but similar sensitivities of the two techniques in the detection of multivessel disease. Obviously, these results are preliminary, and larger published series must be evaluated before conclusions can be drawn.

Although the data are currently inadequate to prove an advantage for qualitative SPECT over quantitative planar thallium imaging, the initial abstracts summarized above point to an increased sensitivity for circumflex disease and a possible increase in specificity for the detection of disease in the other vessels. The evidence for SPECT superiority is more convincing compared with qualitative planar imaging. The published reports demonstrate an improvement in both sensitivity and specificity for detecting CAD in all coronary arteries with the most dramatic improvement in the left circumflex distribution. This is presumably because SPECT eliminates the overlap of other vascular distributions in viewing the LCX area. This increased detection rate for individual vessels carries over to an increased sensitivity and specificity for multivessel disease. Detection of moderate disease as we have described remains suboptimal. Also a study of right ventricular fixed or reversible defects as an indicator of significant RCA disease shows that SPECT is not significantly better than qualitative planar thallium images in detecting these lesions.[70]

NONCORONARY DISEASE

The qualitative SPECT imaging method for thallium appears to have a role in identification of other cardiac conditions than CAD. Suzuki et al.[71] identified patterns of hypertrophic myocardopathies and correlated these with echocardiography. SPECT has an advantage over two-dimensional sector scanning in the detection of apical hypertrophy.

Suzuki and co-workers point out, however, that no reliable SPECT criteria exist for distinguishing obstructive from nonobstructive hypertrophic cardiomyopathies.[71] Kirsch et al.[2] identified a pattern they came to associate with a hypertrophic cardiomyopathy.

Problems and Solutions

Although SPECT has been a valuable clinical tool in ^{201}Tl imaging, some limitations to SPECT must be addressed. Photon attenuation must be considered. The wide variation of attenuation effects in the chest wall, lungs, and ribs makes the problem very complex for thallium. While these attenuation effects can be seen on qualitative SPECT thallium images as reduced relative count rates in some areas of the heart, these are not so severe as to negate the clinical value of the images. However, attenuation must be considered and corrected for if accurate quantification is needed.[72] Different approaches have been devised,[72–75] and current software packages usually include some method for this correction.

Attenuation is only one problem to overcome in SPECT imaging. Scatter of photons must be considered as well. It is optimal to try to correct scatter physically by altering the energy window, but we have discussed the inhomogeneity and potential for artifacts that can result with this method.[35] This problem will be lessened as the energy resolution of the detectors is improved and collimators are designed to better exclude scatter.[76] For now, one method proposed is to subtract a predefined percentage of counts collected in a Compton scatter window from counts obtained in the photopeak pulse-height window.[77] This would be applied before attenuation correction. Because this correction is applied after the collection of data, however, the signal-to-noise (S/N) ratio is degraded.

Resolution of the camera systems could be improved. The point-spread function of the gamma camera is depth dependent, and resolution falls off with distance. Thus, getting close to the patient is helpful, and further refinements of camera motion and noncircular or body contour orbits that allow the camera head to stay closer to the body surface will improve resolution.[20] The use of noncircular motion has the additional advantage of reducing bull's-eye and concentric circle nonuniformity artifacts.[78] State-of-the-art SPECT units provide the hardware and software to perform these noncircular orbits. Either the imaging table moves as the camera continues a circular orbit, or both the camera and table move. An improvement in collimator design to optimize resolution at depth may help the depth resolution problem as well.

Although the backprojection algorithm for ECT data reconstruction is the process now being used clinically, others have been proposed. Miller et al.[79] proposed a maximum likelihood method for image-data reconstruction. This method would incorporate actual absorption measurements obtained by detecting count attenuation through the body from an external transmission source. This is potentially the most accurate method to correct for scatter and attenuation in the chest. Currently, computers used in nuclear medicine would take a prohibitively long time to process these data, but if microprocessors can be developed to speed this process, it may be feasible.

WEIGHING THE DECISION TO BUY SPECT

Although the clinical evidence that thallium SPECT imaging is a highly sensitive and specific method for evaluating myocardial perfusion is compelling, the prospective purchaser of such a system must balance several factors when making the decision to buy.

Naturally, the unit will perform emission tomographic imaging of other organs,[80] but we are especially enthusiastic about its contribution to thallium myocardial imaging and would recommend its purchase for this purpose alone.

This is a more expensive unit than the standard gamma camera, with prices ranging from approximately $160,000 to $200,000. Furthermore, if a computer must be purchased or upgraded by hardware such as an array processor or additional archival storage, the total price of the package can reach $200,000 to $250,.000. In addition, service calls in our experience are more numerous and costly than with standard cameras and the service contract fees reflect this.

For this increased cost, however, the technologist and clinician have a unit that can perform all tests that a standard camera can. In fact, the need for excellent total system uniformity in SPECT reconstructions ensures that the best possible planar images are obtained by these units. The technologist finds that the counterbalanced heads of the ECT camera make positioning for planar imaging easier than those of many vendors' standard cameras. The room size requirements are not significantly different from those for standard cameras. Nevertheless, it should be understood that the acceptance testing, ongoing quality-control procedures, patient setup, and the processing and interpretation of images all will take more time than is generally expended on planar imaging.

The physician should be prepared to spend 10 to 15 minutes per case initially to gain familiarity with the technique. Even when experienced, studying 30 to 40 images per case takes longer than planar interpretations. When SPECT thallium imaging is initiated in a laboratory, comparison with the previous planar format images should be performed until confidence is gained that the results are consistent with previous validated techniques. This requires the performance, processing, and interpretation of two examinations, but the time spent is worthwhile.

The reward for this increased investment in money and time is the performance of an inherently superior study for the evaluation of myocardial perfusion. The increased image contrast and the three-dimensional nature of transaxial tomographic imaging that permits evaluation of the heart from multiple aspects are translated into increased sensitivity and specificity for myocardial perfusion defects. Furthermore, it has been our experience and that of others that there is greater confidence in interpretation and less interobserver error than with planar imaging.[3] The potential for quantification is present in the SPECT data, if some problems can be solved. Some investigators have found good correlation with size measurements of myocardial infarcts[10] and others with regional blood flow,[81] but this work is clearly preliminary. Even though the interpreter of these images must be on guard for artifacts of system nonuniformity, patient motion, and improper processing and display, the current clinical application would appear to make a SPECT system a good investment.

CONCLUSION

Although problems in hardware and software remain to be overcome, SPECT technology has made a positive impact on thallium myocardial imaging. If the equipment is correctly maintained with attention to the additional quality control procedures necessary and the examinations are performed and interpreted with care for detail and reproducibility, then superior results are obtainable. These results are within the reach of any laboratory that is willing to make this commitment.

ACKNOWLEDGMENTS

I wish to thank the technologists who perform these studies everyday for their dedication to excellence in their work. I would also like to thank Dr. Tom Miller for his thoughtful comments on this manuscript during its preparation.

REFERENCES

1. Prigent FM, Maddahi J, Garcia E, et al: Thallium-201 stress-redistribution myocardial rotational tomography: Development of criteria for visual interpretation. Am Heart J 109:274, 1985
2. Kirsch CM, Doliwa R, Buell U, Roedler D: Detection of severe coronary heart disease with Tl-201: Comparison of resting single photon emission tomography with invasive arteriography. J Nucl Med 24:761, 1983
3. Maublant J, Cassagnes J, LeJeune JJ, et al: A comparison between conventional scintigraphy and emission tomography with thallium-201 in the detection of myocardial infarction: Concise communication. J Nucl Med 23:204, 1982
4. Tamaki N, Yonekura Y, Mukai T, et al: Segmental analysis of stress thallium myocardial emission tomography for localization of coronary artery disease. Eur J Nucl Med 9:99, 1984
5. Croft BY: Single-Photon Emission Computed Tomography. Year Book Medical Publishers, Chicago, 1986, p. 168
6. Maublant J, Cassagnes J, Jourde M, et al: Myocardial emission tomography with thallium-201. Eur J Nucl Med 6:289, 1981
7. Ritchie JL, Larsson S, Israelson A, et al: Single photon tomographic imaging of a standard heart phantom with ^{201}Tl: A gamma camera based system. Eur J Nucl Med 7:254, 1982
8. Borrello JA, Clinthorne NE, Rogers WC, et al: Oblique-angle tomography: A restructuring algorithm for transaxial tomographic data. J Nucl Med 22:471, 1981
9. Ritchie JL, Williams DL, Harp D, et al: Transaxial tomography with thallium-201 for detecting remote myocardial infarction: Com-

parison with planar imaging. Am J Cardiol 50:1236, 1982

10. Tamaki S, Nakajima H, Murakami T, et al: Estimation of infarct size by myocardial emission computed tomography with thallium-201 and its relation to creatine kinase-MB release after myocardial infarction in man. Circulation 66:994, 1982

11. Caldwell JH, Williams AL, Hamilton GW, et al: Regional distribution of myocardial blood flow measured by single-photon emission computed tomography: Comparison with in vitro counting. J. Nucl Med 23:490, 1982

12. Malko JA, Eisner RL, Engdahl JC, et al: A threshold method of volume determination from tomographic reconstructions. J Nucl Med 24:P19, 1983 (abst)

13. Vogel RA, Kirch DL, LeFree MT, et al: A new method of multiplanar emission tomography using a seven pinhole collimator and an Anger scintillation camera. J Nucl Med 19:648, 1978

14. Vogel RA, Kirch DL, LeFree MT, et al: Thallium-201 myocardial perfusion scintigraphy: Results of standard and multi-pinhole tomographic techniques. Am J Cardiol 43:787, 1979

15. Muehllehner G: A tomographic scintillation camera. Phys Med Biol 16:87, 1971

16. Starling MR, Dehmer GH, Lancaster JL, et al: Segmental coronary artery disease: Detection by rotating slant-hole collimator tomography and planar thallium-201 myocardial scintigraphy. Radiology 157:231, 1985

17. Tamaki N, Mukai T, Ishii Y, et al: Clinical evaluation of thallium-201 emission myocardial tomography using a rotating gamma camera: Comparison with seven-pinhole tomography. J Nucl Med 22:849, 1981

18. Mills JA, Flint J, Taylor DN, et al: Thallium-201 scintigraphy for ischaemic heart disease and infarct detection: Comparison of rotating slant-hole tomography and planar imaging. Br J Radiol 58:625, 1985

19. Williams DL, Ritchie JL, Harp GD, et al: In vivo simulation of thallium-201 myocardial scintigraphy by seven-pinhole emission tomography. J Nucl Med 21:821, 1980

20. Eisner RL: Principles of instrumentation in SPECT. J Nucl Med Technol 13:23, 1985

21. Prigent F, Maddahi J, Garcia E, et al: Noninvasive quantification of the extent of jeopardized myocardium in patients with single-vessel coronary disease by stress thallium-201 single photon emission computerized rotational tomography. Am Heart J 111:578, 1985

22. Brooks RA, DiChiro G: Theory of image reconstruction in computed tomography. Radiology 117:561, 1975

23. Galt JR, Hise HL, Garcia E, et al: Filtering in frequency space. J Nucl Med Technol 14:152, 1986

24. Madsen MT, Park CH: Enhancement of SPECT images by Fourier filtering the projection image set. J Nucl Med 26:395, 1985

25. Harkness BA, Rogers WL, Clinthorne NH, Keyes JW Jr: SPECT: Quality control procedures and artifact identification. J Nucl Med Technol 11:55, 1983

26. Rogers WL, Clinthorne NH, Harkness BA, et al: Field-flood requirements for emission computed tomography with an Anger camera. J Nucl Med 23:162, 1982

27. Croft BY: Single-Photon Emission Computed Tomography. Year Book Medical Publishers, Chicago, 1986, p. 193

28. Oppenheim BE and Appledorn CR: Uniformity correction for SPECT using a mapped cobalt-57 sheet source. J Nucl Med 26:409, 1985

29. Greer K, Jaszczak R, Harris C, Coleman RE: Quality control in SPECT. J Nucl Med Technol 13:76, 1985

30. Farrell TJ, Cradduck TD: SPECT imaging: Experimental determination of the effect of camera head tilt and appropriate quality control protocol. J Nucl Med 26:P51, 1985 (abst)

31. Cradduck TD, Teresinska A: Head tilt and its effect on resolution orthogonal to transverse slices in SPECT. J Nucl Med 27:960, 1986 (abst)

32. Graham MM: Introduction to single-photon emission computed tomography. p. 212. In Williams AG, Eckel CG (eds): Practical Computer Applications in Radionuclide Imaging. Churchill Livingstone, New York, 1987

33. Croft BY: Single-Photon Emission Computed Tomography. Year Book Medical Publishers, Chicago, 1986, p. 221

34. Areeda J, Chapman D, Garcia E, et al: Quality control for rotational single photon emission computed tomography. Informatek Users Group Newl Sept: 6, 1984

35. LaFontaine R, Graham LS, Stein MA: Effects of assymetric photopeak windows on flood field uniformity and spatial resolution for

scintillation cameras. J Nucl Med 25:P22, 1984 (abst)

36. Coleman RE, Jaszczak RJ, Cobb FR: Comparison of 180° and 360° data collection in thallium-201 imaging using single-photon emission computerized tomography (SPECT). (Concise communication.) J Nucl Med 23:655, 1982

37. Go RT, MacIntyre WJ, O'Donnell JK, et al: Transaxial single photon emission computed tomographic mycardial imaging with 201-Tl: Instrumentation, technical and clinical aspects. p. 233. In Freeman LM, Weissmann HS (eds): Nuclear Medicine Annual. Raven Press, New York, 1985

38. Hoffman EJ: 180° compared with 360° sampling in SPECT. J Nucl Med 23:745, 1982

39. Eisner RL, Nowak DJ, Pettigrew R, Fajman W: Fundamentals of 180° acquisition and reconstruction in SPECT imaging. J Nucl Med 27:1717, 1986

40. Tamaki N, Mukai T, Ishii Y, et al: Comparative study of thallium emission myocardial tomography with 180° and 360° data collection. J Nucl Med 23:661, 1982

41. Rothendler JA, Okada RD, Wilson RA, et al: Effect of a delay in commencing imaging on the ability to detect transient thallium defects. J Nucl Med 26:880, 1985

42. Schwartz JS, Ponto R, Caryle P, et al: Early redistribution of thallium-201 after temporary ischemia. Circulation 57:332, 1978

43. Snyder, DL, Cox JR Jr: An overview of reconstructive tomography and limitations imposed by a finite number of projections. p. 3. In Ter-Pogossian (ed): Reconstruction Tomography in Diagnostic Radiology and Nuclear Medicine University Park Press, Baltimore, 1977

44. King MA, Doherty PW, Schwinger RB, et al: Fast count-dependent digital filtering of nuclear medicine images. (Concise communication.) J Nucl Med 24:1039, 1983

45. Croft BY: Single-Photon Emission Computed Tomography. p. 155. Year Book Medical Publishers, Chicago, 1986

46. Croft BY: Single-Photon Emission Computed Tomography. Year Book Medical Publishers, Chicago, 1986, p. 144

47. Prigent F, Maddahi J, Berman DS: Quantitative stress-redistribution Tl-201 single photon emission tomography (SPECT): Development of a scheme for localization of coronary artery disease. J Nucl Med 27:997, 1986 (abst)

48. James TN: Anatomy of the coronary arteries and veins. p. 631. In Hurst JW, Logue RB (eds): The Heart. McGraw-Hill, New York, 1966

49. Tamaki N, Yoshiharu Y, Mukai T, et al: Stress thallium-201 transaxial emission computed tomography: Quantitative versus qualitative analysis for evaluation of coronary artery disease. J Am Coll Cardiol 4:1213, 1984

50. Garver PR, Wasnich RD, Shibuya AM, Yeh F: Appearance of breast attenuation artifacts with thallium myocardial SPECT imaging. Clin Nucl Med 10:694, 1985

51. Clausen M, Bice AN, Civelek AC, et al: Circumferential wall thickness measurements of the human left ventricle: Reference data for thallium-201 single-photon emission computed tomography. Am J Cardiol 58:827, 1986

52. Friedman J, Van Train K, Maddahi J, et al: "Upward Creep" of the heart: A frequent source of false-positive reversible defects on Tl-201 stress-redistribution SPECT. J Nucl Med 27:899, 1986 (abst)

53. Morton KA, Alazraki NP, Taylor AT, Datz FL: SPECT thallium-201 scintigraphy for the detection of left-ventricular aneurysm. J Nucl Med 28:168, 1987

54. Kotler J, Trobaugh GB, Williams DL, et al: Demonstration of a right ventricular infarction with tomographic thallium myocardial imaging. J Nucl Med 23:1111, 1982

55. Rich MW, Keller A, Chouhan L, Fischer K: Exercise-induced hypotension as a manifestation of right ventricular ischemia. Am Heart J 115:184, 1988

56. Chouhan LK, Fischer KC, Krone RJ, et al: The value of tomographic thallium imaging of the right ventricle in the detection of right coronary artery disease. Presented at the Sixtieth Scientific Session of the American Heart Association, Anaheim, CA, Nov. 1987

57. Tamaki S, Kambara H, Kadota K, et al: Improved detection of myocardial infarction by emission computed tomography with thallium-201: Relation to infarct size. Br Heart J 52:621, 1984

58. Tamaki N, Yonekura Y, Minato K, et al:

Evaluation of nontransmural myocardial infarction by Tl single-photon emission CT. J Nucl Med 24:P18, 1983 (abst)

59. Massie BM, Botvinick EH, Brundage BH: Correlation of thallium-201 scintigrams with coronary anatomy: Factors affecting region by region sensitivity. Am J Cardiol 44:616, 1979

60. Rigo P, Bailey IK, Griffith LSC, et al: Value and limitations of segmental analysis of stress thallium myocardial imaging for localization of coronary artery disease. Circulation 61:973, 1980

61. McKillop JH, Murray RG, Turner JG, et al: Can the extent of coronary artery disease be predicted from thallium-201 myocardial images? J Nucl Med 20:715, 1979

62. Maddahi J, Garcia EV, Berman DS, et al: Improved noninvasive assessment of coronary artery disease by quantitative analysis of regional stress myocardial distribution and washout of thallium-201. Circulation 64:924, 1981

63. Trobaugh GB, Wackers FJ, Sokole EB, et al: Thallium-201 myocardial imaging: An interinstitutional study of observer variability. J Nucl Med 19:359, 1978

64. Go RT, Cook SA, MacIntyre D, et al: Comparative accuracy of stress and redistribution thallium-201 cardiac single photon emission transaxial tomography and planar imaging in the diagnosis of myocardial ischemia. J Nucl Med 23:P25, 1982 (abst)

65. Links JM, Fintel DF, Becker LL, Wagner HN Jr: Comparison of planar and SPECT thallium imaging in men and women. J Nucl Med 26:P49, 1985 (abst)

66. Nohara R, Kambara H, Suzuki Y, et al: Stress scintigraphy using single-photon emission computed tomography in the evaluation of coronary artery disease. Am J Cardiol 53:1250, 1984

67. Prigent F, Friedman J, Maddahi J, et al: Comparison of rotational tomography with planar imaging for thallium-201 stress myocardial scintigraphy. J Nucl Med 24:P18, 1983 (abst)

68. Hung G, Siegel ME, McKay CR, et al: Detection of coronary artery disease by planar, circumferential analysis and SPECT-201 scintigraphy. p. 37. Presented at the Seventy-second RSNA Scientific Program 1986 (abst)

69. Mahmarian JJ, Jain A, Roberts R, et al: Single photon emission computerized tomography with thallium-201 during exercise in the diagnosis of coronary artery disease: Comparison with quantitative planar imaging. p. 34. Presented at the 33rd Annual Meeting of the Society of Nuclear Medicine, Washington, DC 1986 (abst)

70. Gutman J, Brachman M, Rozanski A, et al: Enhanced detection of proximal right coronary artery stenosis with the additional analysis of right ventricular thallium-201 uptake in stress scintigraphy. Am J Cardiol 51:1256, 1983

71. Suzuki Y, Kadota K, Nohara R, et al: Recognition of regional hypertrophy in hypertrophic cardiomyopathy using thallium-201 emission-computed tomography: Comparison with two-dimensional echocardiography. Am J Cardiol 53:1095, 1984

72. Chang W, Henkin RE: Photon attenuation in Tl-201 myocardial SPECT and quantitation through am empirical correction. p. 123. In Esser PD (ed): Emission Computed Tomography. Society of Nuclear Medicine, New York, 1983

73. Chang LT: A method for attenuation correction in radionuclide computed tomography. IEEE Trans Nucl Sci NS-25:638, 1978

74. Budinger TF, Gullberg GT, Huesman RH: Emission computed tomography. p. 147. In Herman GT (ed): Image Reconstruction from Projections: Implementation and Applications. Springer-Verlag, New York, 1979

75. Gullberg GT, Budinger TF: The use of filtering methods to compensate for constant attenuation in single-photon emission computed tomography. IEEE Trans Biomed Eng BME-28:1421, 1981

76. Todd-Pokropek AE: The mathematics and physics of emission computerized tomography (ECT) p. 3. In Esser PD (ed): Emission Computed Tomography. Society of Nuclear Medicine, New York, 1983

77. Jaszczak RJ, Greer KL, Floyd CE, et al: Improved SPECT quantification using compensation for scattered photons. J Nucl Med 25:893, 1984

78. Todd-Pokropek AE: Non-circular orbits for the reduction of uniformity artifacts in SPECT. Phys Med Biol 28:309, 1983

79. Miller MI, Snyder DL, Miller TR: Maximum-likelihood reconstruction for single-photon emission computed-tomography. IEEE Trans Nucl Sci NS-32:769, 1985

80. Dillehay GL, Henkin RE: Noncardiac single-photon emission computed tomography. p. 255. In Williams AG, Eckel CG (eds): Practical Computer Applications in Radionuclide Imaging. Churchill Livingstone, New York, 1987

81. Caldwell JH, Williams DL, Hamilton GW, et al: Regional distribution of myocardial blood flow measured by single photon emission tomography: Comparison with in vivo counting. J Nucl Med 23:490, 1982

9

Quantitative SPECT Thallium Imaging

E. Gordon DePuey
Ernest V. Garcia

Sequential ^{201}Tl imaging following injection at peak exercise is a useful noninvasive method for detecting and evaluating patients with significant coronary artery disease (CAD). Visual interpretation of ^{201}Tl scintigrams or tomograms, even by experienced observers, is subject to substantial variability.[1] This approach is further limited by dependence on the quality of the final display and inability to compensate accurately for background activity or attenuation. Finally, although the myocardial ^{201}Tl regional washout characteristics contain important diagnostic information, these can be difficult to detect by visual inspection.

Several approaches have contributed significantly to the quantitation of initial distribution and washout of myocardial ^{201}Tl from both planar scintigraphic projections[2-5] and tomographic sections.[6-10] This chapter describes the algorithms involved in quantifying stress–redistribution ^{201}Tl tomographic

studies, their limitations, and their clinical applications.

TOMOGRAPHIC METHODS

Preliminary investigations have suggested that rotational myocardial tomography following injection of ^{201}Tl at peak exercise is significantly better than planar scintigraphy for the detection and localization of myocardial ischemia.[11,12] Rotational ^{201}Tl tomography at rest has also been reported to be better than planar imaging for detection and localization of myocardial infarction and for estimating the extent of infarcted myocardium.[13,14] Several investigators[7,9,15] have used extensions of the planar quantitation concept to quantify the three-dimensional distribution of myocardial ^{201}Tl at stress and redistribution from rotational tomograms. These algorithms express the percentage of the myocardium that is involved with a perfusion defect, washout abnormality, and/or reversible abnormality.

PROTOCOL

In the approach implemented at Emory University,[8,9] the patient undergoes the same exercise protocol described for planar imaging, with the exception that a thallium dose of 3.5 mCi is used. The standard 2.0-mCi dose yields suboptimal counting statistics with consequent poor image quality and frequent image artifacts. This limitation is particularly marked in delayed images and in obese patients with accentuated soft tissue attenuation. Acquisition consists of obtaining 32 projections for 40 seconds each over the 180-degree arc extending from the 45-degree right anterior oblique to the 45-degree left posterior oblique projection. Each of the 32 projections is corrected for misalignment of the mechanical center of rotation with respect to the reconstruction matrix. A 30 million count flood field obtained using a ^{57}Co flat source is used to correct field nonuniformity. The projections are prefiltered prior to back-projection using a Hanning filter with a cutoff frequency of 0.822 cycles/cm. Filtered back-projection is then performed to reconstruct the transverse axial tomograms (of 6 mm each) encompassing the entire heart. Oblique tomograms parallel to the vertical and horizontal long axis and the short axis of the left ventricle are extracted from the filtered transaxial tomograms by performing a coordinate transformation with appropriate interpolation.[16] The tomograms are reconstructed without scatter or attenuation correction due to the difficulties involved in correcting for the variable attenuation of the ^{201}Tl 80-keV x-rays through the thorax. These effects are accounted for in part by comparison of each patient's thallium distribution to distribution files of normal patients exhibiting similar effects as detailed below.

THREE-DIMENSIONAL QUANTIFICATION

In the method developed at Emory University, the short-axis slices to be quantified are selected by an operator following a strict protocol. Using the long-axis slice with the largest cavity length, the operator selects the short-axis cuts for quantification to extend from the base of the left ventricle (LV) to the apical cap. On the short-axis cut falling halfway between the apex and base, the operator then defines the center of the LV cavity and the radius of search (Fig. 9-1A). The maximal count circumferential profiles (CP) for each short-axis cut are then generated automatically from the most apical to the most basal cut (Fig. 9-2A). The actual raw counts are extracted and used without normalization. This procedure is performed for each stress and each delayed tomographic study. Percentage washout CP are also calculated, using the profiles of the corresponding anatomic cut at stress and delayed tomography, respectively.

Alternating short-axis slices of the left ventricle are displayed from base to apex in Figure 9-1A. Approximately 12 slices are obtained from a normal sized heart. In this example, a defect in the septum is highlighted in the middle slice. This slice has been divided into 40 sectors of 9 degrees each (Fig. 9-1B). The septum is represented by the sectors from 90 to 180 degrees. The maximal counts per pixel (mcp) within each sector are determined. These 40 values have been plotted as a circumferential profile of the mcp-versus-angular location (Fig. 9-2A). A similar profile is constructed for each slice, except for the first two containing the apex, which are represented by a single value representing the mcp within the entire slice. To take into account variations in the number of slices per study, these curves are interpolated to produce a total of 15 profiles. Each of the

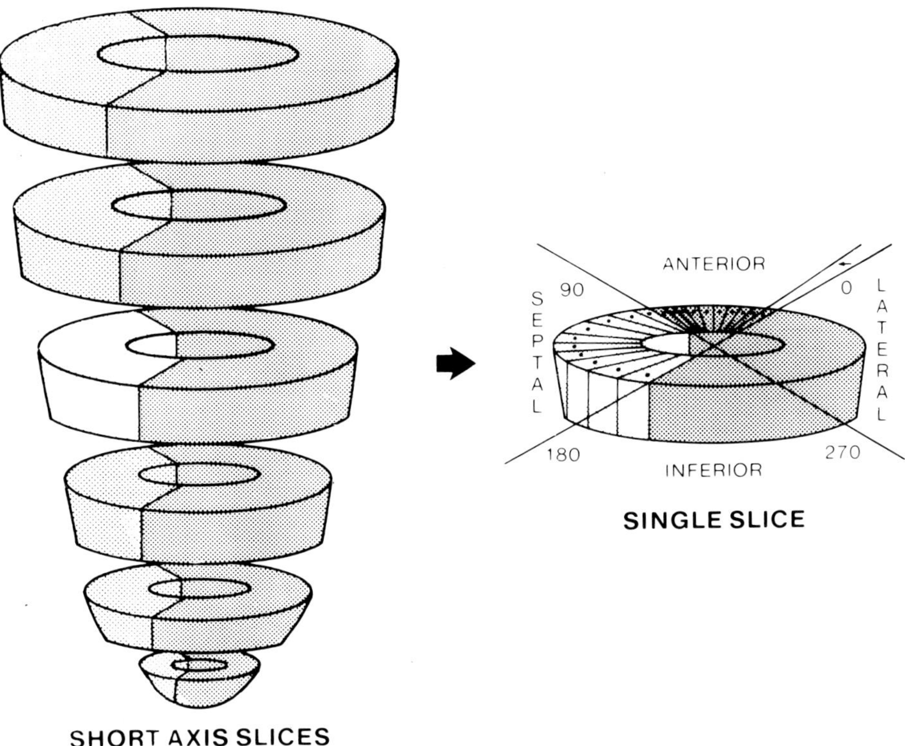

Fig. 9-1 Diagrammatic representation of short-axis slices of the left ventricle from base to apex. **(A)** A septal myocardial perfusion defect, extending from the base to the apex, is represented as a shaded area. **(B)** Each short-axis slice is divided into 40 sectors, 9 degrees each. The high lateral wall is arbitrarily assigned 0 degrees, with the sectors proceeding in a counterclockwise direction. (From DePasquale et al.,[9] with permission.)

rectangular coordinate profiles is translated into a polar coordinate profile (Fig. 9-2B), which displays the curve as a circle composed of 40 pixels. These data are displayed as a polar map, called a *bull's-eye plot,* which consists of a series of 15 concentric circles with the apex at the center and the base at the periphery (Fig. 9-2C). Individual bull's-eyes are constructed for the stress and delayed images as well as for percentage washout. In this display format, the stress and delayed bull's-eyes are adjusted by multiplying each pixel in the delayed bull's-eye by the ratio of the mcp in the stress bull's-eye to the mcp in the delayed bull's-eye.

Normalization occurs only when the profiles are compared with the gender-matched normal files developed from the low probability of disease group, in which the mean values and standard deviations (SD) were established from the pooled data for each of the angular locations in each of the 15 profiles.[17] This was accomplished by dividing each bull's-eye into four regions, 90 degrees each (anterior, septal, inferior, and lateral), from profiles 4 through 12 and determining the ratio of the average counts per pixel in each region of the patient's bull's-eye to the same region in the appropriate normal file. The region with the highest ratio was assumed

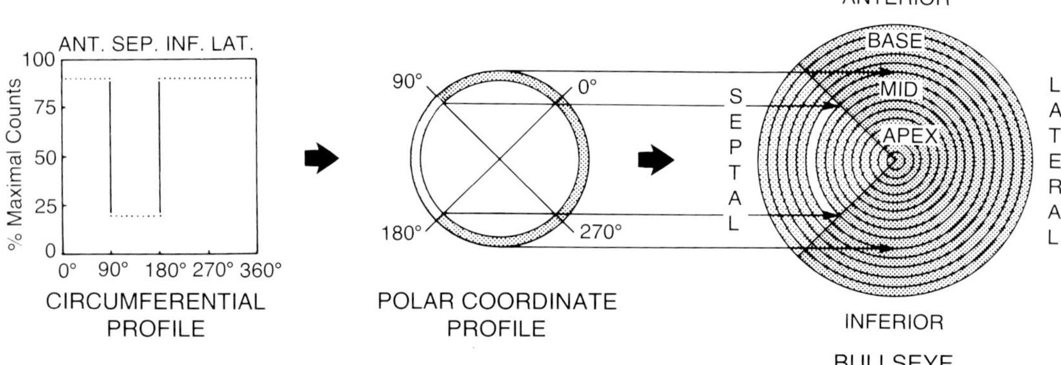

Fig. 9-2 Circumferential profile from the short-axis slice in Figure 9-1B plotted in rectangular coordinates. Note a marked decrease in count density (percentage maximum counts) between 90 and 180 degrees in the region of the septal perfusion defect. **(B)** Circumferential profile replotted in polar coordinates. **(C)** Each of the polar coordinates profiles is positioned in a bull's-eye plot. The apical circumferential profile is plotted at the center of the bull's-eye. Profiles for slices proceeding toward the base are plotted concentrically, proceeding from the center to the periphery of the bull's-eye plot. (From DePasquale et al,[9] with permission.)

to be normal, and each pixel in the patient's bull's-eye was multiplied by the reciprocal of this ratio. Before comparing the washout profiles with the corresponding normal profiles, the normal curves were adjusted to correspond to the same acquisition interval as the patient's study by moving the values in the normal curves along a monoexponential curve.

Each individual patient's bull's-eye was compared with a gender-matched normal file. The male and female normal files consisted of patients referred for ^{201}Tl SPECT, but with a less than 5 percent probability of coronary artery disease by analysis of risk factors. Of note, normal volunteers were not included, since their exercise capacity and, in most cases, their body habitus, differ significantly from those of a typical patient population. Likewise, patients referred for coronary arteriography, but with angiographically normal arteries were not included, since a high likelihood of disease usually directed them to catheterization; thus, coronary

spasm or small vessel disease not detectable angiographically would be possible causes for symptoms.

Comparison of patient data with normal limits resulted in the conversion of the bull's-eye plot into a standard deviation map displaying pixels color coded to the number of SD below normal (see Plates 9-2, 9-3, 9-6, 9-7, and 9-9). Pixels 1 to 2 SD below mean normal are coded in tan, pixels 2 to 3 SD below normal are coded in brown, pixels 3 to 5 SD below normal in blue, 5 to 7 SD below normal in green, and pixels more than 7 SD below normal in black. This analysis resulted in establishing additional profile curves representing 2.5 SD below the mean normal response as the threshold for defect detection. Points falling below this established normal limit are plotted in a blackout bull's-eye, in which the black region within the bull's-eye plot defines the extent of the perfusion abnormality. The location, size, and shape of these blacked-out regions are used in conjunction with heuristic rules de-

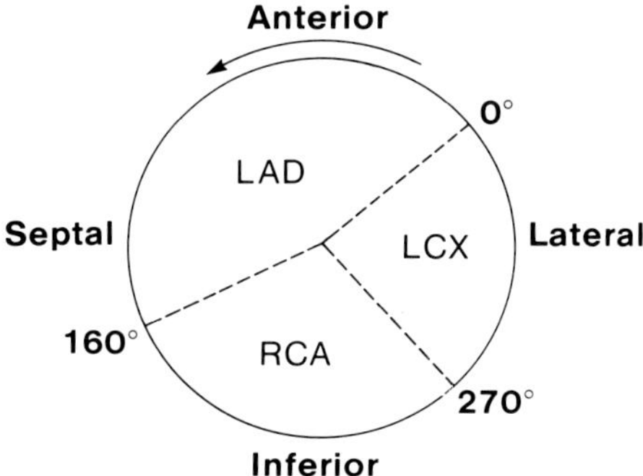

Fig. 9-3 Diagrammatic representation of approximate distribution of left anterior descending (LAD), left circumflex (LCX), and right coronary arteries (RCA). (From DePasquale et al.,[9] with permission.)

veloped from the pilot group to identify the stenosed coronary artery associated with specific patterns of perfusion abnormality. Figure 9-3 illustrates the approximate location on a bull's-eye plot of the regions perfused by specific coronaries.

OTHER APPROACHES

Other investigators have also used circumferential profiles to extract the initial ^{201}Tl myocardial distribution and washout rate. N. Tamaki et al.[15] assessed the myocardium by using circumferential profiles from three short-axis sections and one middle right anterior oblique (RAO) long-axis section. The main difference in other approaches has been in how the CP are normalized. Caldwell et al.[18] scaled the CP to a percentage of maximal counts in the entire left ventricular region of interest. In the method developed at Cedars-Sinai Hospital, Los Angeles, California,[7] each profile is normalized to the maximum pixel value for that profile.

In the Cedars approach, arcs of 60 to 120 degrees of each vertical long-axis cut are mapped into the central region of the display to depict the apical ^{201}Tl distribution. Immediately surrounding the apical region, the entire most apical short-axis stress profile (0 to 360 degrees) is mapped, with all the following short-axis CP in increasingly larger

circles until the most basal CP is reached. In the two-dimensional Cedars polar map, the size of the display always remains the same, so the size of the LV is reflected by the number of CP mapped. Thus, in a larger LV, the band representing each slice is thinner than with a smaller LV.

QUANTIFICATION OF DEFECTS: THALLIUM SCORE

The severity of a perfusion defect in a thallium tomographic study may be objectified when patient data are compared with gender-matched normal files. Through clinical experience and comparison with coronary angiography,[9] the investigators at Emory University have realized optimum accuracy in the diagnosis of coronary artery disease if bull's-eye abnormalities only greater than 2.5 SD below normal limits are judged abnormal. Such abnormalities may be characterized in terms of severity, using a thallium score. This thallium score is derived by identifying all pixels in the bull's-eye plot that are more than 2.5 SD below gender-matched normal limits. For each of these pixels, the number of standard deviations below normal limits is then determined. Figure 9-4 illustrates how the ischemic score is calculated as the sum of standard deviations below mean normal for all pixels greater than 2.5 SD. A thallium

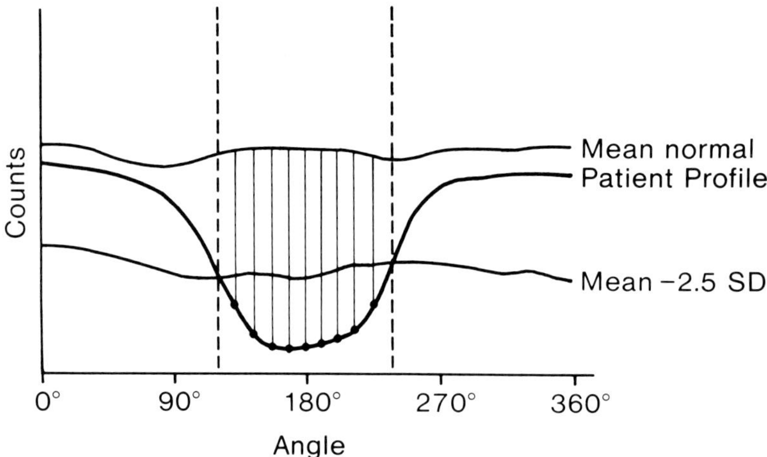

Fig. 9-4 Representation of the method used to calculate the thallium score. Pixels greater than 2.5 SD below normal are identified as indicated. The sum of the standard deviations below normal of these pixels is then calculated. (From DePuey et al.,[19] with permission.)

score may be determined for the entire bull's-eye plot or for individual territories.

The applications of an objective measure of either myocardial ischemia or scarring, or both, are manifold; however, some important limitations and potential errors of this quantitative method must be emphasized. The bull's-eye plot is dependent on an observer's correct selection of the apex and the base of the LV from oblique tomographic slices. If the slices extend too far past the actual base or apex, there will be a rim of apparently decreased tracer concentration at the periphery of the bull's-eye or a localized central defect near the apex, respectively (Plate 9-1). Recalling that the basal portion of the ventricle is relatively magnified in the bull's-eye plot and regions near the apex are minified, basal perfusion abnormalities will appear larger than equivalent defects in the mid- and distal portions of the LV.

With due consideration of the limitations in the quantitative analysis of thallium bull's-eye plots, this method serves as a useful tool to determine the severity of myocardial isch-emia and the amount of myocardium in jeopardy in patients with CAD. In the experience at Emory, a thallium score of greater than 40 is considered to represent a true perfusion defect. Patients with more severe and extensive coronary artery disease demonstrate more markedly abnormal thallium scores.

CLINICAL APPLICATIONS

Application of the Emory bull's-eye quantitative technique to a prospective group of 210 patients (179 with and 31 without CAD) resulted in an overall sensitivity of 95 percent, specificity of 74 percent, and an accuracy of 92 percent for detecting the presence or absence of CAD. The ability of this analysis to identify individual coronary stenoses is displayed in Figure 9-5 for each major coronary artery and for the left circumflex and right coronary arteries combined. The results of this prospective evaluation of the method demonstrate a high sensitivity and specificity for the detection of CAD in patients and in individual coronary stenoses.[9]

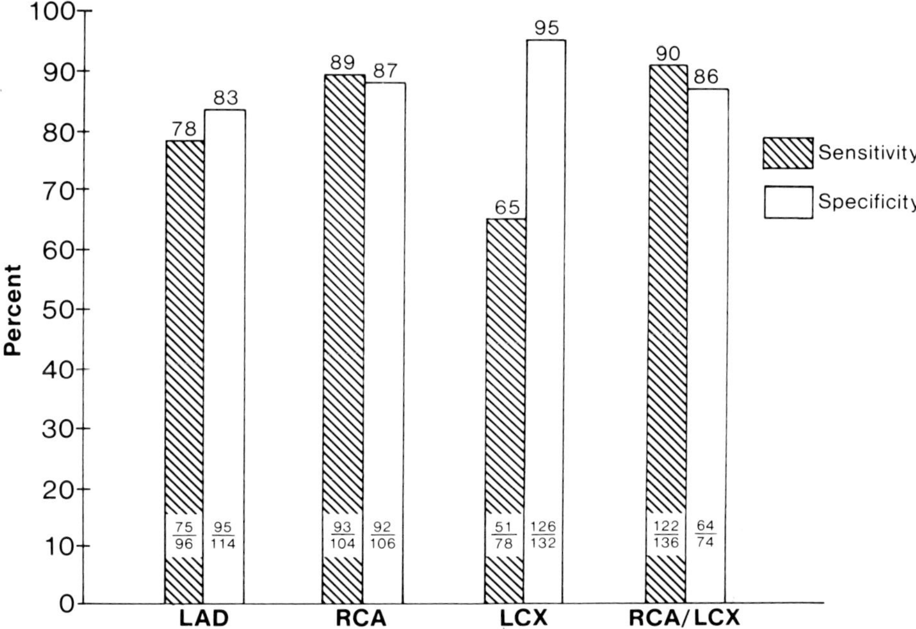

Fig. 9-5 Performance parameters of ^{201}Tl SPECT with bull's-eye plot analysis in the detection of individual coronary stenoses. (From DePasquale et al.,[9] with permission.)

ASSESSMENT OF MEDICAL THERAPY

Quantitative thallium tomography has also been helpful in following the response to medical therapy of patients with CAD (Plate 9-2). Sequential thallium studies may be helpful in patients in whom angina is controlled with β-blockers, nitroglycerin, or calcium channel blockers to assess the adequacy of therapy in abolishing or ameliorating ischemia. In patients undergoing cardiac rehabilitation, thallium tomography may also be useful in determining the level of exercise safe for a patient without subjecting him to undue coronary ischemia.

ASSESSMENT OF PTCA

Quantitative ^{201}Tl tomography has been performed in patients before and 1 to 2 days after PTCA (Plate 9-3). In order to determine which hemodynamic and angiographic variables measured during coronary artery dilation correlate best with the improvement in myocardial perfusion afforded by PTCA as measured by thallium tomography, 158 patients were studied before and after PTCA.[19] In these patients, myocardial perfusion abnormalities in the distribution of the diseased coronary artery were detected in 147 patients (93 percent). Following PTCA, thallium tomography demonstrated improvement or normalization of myocardial perfusion in 111 of 147 patients (76 percent). Scan findings demonstrated no improvement or even worsening of perfusion in the remaining 36 patients (24 percent). The improvement in thallium score post-PTCA was correlated with a variety of noncontinuous and continuous hemodynamic and angiographic variables, such as lesion length, eccentricity, calcification, and translesional pressure gradients. Improvement in a thallium score in the immediate postexercise images was shown to be related to localization of the coronary artery abnormality to the left anterior descending coronary artery, the change in stenosis afforded by PTCA, and the degree of stenosis present prior to PTCA. It is not surprising that patients undergoing dilation of the most severe lesions derive the greatest benefit from PTCA and that lesions in which the degree of stenosis is most reduced are afforded a greater improvement in perfusion. Importantly, however, although the improvement in thallium score was positively associated with the change in stenosis afforded by PTCA, the correlation was weak ($r = 0.41$). This weak correlation indicates that early after PTCA, ^{201}Tl SPECT and coronary arteriography provide independent assessments of myocardial perfusion in the distribution of the dilated artery.

Quantitative thallium tomography has also been used at Emory University to monitor the progressive improvement in myocardial perfusion afforded by sequential PTCA.[20] Many patients cannot tolerate dilation of multiple coronary arteries during a single procedure. In others, due to questionable success of the first vessel dilated, a second vessel is not attempted in a single procedure. By performing quantitative thallium tomography before and after the first PTCA procedure and again following the second PTCA procedure, we have demonstrated a progressive improvement in myocardial perfusion as manifested by a progressive decrease in thallium score.

NONCORONARY DISEASE STATES THAT ALTER [201]TI DISTRIBUTION

Tracer distribution departs from the normal pattern not only in patients with coronary artery disease but in several noncoronary disease states affecting the myocardium as well. It is important to identify such patients, since ^{201}Tl SPECT studies may be falsely positive for coronary artery disease, thereby decreasing test specificity. When ^{201}Tl studies are analyzed quantitatively and compared with normal files, these alterations in tracer distribution become more apparent.

In patients with asymmetric septal hypertrophy, there is a marked increase in tracer concentration in the thickened septum. This finding was previously described with planar imaging.[21,22] However, the alteration in tracer distribution is more apparent in SPECT studies due to improved image contrast and the ability to isolate the septum in long-axis tomographic slices. In the horizontal long-axis slices, the extent of septal involvement is most readily apparent.

We have also noted a marked alteration in myocardial distribution of ^{201}Tl in patients with long-standing systemic hypertension and concentric myocardial hypertrophy.[23] To investigate the magnitude of this problem in decreasing test specificity for CAD, the Emory group studied 100 patients with end-stage renal disease and chronic systemic hypertension. The likelihood of coronary disease in these patients was minimized by excluding patients with cardiac symptoms or prior myocardial infarction. Hypertensive patients who underwent cardiac catherization (often due to false-positive ^{201}Tl studies) and demonstrated greater than 20 percent luminal diameter narrowing of any coronary artery were excluded. All patients were being treated for hypertension, so few were actually more than mildly hypertensive at the time of the study.

For comparison and defect quantification, 35 normotensive control subjects were studied, including 20 males and 15 females, each with a less than 5 percent likelihood of coronary disease determined by analysis of risk factors. All 35 control subjects and 70 of the hypertensive patients underwent symptom-limited graded treadmill exercise to at least 85 percent of their age-predicted maximal heart rate.

Thirty patients who were unable to exercise adequately or who were unable to achieve their maximal predicted heart rate, usually due to β-blocker therapy, received intravenous dipyridamole, 0.71 mg/kg infused over 5 minutes. Alterations in count density of the septum were anticipated in the hypertensive patients. Therefore, by means of standardized computer-generated regions of interest, the ratio of the lateral to septal count densities (L/S CD ratio) was determined for both the hypertensive patients and control subjects.

A consistent finding in hypertensive patients was a fixed decrease in the L/S CD ratio as compared with normal controls (Table 9-1). No significant difference in the L/S CD ratio was present in hypertensive patients undergoing treadmill versus dipyridamole intervention. In 35 of the 100 patients, the L/S CD ratio was greater than 2.0 SD below normal, creating the impression of a fixed lateral wall defect (Plate 9-4). Frequently, lateral defects appeared to extend to the contiguous anterior and inferior walls. Twelve of the hypertensive patients enrolled in this study also underwent two-dimensional echocardiography. Measurements of myocardial wall thickness were taken from the short-axis view immediately below the tips of the mitral valve leaflets. In all patients, the thickness of the septal wall and lateral wall was increased (greater than 11 mm). However, in no patient was the L/S ratio less than 0.76, to indicate selective septal hypertrophy.

TABLE 9-1 Lateral to Septal Wall ^{201}Tl Count Density Ratios in Patients with Long-standing Hypertension and Normal Control Subjects

Controls (N = 35)	Hypertensive Patients (N = 100)	P
1.17 ± 0.08	1.03 ± 0.10	<0.00001
1.11 ± 0.08	1.03 ± 0.08	<0.00001

Thus, from this study we concluded that alterations in ^{201}Tl myocardial count density occur frequently in patients with chronic hypertension and myocardial hypertrophy. In comparison with normotensive control subjects, there is a relative increase in septal wall count density. This finding does not necessarily indicate selective septal hypertrophy. Without knowledge of this common scan pattern in hypertensive patients, nuclear medicine physicians may incorrectly interpret ^{201}Tl SPECT studies to be indicative of lateral wall myocardial infarction. Since hypertension is a major risk factor for CAD, hypertensive patients are frequently referred for ^{201}Tl myocardial perfusion scintigraphy.

Another patient group frequently encountered in the nuclear cardiology laboratory are patients with left bundle branch block (LBBB). Since electrocardiographic (ECG) testing is indeterminate in patients with LBBB, a noninvasive diagnosis of CAD is frequently sought by means of ^{201}Tl imaging. Septal perfusion abnormalities in planar ^{201}Tl imaging have been described in patients with LBBB but with no demonstrable coronary disease.[24] To investigate the sensitivity and specificity of ^{201}Tl SPECT in patients with LBBB, 24 patients with LBBB underwent immediate postexercise and 4-hour delayed ^{201}Tl SPECT imaging with quantitative analysis using bull's-eye polar maps.[25] In 14 patients who underwent arteriography, test performance in detecting individual coronary artery stenoses greater than or equal to 50 percent was excellent for the circumflex and right coronary artery but was very poor (specificity = 10 percent) for the left anterior descending coronary artery (Table 9-2). Despite excellent sensitivity, the 10 percent specificity for LAD disease is much lower than reported values of 80 to 85 percent for patients with normal intraventricular conduction, as three of four patients with LAD stenosis and also 9 of 10 patients with normal coronary arteries had immediate septal perfusion defects with redistribution at 4 hours

TABLE 9-2 Sensitivity and Specificity of ^{201}Tl SPECT in Diagnosing Coronary Artery Disease in Patients with LBBB

	LAD		LCX		RCA	
	N	*%*	*N*	*%*	*N*	*%*
Sensitivity	4/4	100	2/2	100	5/5	100
Specificity	1/10	10	12/12	100	7/9	7/8

LBBB, left bundle branch block; LAD, left anterior descending; LCX, left circumflex; RCA, right coronary artery.

(Plate 9-5). All 10 patients without arteriographic correlation had reversible septal defects. The L/S count density ratio was calculated in the 10 LBBB patients with normal coronary arteries and in 35 control subjects with normal intraventricular conduction (Table 9-3). In the LBBB patients, the L/S CD ratio was significantly increased as compared with normal in the immediate images, but not significantly different from normal in the delayed images.

Thus, with LBBB, ^{201}Tl SPECT is indeterminate for LAD disease due to reversible septal perfusion defects. Decreased coronary flow due to altered septal relaxation has been proposed as an explanation for this phenomenon.[24] We believe that ^{201}Tl scintigraphy is still of value in these patients, since accuracy in detecting disease of the right and circumflex coronary arteries is excellent. However, if abnormalities are present only in the LAD distribution, the scan is indeterminate for coronary artery disease, and the patient should be directed to cardiac cather-

TABLE 9-3 Lateral to Septal Wall [201]Tl Count Density Ratios in Patients with LBBB and Normal Control Subjects

Response	LBBB	Normal	*P*
immediate	1.27 ± 0.16	1.17 ± 0.08	<0.05
4-hr delay	1.13 ± 0.06	1.11 ± 0.08	NS

LBBB, left bundle branch block.

ization for a definitive diagnosis of coronary artery disease.

INTRAVENOUS AND ORAL DIPYRIDAMOLE USED IN CONJUNCTION WITH QUANTITATIVE [201]TI SPECT

The use of dipyridamole as an alternative to exercise in patients suspected of having coronary artery disease is detailed in Chapter 7. Quantitative analysis of dipyridamole-SPECT ^{201}Tl studies is also of value in the detection of CAD. Unlike exercise, a great degree of patient-to-patient variability in the amount of coronary vasodilation is present with dipyridamole. Therefore, analysis of myocardial washout curves has proved to be of little diagnostic value. It has also been postulated that the distribution of ^{201}Tl within the myocardium following intravenous dipyridamole coronary vasodilation differs from that with exercise. Therefore, some investigators have cautioned that normal exercise files should not be used for comparison with dipyridamole patient data. Using planar ^{201}Tl imaging, Berman et al.[26] noted a decreased specificity when dipyridamole data were compared with exercise files (42 percent versus 73 percent) due to a high incidence of false-positive studies.

In our experience with the gender-matched normal exercise files obtained at Emory University, dipyridamole-^{201}Tl SPECT test sensitivity has been quite acceptable. Seventy-six patients who were unable to exercise adequately underwent ^{201}Tl SPECT and quantitative analysis with bull's-eye polar maps both immediately after dipyridamole infusion and 4 hours later.[27] All dipyridamole patients underwent coronary arteriography, which was interpreted independently. Twenty-five patients had three-vessel disease, 24 had two-vessel disease, 12 had single-vessel disease, and 15 had no luminal diameter stenosis greater than 50 percent. Test per-

TABLE 9-4 Test Performance Parameters of ^{201}Tl SPECT After IV Dipyridamole in the Diagnosis of Coronary Artery Disease

	CAD (%)	LAD (%)	LCX (%)	RCA (%)
Sensitivity	89	73	82	74
Specificity	43	83	83	88
Accuracy	79	78	86	80

CAD, coronary artery disease; LAD, left anterior descending; LCX, left circumflex; RCA, right coronary artery.

formance parameters to detect CAD and individual coronary stenoses are detailed in Table 9-4. Sensitivity in detecting individual coronary stenoses is only slightly reduced compared with data reported previously for exercise ^{201}Tl SPECT. Specificity for CAD (43 percent) was decreased, since most patients were referred for arteriography on the basis of ^{201}Tl SPECT results. Also, five of the eight patients with false-positive ^{201}Tl SPECT had subcritical (30 to 40 percent) stenoses. Thus, in our experience, dipyridamole is a satisfactory alternative to exercise for ^{201}Tl SPECT; individual coronary stenoses are accurately detected by comparison of dipyridamole patient data with normal exercise files.

IMAGE ARTIFACTS THAT DECREASE ^{201}Tl SPECT SPECIFICITY

Sensitivities of greater than 90 percent in detecting individual coronary stenoses have been reported using ^{201}Tl SPECT data analysis with bull's-eye polar maps and comparison with gender-matched normal files. However, the specificity of this method has been reported to be as low as 75 percent.[9] With increasing experience with ^{201}Tl SPECT, having now studied more than 7,000 patients, we have come to realize that image artifacts significantly decrease test specificity.[28] The artifacts described below are present in

oblique tomographic slices but are more graphically portrayed and easily recognized in bull's-eye polar maps, particularly when patient data are compared with normal files.

Soft Tissue Attenuation

The most common artifact encountered is soft tissue attenuation by the female breast and by the left hemidiaphragm in both men and women. Breasts vary in size, position, and density, thereby having a variable attenuation effect on photons emanating from the left ventricular myocardium. Normal female data files primarily include women with average sized breasts which are anteriorly positioned. Women with unusually large or dense breasts will be noted to have fixed anterior scan defects (Plate 9-6). If the breasts are pendulous, lying over the lateral chest wall, the defect will appear to involve more of the anterolateral wall, often extending posterolaterally. Slight imprecision in breast repositioning in the delayed images gives the false impression of anterior redistribution and thus ischemia. False-positive studies due to breast attenuation can be minimized by knowing the patient's chest circumference and the position and configuration of her breasts. Occasionally, smaller breast will be quite dense, causing marked attenuation. Inspection of rotating planar images aids in determination of breast density in the region of the myocardium that has been eclipsed. Errors in breast repositioning can be minimized by ensuring that the patient wears the same type of clothing in both the immediate and delayed studies.

A less frequently encountered problem is ^{201}Tl SPECT artifacts due to small or absent breasts, causing an inferior defect when compared to normal female files. In the normal female file, anterior count density is relatively less than that of the inferior wall due to physiologic breast attenuation. In patients with small breasts or following mastectomy, the count distribution pattern is more similar to that of the male, with inferior attenuation due to the left hemidiaphragm. When patient data are compared with the normal female file, the inferior wall is relatively count poor, causing an apparent fixed inferior wall defect. Therefore, ^{201}Tl SPECT in women with small or absent breasts should instead be compared with the normal male file (Plate 9-7).

In both men and women, elevation of the left hemidiaphragm will result in inferior wall attenuation, mimicking inferior myocardial infarction. This phenomenon is particularly marked in patients with cardiomegaly, where the heart "sinks" below the diaphram (Plate 9-8). This artifact is a major cause of test nonspecificity. Determination of diaphragmatic height on chest radiographs is sometimes helpful. In our experience, inspection of rotating planar images has been of little value. Evaluation of inferior wall motion by radionuclide ventriculography or two-dimensional echocardiography can confirm the presence of infarction. However, subendocardial infarction resulting in scan abnormalities often may not result in a wall motion abnormality.

Superimposition of Other Tracer-Avid Structures

Considerable tracer accumulation may occur in the liver, stomach, or bowel, which may overlie the inferior wall of the left ventricle. Since with exercise studies, extracardiac accumulation is most marked in the delayed images, this phenomenon may result in apparent tracer redistribution into the inferior wall (Plate 9-9). Inspection of the rotating planar images is crucial to detect extracardiac tracer concentration.

Cardiac Dextrorotation and Levorotation

For a 180-degree SPECT acquisition, the camera rotates from the 45-degree right anterior oblique (RAO) to the 45-degree left posterior oblique (LPO) positions. In a normal individual, the bull's-eye plot demonstrates a L/S CD ratio of approximately 1.17. With progressive cardiac dextrorotation, the L/S CD ratio decreases. Conversely, levorotation causes an increase in this ratio (Plate 9-10). Thus, with dextrorotation, there is an apparent fixed lateral wall defect when patient data are compared with normal files. With levorotation, a fixed septal wall abnormality may be apparent. Inspection of rotating planar images helps determine the axis of the heart and identify patients with either marked dextrorotation or levorotation.

Center of Rotation Errors

Errors in the determination of the camera center of rotation create comma-shaped artifacts, best seen when bull's-eye plots are compared with normal files. With errors in the center of rotation in the positive direction ($+1$ to $+4$ pixels), the artifact appears posteroapically. With negative errors (-1 to -4 pixels), the artifact appears anteroseptally (Plate 9-11). There is no way to identify with certainty an error in the center of rotation as a cause of a SPECT image abnormality by inspection of either planar, oblique, or bull's-eye images. Rigorous camera quality control is essential to prevent such artifacts.

Miscellaneous SPECT Artifacts

Other common causes of SPECT image artifacts include arm motion across the chest during image acquisition and metallic attenuators such as medallions and pacemakers. These artifacts are easily recognized by inspection of the rotating planar images. Flood-field nonuniformity will also result in significant image artifacts; therefore, inspection of the daily 30 million count flood field is essential. Patient motion is not uncommon, since for SPECT image acquisition the patient is required to remain motionless under the camera with arms extended over the head, a position that is quite uncomfortable. Artifacts resulting from patient motion are variable

Color Plates

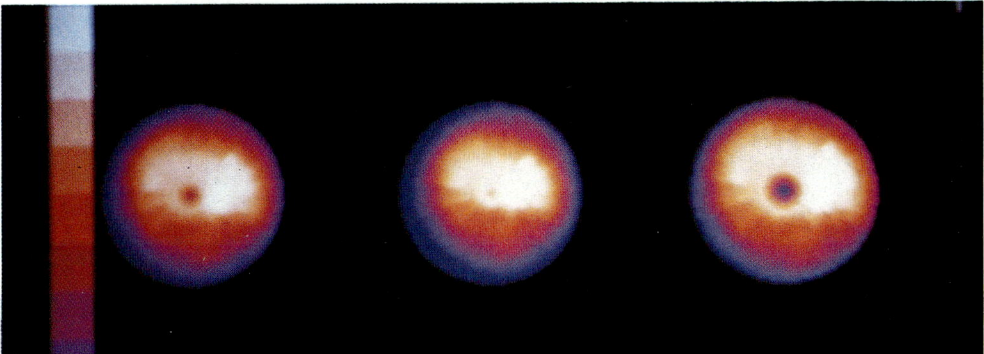

Plate 9-1

Plate 9-1 Correct slice selection for bull's-eye plot reconstruction produces a bull's-eye plot with a slight decrease in count density at the apex and around the rim of the bull's-eye, particularly in the septal and inferior regions (left). If slices extend too far past the base (toward the left atrium), the rim of decreased count density at the periphery of the bull's-eye will be accentuated (middle). Conversely, if slices extend too far past he apex, an apical defect will be created (right).

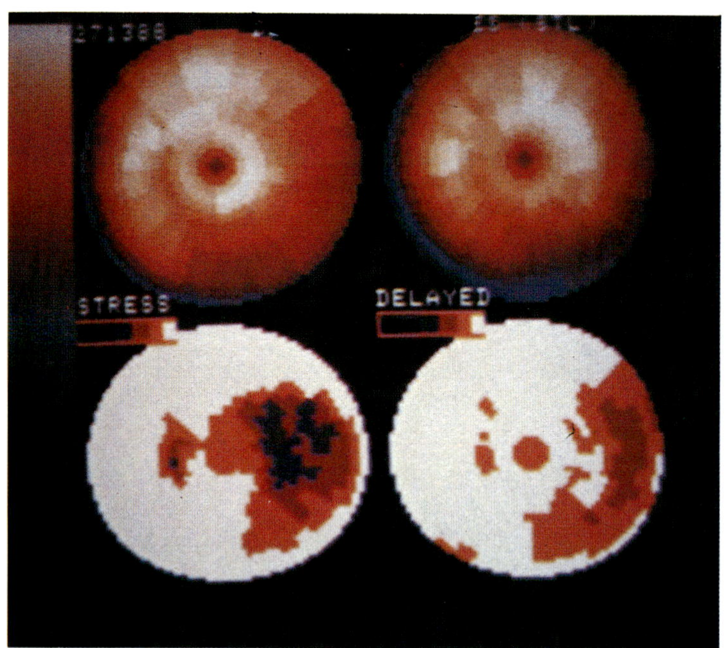

Plate 9-2A

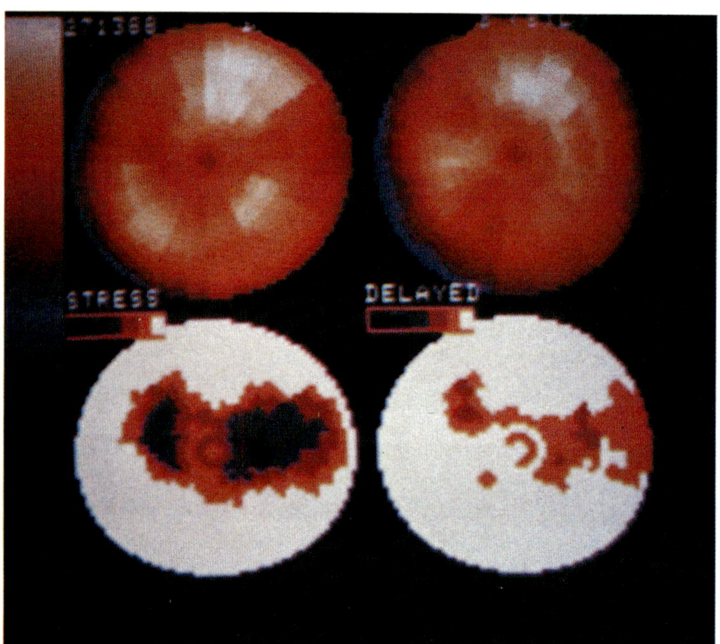

Plate 9-2B

Study	LAD	LCX	Total
initial (fig. 9-2A)	7	122	129
follow-up (fig. 9-2B)	130	339	469

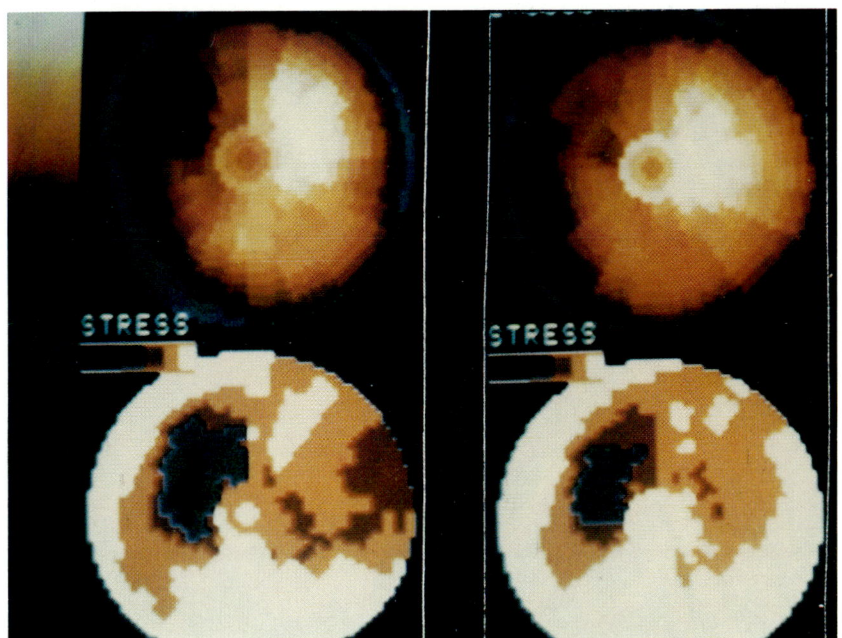

Plate 9-3

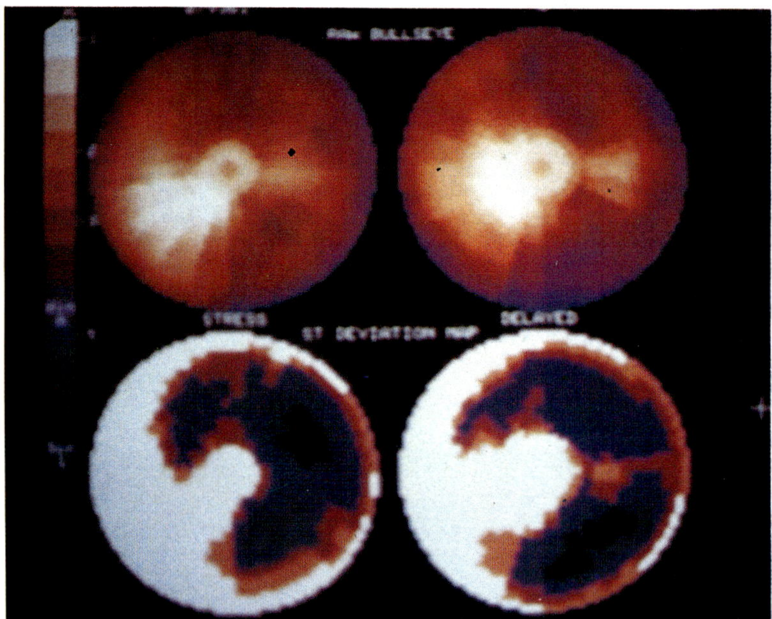

Plate 9-4

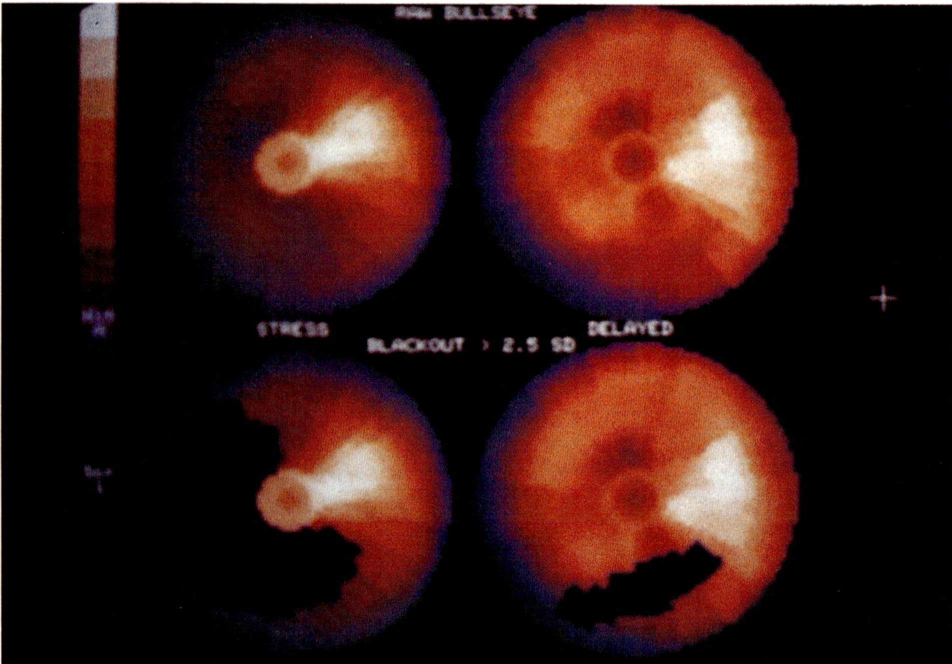

Plate 9-5

Plate 9-4 In this patient with long-standing systemic hypertension but normal coronary arteries, there is reversal of the normal lateral-to-septal wall count density (L/S CD) ratio, with a relative decrease in count density of the lateral wall. This finding mimicks lateral wall myocardial infarction.

Plate 9-5 Reversible septal perfusion abnormality in a patient with LBBB and normal coronary arteries. The lateral-to-septal wall count density (L/S CD) ratio in the stress image (left) is 1.54 (normal = 1.17 ± 0.08). In the delayed image (right), the ratio is 1.21

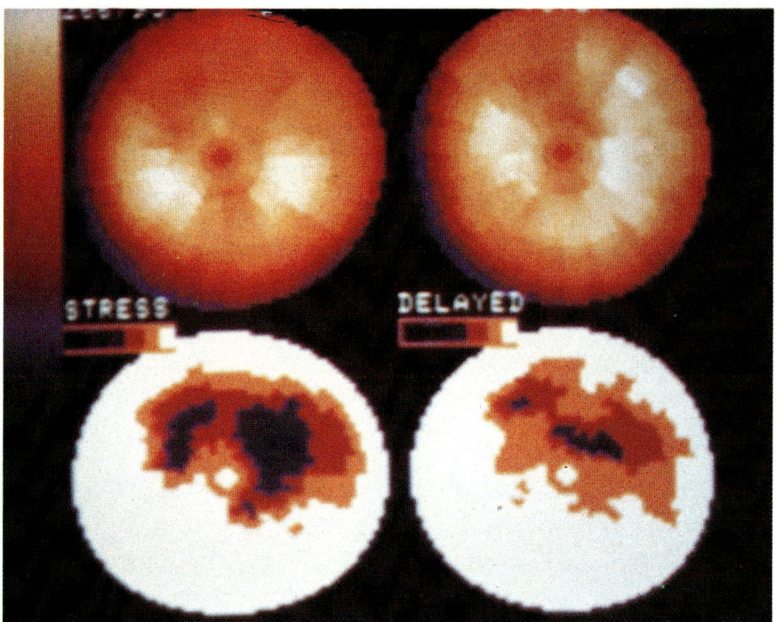

Plate 9-6

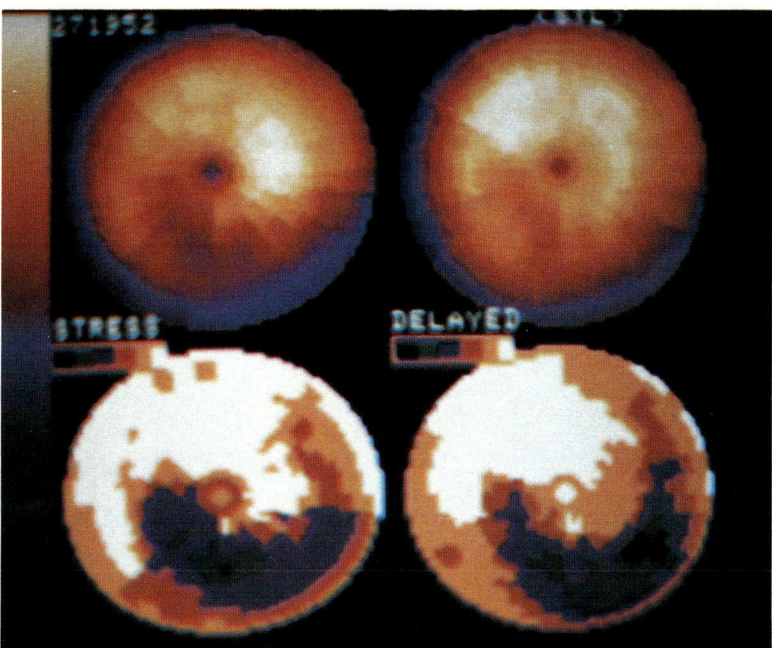

Plate 9-7

Plate 9-6 In this patient with large dense breasts, an apparent fixed anterior wall perfusion defect is attributable to photon attenuation.

Plate 9-7 In this patient, following bilateral mastectomy, the inferior wall of the left ventricle appears relatively count poor compared with the normal female file. An inferior wall myocardial infarction is mimicked by this artifact.

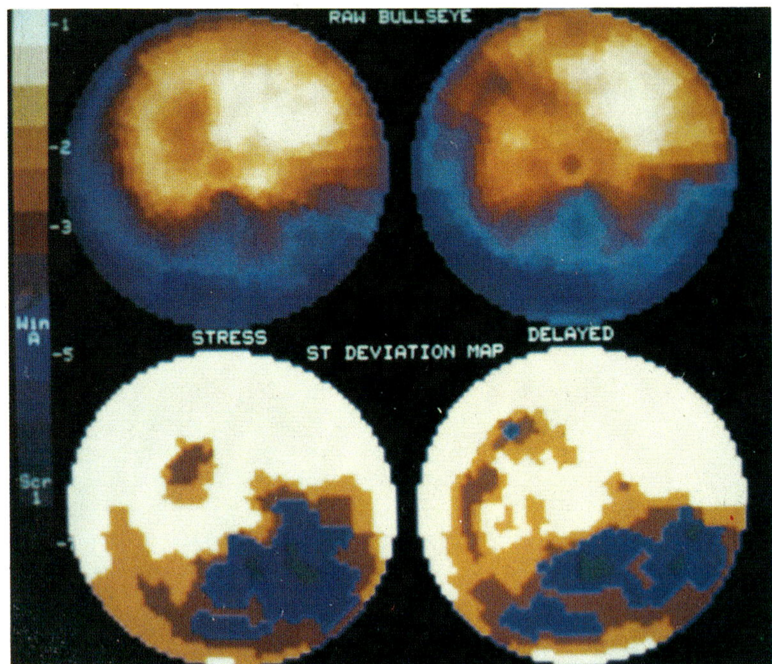

Plate 9-8

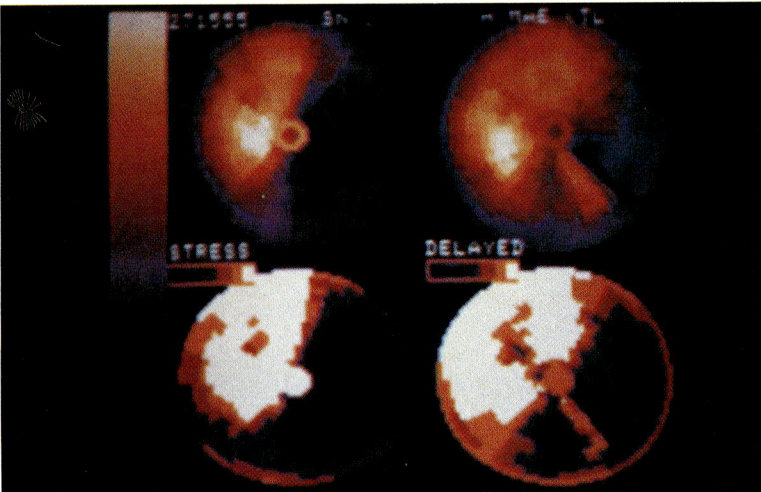

Plate 9-9

Plate 9-8 In this patient with cardiomegaly and an elevated left hemidiaphragm, there is an apparent fixed inferior wall defect attributable to photon attentuation by the left hemidiaphragm, mimicking inferior wall myocardial infarction.

Plate 9-9 In this patient with an extensive lateral and inferior wall myocardial infarction, there is apparent tracer redistribution into the inferolateral wall due to tracer concentration in a loop of bowel overlying the inferior wall of the left ventricle in delayed images.

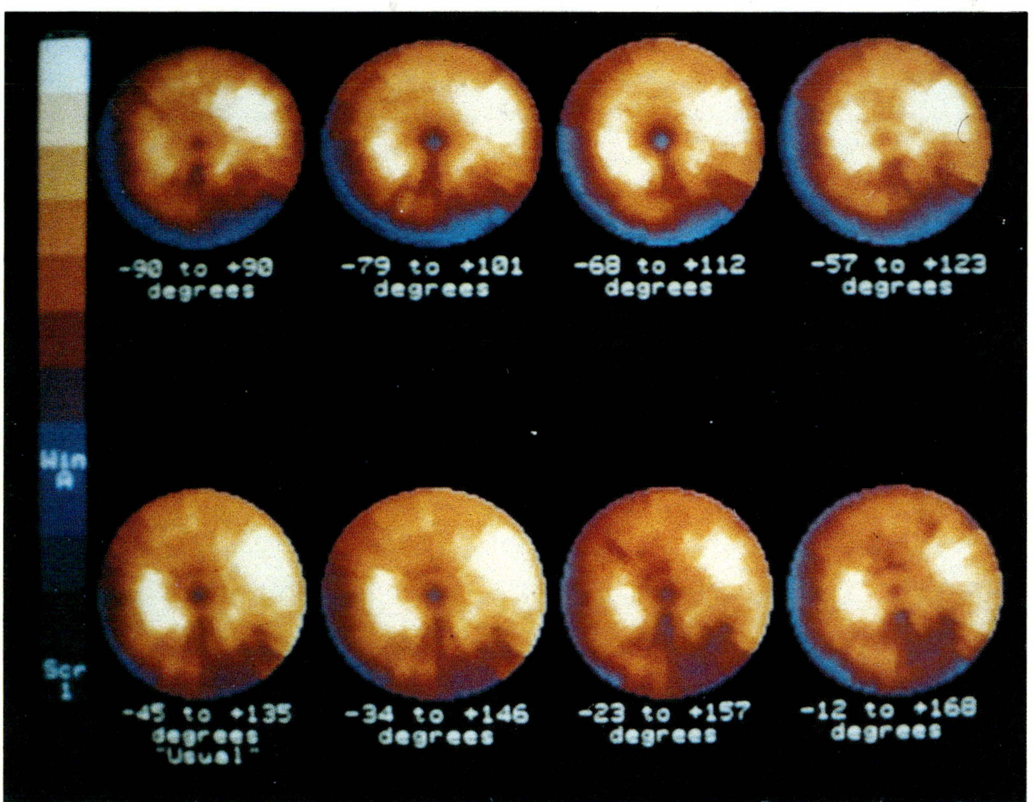

Plate 9-10

Plate 9-10 By varying the starting and ending points of the 180–degree arc used for ^{201}Tl SPECT, cardiac levorotation and dextrorotation are simulated. With progressive cardiac levorotation (moving leftward in the upper row of images), there is a progressive decrease in septal count density. With progressive dextrorotation (moving rightward in the bottom row of images), there is a progressive decrease in lateral wall count density. (From DePuey and Garcia,[28] with permission.)

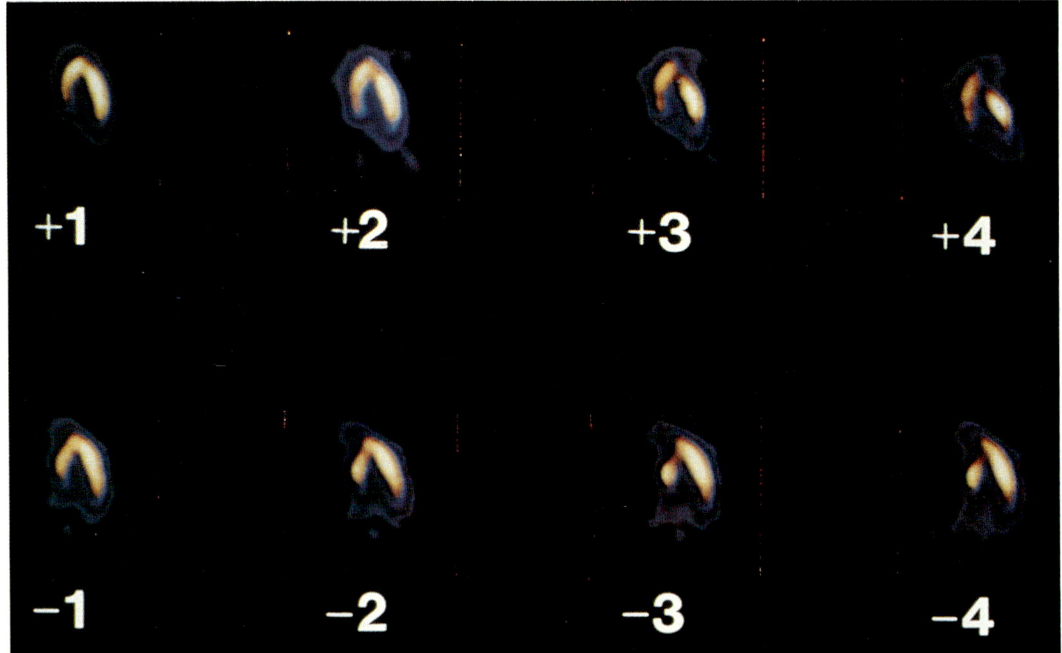

Plate 9-11A

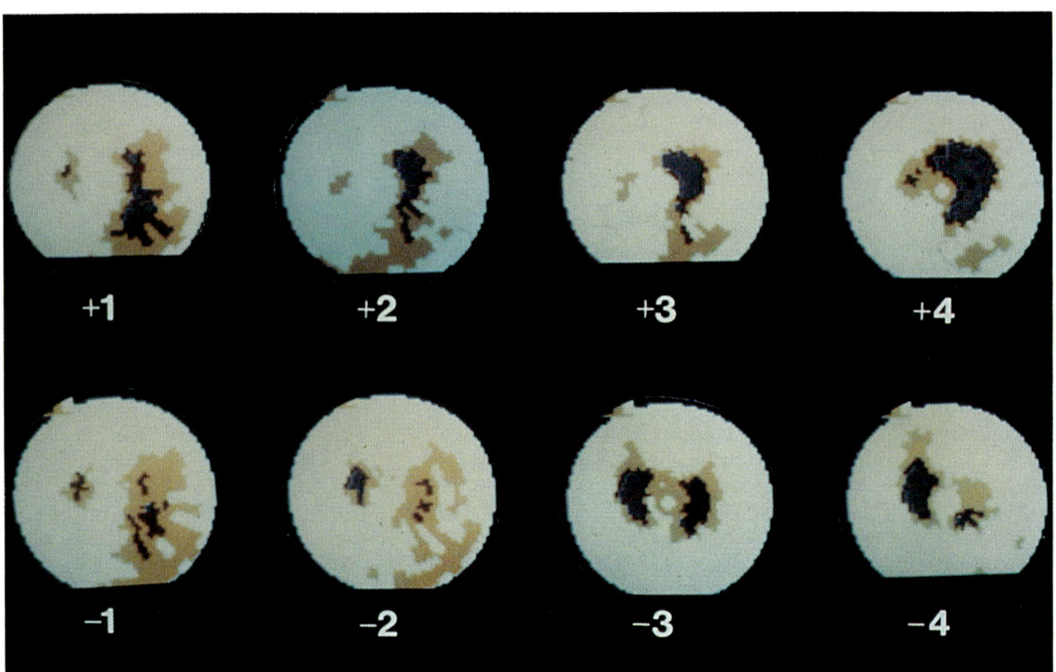

Plate 9-11B

Plate 9-11 With errors in the center of rotation, comma-shaped artifacts are created. Posteroapical defects occur with errors in the positive direction, and septal artifacts occur with errors in the negative direction. Abnormalities are most noticeable in horizontal long axis slices **(A)** and bull's-eye plots compared with gender-matched normal files **(B)**. (From DePuey and Garcia,[28] with permission.)

in appearance and are difficult to identify as such in either oblique tomographic slices or the bull's-eye plots. Inspection of the acquisition sinogram and rotating planar images is essential to detect patient motion. Point sources may be placed to the right of the patient's sternum above and below the heart as a further aid in detecting motion. When the rotating planar images are summed, the point source should appear as a straight horizontal line across the image. Patient motion is detected as a deviation of this line from the exact horizontal.

Planar Versus Tomography

Quantification of either planar or tomographic ^{201}Tl myocardial studies affords the advantage of objectivity over visual analysis. Moreover, comparison of patient profiles with lower limits of normal gives the nonexpert reader a sense of confidence that can be used in interpreting these studies and, more importantly, in developing expertise. Quantification of planar scintigrams aids in overcoming the lack of contrast resolution inherent to washout rate determinations. Thus, in patients who do not exhibit a reduction in counts in the myocardium at stress due to low-contrast resolution, the slow washout criterion may identify the perfusion defect. By contrast, tomography has excellent contrast resolution and, in our experience, identifies most stress perfusion defects without the need for using the slow washout criterion. Moreover, with the use of polar displays such as the bull's-eye map, the perfusion defect is better characterized by tomography in terms of its location, shape, and size. The main caveat in the use of tomography is that it is technically demanding; if a technical problem does occur, the physician interpreting the study can be so removed from the raw data as to make detection of the error difficult. The decision as to which method to use depends largely on the application and on the instrumentation and technical expertise available.

CONCLUSIONS

Quantitative ^{201}Tl SPECT has provided improved accuracy in the diagnosis of coronary artery disease as compared with conventional methods. Comparison with normal patient files highlights abnormalities and helps the inexperienced observer gain expertise more rapidly. However, as with any other nuclear medicine study, the physician must be intimately aware of technical and physiologic artifacts that affect tracer distribution. Familiarity with such alterations in tracer distribution increases test specificity and the overall accuracy of this useful noninvasive method to detect coronary artery disease.

REFERENCES

1. Trobaugh BB, Wackers FJT, Sokole EB, et al: Thallium-201 myocardial imaging: An interinstitutional study of observer variability. J Nucl Med 19:359, 1978
2. Garcia EV, Maddahi J, Berman DS, Waxman A: Space-time quantitation of thallium-201 myocardial scintigraphy. J Nucl Med 22:309, 1981
3. Meade RC, Bamrah VS, Horgan JD, et al: Quantitative methods in the evaluation of thallium-201 myocardial perfusion images. J Nucl Med 19:1175, 1978
4. Burow RD, Pond M, Schafer AW, Becker L: Circumferential profiles: A new method for computer analysis of thallium-201 myocardial perfusion images. J Nucl Med 20:771, 1979
5. Watson DD, Campbell NP, Read EK, et al: Spatial and temporal quantitation of plane thallium myocardial images. J Nucl Med 22:577, 1981
6. Vogel RA, Kirch DL, LeFree MT, et al: Thallium 201 myocardial perfusion scintigraphy: Results of standard and multi-pinhole tomographic techniques. Am J Cardiol 43:787, 1979
7. Garcia EV, Van Train K, Maddahi J, et al: Quantification of rotational thallium-201 myocardial tomography. J Nucl Med 26:17, 1985

8. Folks R, Banks L, Plankey M, et al: Cardio-vascular SPECT. J Nucl Med Technol 13:150, 1985

9. DePasquale E, Nody A, DePuey G, et al: Quantitative rotational thallium-201 tomography for identifying and localizing coronary artery disease. Circulation 77:316, 1988

10. Caldwell J, Williams D, Richie J: Single photon emission computed tomography: Validation and application for myocardial perfusion imaging. p. 115. In Pohost G, Higgins C, Morganroth J, et al: (eds): New Concepts in Cardiac Imaging 1985. GK Hall, Boston, 1985

11. Go RT, Cook SA, MacIntyre WJ, et al: Comparative accuracy of stress and redistribution thallium-201 cardiac single photon emission transaxial tomography and planar imaging in the diagnosis of myocardial ischemia. J Nucl Med 23:24, 1982 (abst)

12. Maddahi J, Van Train KF, Wong C, et al: Comparison of thallium-201 SPECT and planar imaging for evaluation of coronary artery disease. J Nucl Med 27:999, 1986 (abst)

13. Tamaki S, Najajima H, Murakami T, et al: Estimation of infarct size by myocardial emission computed tomography with thallium-201 and its relation to creatine kinase-MB release after myocardial infarction in man. Circulation 66:994, 1982

14. Ritchie JL, Williams DL, Harp G, et al: Transaxial tomography with thallium-201 for detecting remote myocardial infarction. Am J Cardiol 50:1236, 1982

15. Tamaki N, Yonekura Y, Kadaa S, et al: Value of quantitative stress thallium-201 emission CT for localization of coronary artery disease: Comparison with qualitative analysis. J Nucl Med 25:61, 1984 (abst)

16. Borello, JA, Clinthorne NH, Rogers WL, et al: Oblique-angle tomography: A restructuring algorithm for transaxial tomographic data. J Nucl Med 22:471, 1981

17. Eisner RL, Gober A, Cerqueira M, et al: Quantitative analysis of normal thallium-201 tomographic studies. J Nucl Med 26:49, 1985 (abst)

18. Caldwell J, Williams D, Harp G, et al: Quantitation of size of relative myocardial perfusion defect by single-photon emission computed tomography. Circulation 70:1048, 1984

19. DePuey EG, Roubin G, Cloninger K, et al: Correlation of transluminal coronary angioplasty parameters and quantitative thallium-201 tomography. J Inv Car 1:40, 1988

20. DePuey EG, DePasquale E, Nody A, et al: Sequential multivessel coronary angioplasty assessed by thallium-201 tomography. Cath Card Diag (in press)

21. Bulkley BH, Roleau J, Strauss HW, Pitt B: Idiopathic hypertrophic subaortic stenosis: Detection by thallium-201 myocardial perfusion imaging. N Engl J Med 293:1113, 1975

22. Rubin KA, Morrison J, Padnick MB, et al: Idiopathic hypertrophic subaortic stenosis: Evaluation of anginal symptoms with thallium-201 myocardial imaging. Am J Cardiol 44:1040, 1979

23. DePuey EG, Krawczynska EG, Perkins JV, et al: Alterations in Tl-201 SPECT distribution in patients with chronic systemic hypertension undergoing single photon emission computed tomography. Am J Cardiol 62:234, 1988

24. Hirzel HO, Senn M, Nuesch K, et al: Thallium-201 scintigraphy in complete left bundle branch block. Am J Cardiol 53:764, 1984

25. DePuey EG, Krawczynska EG, Robbins WL: Thallium-201 SPECT in patients with LBBB. J Nucl Med 29:1479, 1988

26. O'Byrne GT, Berman D, Van Train KF, et al: Quantitative assessment of dipyridamole thallium-201 planar scintigrams: Comparison of dipyridamole specific to stress normal limits. J Nucl Med 27:944, 1986 (abst)

27. DePuey EG, Krawczynska EG, D'Amato PH, Patterson RE: Thallium-201 SPECT with dipyridamole to diagnose coronary disease. J Nucl Med 28:642, 1987 (abst)

28. DePuey EG, Garcia EV: Optimal specificity of thallium-201 SPECT through recognition of imaging artifacts. J Nucl Med 30:441, 1989

10

Prognostication and Risk Stratification in Coronary Artery Disease

Milton J. Guiberteau

Early in the course of the development of noninvasive tests to evaluate myocardial perfusion and ventricular pump function, emphasis was given to the diagnosis of cardiac disease, most notably that of coronary artery origin. More recently, however, considerable attention has been directed to the use of these procedures in assessing risk and prognosis in patients already known to have heart disease, in hope of aiding the direction of clinical management decisions. This thrust has been fueled considerably by the advent of new therapies in cardiology as well as by the economic considerations that mandate their judicious use. Radionuclide tests of cardiac perfusion and function have come to play an important role in selecting among the growing alternative forms of medical and surgical treatment and in judging the efficacy of a particular therapy, once it has become instituted. In these respects, radionuclide-based risk stratification and prognostication provide crucial information that cannot be obtained on clinical or routine diagnostic evaluation alone.

Radionuclide tests selected to evaluate the patient with known coronary artery disease (CAD) depend greatly on the precise nature of the disease, the information needed for management decision-making and on the confidence of the referring and/or imaging physician in the various nuclear imaging alternatives at a given institution. Frequently, the information required about a patient's disease can be acquired by more than one approach. In many cases, this permits the choice of an examination for which the patient's physicians have a philosophical or technical bias. Thus, considerable interinstitutional, and even intrainstitutional, variation exists in the approach to assessing a particular disease.

For the practicing nuclear medicine physician, perhaps the simplest organizational approach to sorting through the information available regarding the evaluation of patients with established CAD is to consider the specific clinical decision-making situations that commonly arise in such a setting.

ACUTE MYOCARDIAL INFARCTION

Early-Postinfarction Period

In the setting of acute myocardial infarction, noninvasive nuclear imaging can provide valuable information at various stages of clinical evolution. This includes the prediction of early stage mortality and morbidity as well as subacute risk stratification and long-term prognosis.

In the early stages of acute myocardial infarction (MI), the occurrence of life-threatening complications, especially ventricular arrhythmias and pump failure, correlates with both the extent of necrosis (infarct size) and the extent of surrounding ischemia (myocardium at risk). As the infarct evolves, the risk of infarct extension with an attendant increase in morbidity and mortality becomes an important consideration. Noninvasive determination of infarct size and residual myocardium at risk have proved to be powerful predictors in these settings.[1-4] In many studies, radionuclide examinations providing data not supplied by routine clinical evaluation have proved superior to clinical and laboratory assessments in predicting early complications of acute MI. When performed during the early hours of infarction, these studies may also indentify patients who are likely to die inhospital. Uniformly, such tests applied during the early postinfarction period do not employ significant exercise or stress but rely primarily on resting parameters.

INFARCT-AVID IMAGING

The value of infarct-avid imaging in acute myocardial injury has been established by extensive work with technetium-99m-pyro-phosphate. It is likely that future work with labeled antimyosin will prove this agent to be similarly valuable, and probably more precise. In addition to being specific for irreversibly damaged myocardium, antimyosin has the advantage of being less influenced by the timing constraints encountered in pyrophosphate imaging, with its peak sensitivity at 48 to 72 hours. With both radiopharmaceuticals, however, the information obtained is limited to an estimate of infarct size, with no assessment of residual myocardial ischemia.

In general, technetium-99m-pyrophosphate imaging appears to predict morbidity and mortality by confirming the direct relationship between infarct size and the likelihood of acute complications. More specifically, abnormal infarct-avid images have been shown to correlate with early infarct complications in two particular settings. First, an extensive infarct (especially a doughnut pattern of increased activity with a central cold area) is predictive of a high incidence of congestive failure (67 percent in one series) and a poor prognosis.[5] Over the long term, a greater than 80 percent 2-year mortality rate has been demonstrated in patients exhibiting the doughnut sign.[6] Second, serial scans demonstrating an enlarging abnormality with increasing intensity correlate with early congestive heart failure (CHF) and mortality.[7] In the postacute setting, technetium-99m-pyrophosphate scans that remain abnormal for more than 3 months are associated with an increased risk of future ischemic events.[8]

RADIONUCLIDE VENTRICULOGRAPHY

Resting left ventricular (LV) function as an indirect measure of infarct size can be easily determined at the bedside by gated radionuclide technique. Left ventricular ejection fraction (LVEF) in early MI has proved a reliable measure of the impact of coronary occlusion on LV function and, as such, an important predictor of prognosis.[1-4] In these patients, an ejection fraction of 0.30 during the first 24 hours postinfarction appears to represent a watershed with approximately half the patients with values at or below this level succumbing to left heart failure and/or death (a nearly ninefold higher mortality than patients with a LVEF greater than 0.30).[2] Conversely, only approximately 2 percent of patients with higher ejection fractions will die acutely. Interestingly, isolated quantitation of right ventricular (RV) function immediately postinfarction has not proved a useful indicator of prognosis, even though it can clearly aid in the diagnosis of RV infarction. However, when a depressed right ventricular ejection fraction (RVEF) (0.38 or less) coexists with a LVEF of 0.30 or less, a threefold higher 1-year mortality rate has been demonstrated than with a low LVEF alone.[9] Optimally, prediction of 90-day mortality in acute MI is embodied by a combination of early LVEF and clinical status as defined by Killip class.[10]

While less quantitative, abnormal regional wall motion has shown to predict early mortality in acute myocardial injury. According to Ong et al.,[1] abnormal contraction of more than 70 percent of LV regions during the first 24 hours of the onset of symptoms post-MI is strongly predictive of a poor prognosis, as measured by 90-day mortality.

MYOCARDIAL PERFUSION IMAGING

Resting imaging with ^{201}Tl in acute myocardial infarction is a measure of locally compromised perfusion, which includes both irreversibly damaged and ischemic myocardium. Most MIs are detectable as defects in patients scanned within 6 hours of the onset of symptoms; the size of the defect in this early stage is a powerful predictor of morbidity and mortality. Various grading systems (defect scores) have been devised to reflect the size of the defect, hence the severity of the event. Regardless of the scoring system employed, it appears that a defect of approximately one-third of the LV myocardial circumference

in a given view distinguishes between high- and low-risk patients. Silverman et al.[11] reported a 46 percent 6-month mortality rate with early defects of 40 percent or more of LV circumference, but only an 8 percent mortality over the same period with smaller defects. These investigators also found this approach to be a more sensitive predictor than initial resting LVEF by gated blood-pool imaging. This may be indicative of the measurement of both infarcted and ischemic but viable tissue by the thallium study and perhaps the maintenance of LVEF in some patients by hyperkinetic unaffected myocardium on the radionuclide ventriculogram.

Convalescent Period

Establishing risk for future cardiac events and mortality in patients in the prehospital discharge convalescent phase of acute MI has special significance in determining therapeutic direction. Once a patient has survived the initial insult, attention is focused on assessing the need for, and rigor of, medical or surgical intervention. For the most part, the merit of such therapy hinges on the demonstration of significant myocardium still at risk. The definition of what is considered significant is frequently relative to the amount of functioning myocardium already lost in a given patient. If salvageable tissue important to the patient's functional status is demonstrated, arteriography and surgical or angioplastic intervention can be recommended.

In short, the goal of risk stratification in this setting is to segregate essentially two groups of acute MI survivors: (1) a low-risk group exhibiting little propensity for future cardiac events and that can be expected to do well under conservative medical management, and (2) a high-risk population with a significantly increased likelihood of recurrent insults when medically managed, such that coronary arteriography and surgical therapy may be indicated.

While radionuclide examinations of the resting heart may provide important data in the convalescent phase of acute MI, predischarge exercise testing employing radionuclide techniques is by far the more sensitive approach. Since such studies are routinely conducted at submaximal exercise, the data provided are uniformly prognostically more significant and reliable than electrocardiogram(ECG)-monitored stress testing alone. Generally, candidates for exercise testing are those with MI uncomplicated by such findings as CHF, unstable angina at rest, or significant dysrhythmias within several days of testing.

INFARCT-AVID IMAGING

As with immediate prognosis, the long-term prognosis of patients suffering MI varies directly with estimates of infarct size. Patients with large areas of focal technetium-99m-pyrophosphate activity are at high risk for unstable angina, recurrent MI, or death following hospital discharge. Comparison of the predictive value of the amount of involved myocardium as mapped by infarct-avid imaging with clinical and laboratory assessment has shown the radionuclide technique to be superior to peak creatinine kinase levels in predicting future complications.[7]

RESTING RADIONUCLIDE VENTRICULOGRAPHY

Left ventricular ejection fraction data acquired early after acute MI have been shown to have prognostic implications beyond those of early inhospital risk. Becker et al.[4] confirmed that early in the course of acute myocardial infarction, LVEF values above or below 0.35 are predictive of intermediate (6-month) mortality. While those patients with LVEF values at or below 0.35 exhibited a 60 percent mortality at 6 months, only 11 percent of those with LVEF values above this level had died. Similarly, this watershed level of resting LVEF has been effective in

segregating high- and low-risk mortality groups during the first year postinfarction. The Multicenter Postinfarction Research Group analysis of 811 infarct survivors confirmed a continuum of the relationship between predischarge resting LVEF and mortality risk during the first year postinfarction.[12] It also further extended the validity of a 0.35 to 0.40 LVEF watershed to 3 years postinfarction. In fact, predischarge LVEF remained the single most reliable indicator of MI mortality risk demonstrating a 2.4 times greater risk of death when the LVEF fell below the 0.40 level. Independently, the demonstration of a LV aneurysm after anterior wall MI appears to represent a distinct high-risk predictor of death the first year postinfarction.

EXERCISE RADIONUCLIDE VENTRICULOGRAPHY

While resting radionuclide ventriculography (RNV) primarily evaluates the functional significance of LV fibrosis (scar) in the post-MI patient, exercise RNV can determine the degree of residual and possibly reversible myocardial ischemia (myocardium at risk). In addition to providing prognostic information, this assessment is critical to the selection of postinfarction therapy. For these purposes, exercise RNV appears to be of greatest clinical value when applied in the late hospital stage of acute MI. Risk stratification may thus be optimized by determining the amount of additional and potentially salvageable myocardium at risk and quantifying its functional impact on an already damaged ventricle.

Since the work of Corbett et al.[14] in the early 1980s, which established postinfarction LVEF response to exercise as an independent accurate predictor of future unstable or refractory angina, recurrent MI, or death, much effort has been expended in refining the use of exercise ventriculography for the prediction of outcome in the post-MI patient. Generally, the collective data generated have confirmed that exercise RNV results give better overall risk descriptors than do arteriography, exercise ECG-monitored treadmill stress, or resting LVEF. As prognostic indicators, parameters of exercise RNV that have been specifically studied include (1) global LVEF response to exercise, (2) absolute LVEF at peak exercise, and (3) induction or worsening of LV wall-motion abnormalities.

In a study by Hung et al.,[15] 117 males were evaluated 3 weeks postinfarction by a variety of noninvasive tests, including LV RNV. Follow-up over approximately 1 year showed that serious cardiac events, including death, were best predicted by LVEF response to exercise and by peak stress workload achieved at exercise. A decrease in LVEF during exercise of 0.05 or greater foretold a 23 percent incidence of major events during the first year postinfarction.

More recently, Borer et al.[16,17] summarized a collaborative study that attempted to refine the use of LVEF response to stress as a risk stratifier by relating these data to early resting LVEF in postinfarction patients. These workers found a resting LVEF to be a valid predictor of death in this population, with a mortality rate of more than 40 percent over 3½ years in patients with resting LVEF values of less than 0.30. However, it appears that patients with resting LVEF greater than 0.30 can be further risk-segregated according to their LVEF response to exercise. In this study, the latter group of patients was found to include no mortalities over 3½ years postinfarction when LVEF response to exercise was normal (greater than or equal to a 0.05 rise from resting values) but to have a 10 percent mortality rate over the same period of time when LVEF response was abnormal, demonstrating residual myocardium at risk.

The absolute value of predischarge exercise LVEF at peak stress was found by Morris et al.[18] to be a potent mortality predictor in 106 acute MI survivors followed for approximately 4 years. In this population, 4-year survival greater than 90 percent was seen in patients with peak exercise LVEF values at or greater than 0.40. Survival of less than 50 percent was seen in those with values less than 0.40. In this study, a peak exercise LVEF of 0.40 again appeared to present a prognostic watershed.

Exercise ventriculography has also been used to predict the angiographic presence of high-risk multivessel coronary artery disease in patients experiencing a single transmural MI. Morris et al.[19] found exercise RNV a more significant predictor in this respect than other clinical and exercise ECG parameters. Using a combination of abnormal LVEF response to exercise and stress-induced wall-motion abnormalities at a distance from the known MI, exercise RNV was found to be 62 percent sensitive and 75 percent specific for predicting multivessel CAD in this population.

In terms of patient management decisions, it would seem that angiography in anticipation of possible surgical intervention could well be justified in high-risk post-MI patients as segregated by exercise RNV findings of an absolute peak exercise LVEF of less than 0.40 or a fall in exercise LVEF of 0.05 or greater from resting values.

EXERCISE THALLIUM-201 IMAGING

The role of predischarge exercise ^{201}Tl imaging in the postinfarction patient is primarily that of risk stratification based on the identification of significant residual peri-infarct ischemia (myocardium at risk) and/or ischemia remote from the acute injury (multivessel disease) with their attendant therapeutic management implications.

High-risk findings indicative of future postinfarction ischemic events include (1) multiple stress-induced defects in more than one vascular distribution compatible with multivessel disease[20]; (2) stress-induced defects that show only partial redistribution, compatible with an infarct with residual peri-infarct ischemia[21]; and (3) abnormally increased pulmonary activity at exercise, reflecting stress-induced LV dysfunction.[22]

Conversely, low-risk findings on exercise ^{201}Tl testing include (1) a normal study[23–25]; and (2) single vascular territory defects at stress that do not change significantly on redistribution views, indicative of no residual peri-infarct ischemia and without abnormal ^{201}Tl lung activity.[26]

Using such criteria, Gibson et al.[27] evaluated 140 consecutive patients with uncomplicated MI. Their group found similar high-risk criteria to be 94 percent sensitive overall as an indicator of future significant cardiac events, more sensitive than submaximal exercise-induced ST-segment depression or chest pain, or angiographic delineation of CAD for nonfatal events, and equally predictive of mortality. Furthermore, in patients with single-vessel disease, evidence of residual ischemia in the infarct zone proved to be 92 percent sensitive for reinfarction or severe angina during 15 months of follow-up. Interestingly, the low-risk criteria were particularly reliable in identifying patients with low postinfarction risk of future cardiac events (6 percent) with a low false-negative rate.

Other studies of postinfarction patients have confirmed that (1) the presence of an exercise thallium scintigraphic defect remote from the vascular distribution of the known MI is perhaps the most reliable indicator of underlying high-risk multivessel or left main CAD[28]; and (2) both the size as well as the degree of redistribution are significant parameters in predicting future cardiac events.[15] Since the high-risk stress ^{201}Tl scintigram is significantly more predictive of future cardiac events related to residual ischemia or multi-

vessel CAD than ECG stress testing in the postinfarction setting,[201]Tl stress testing offers a more sensitive method of segregating high-risk patients for angiographic evaluation and possible bypass surgery.

DIPYRIDAMOLE-THALLIUM-201 IMAGING

As an alternative to stress ^{201}Tl scintigraphy, dipyridamole-^{201}Tl imaging may safely provide significant predictive data. Using this technique in 51 asymptomatic postinfarction patients studied before discharge, Leppo et al.[29] demonstrated a greater than 90 percent sensitivity of this technique, which revealed an approximate six times greater chance of subsequent cardiac events over 19 months when reversible dipyridamole-induced hypoperfusion was identified. Because this examination eliminates the need for exercise, it may prove of great benefit in a subpopulation of post-MI patients with a reduced tolerance for exercise, permitting the segregation of an otherwise unidentifiable subgroup of asymptomatic post-MI patients at higher risk of adverse events.

EXERCISE RNV VERSUS EXERCISE THALLIUM-201 IMAGING

Both examinations have proved to be efficacious in segregating high- and low-risk groups and in predicting subsequent events when used in a setting of predischarge evaluation of post-MI patients. Currently, there is no clear evidence to recommend one examination over the other, since sufficient detailed comparisons in a given patient population are lacking. Choice of examination generally is left to the biases of the referring and imaging physicians at a given institution.

Since both techniques have shown to be generally more sensitive for risk stratification purposes in post-MI patients than either routine exercise ECG or coronary arteriography, incorporation of one or the other into protocols for the evaluation of patients during the postinfarction period will greatly enhance the efficacy of such an effort.

CHRONIC SYMPTOMATIC OR KNOWN CORONARY ARTERY DISEASE

The risk of MI in patients with known CAD is related primarily to (1) the severity of compromised blood flow, and (2) the amount of potentially jeopardized cardiac muscle. Detection and semiquantitation of these parameters is basic to the concept of risk stratification in this population, hence to the determination of therapeutic course. In this respect, exercise radionuclide testing of LV myocardial perfusion and function frequently provides the most reliable noninvasive means of obtaining such information. Approaches and techniques may vary but, when used in the appropriate setting, stress ^{201}Tl perfusion imaging, exercise gated ventriculography, and radionuclide scintiangiography at exercise are each of significant value.

Coronary arteriography, traditionally thought of as the gold standard for the evaluation of CAD, has recently been rivaled, and in some respects eclipsed, by noninvasive radionuclide techniques in providing prognostically significant information regarding the severity and extent of compromised myocardial blood flow reserve. The well-demonstrated potential for discordancy between the number, distribution, and degree of coronary artery stenoses as demonstrated angiographically and the amount and location of jeopardized myocardium shown on exercise radionuclide studies provides a rationale for the use of such noninvasive examinations not only to assess the significance of coronary angiographic findings, but for their employment as the initial test to predict risk and determine the need for further angiographic evaluation.

Specific risk and decision-making implications of these diagnostic capabilities are discussed below.

Exercise (Stress) Thallium-201 Scintigraphy

As a direct measure of the degree and distribution of impaired myocardial perfusion at stress, ^{201}Tl imaging has been substantiated by numerous studies as an effective technology for assessing risk of future cardiac events in patients with presumed chronic or known CAD.

Several recent studies have confirmed the negative predictive value of normal maximal exercise ^{201}Tl studies in patients with chest pain or suspected CAD when adequate heart rates are achieved.[23–25, 30] In general, cardiac event rates in this population are less than 1 percent per year. This rate is virtually indistinguishable from that seen in patients with normal coronary arteriograms. In addition, several studies have indicated a good short-term prognosis in patients with positive exercise ECG findings but normal exercise ^{201}Tl images.[25,31]

Findings on abnormal ^{201}Tl stress imaging that have been found to represent potent prognosticators of future cardiac events have also been identified. Included among such risk stratifiers are the following:

1. Number of reversible thallium defects (an indicator of multivessel disease)
2. Initial size and severity of the reversible defect
3. Reversible defects in the left main coronary artery distribution
4. Abnormal lung accumulation of [201]Tl

Since in general, diminished exercise tolerance is a poor prognostic sign in patients with coronary artery disease, the occurrence of any of the above findings at low levels of stress, as reflected by heart rate may magnify their significance implying a worse prognosis.[32]

NUMBER OF REVERSIBLE THALLIUM DEFECTS

The risk of mortality in patients in CAD is directly related to the number of stenotic vessels and the severity of those stenoses. While coronary arteriography can define the anatomic distribution of disease, it cannot directly determine the significance of the stenosis with respect to its potential for producing ischemia. Because exercise-redistribution ^{201}Tl imaging provides a direct sensitive marker of myocardial perfusion and ischemia and has a high specificity for individual coronary vessels (especially with computer-assisted quantitative analysis), the finding of ^{201}Tl perfusion defects in a multivascular distribution gives reliable evidence of significant multivessel CAD. Tomographic imaging permits better contrast resolution of thallium defects and therefore appears to improve the definition of multivessel CAD. In a study of 568 patients, Staniloff et al.[33] reported a 1-year cardiac event rate of 16 percent in patients with multiple reversible thallium defects and a rate of 21 percent with severe thallium defects, as defined by their criteria. Brown et al.[20] suggested that the identification of multiple regions of reversible myocardial ischemia at exercise ^{201}Tl imaging (suggestive of multivessel disease) may be a better predictor of a poor clinical prognosis than coronary arteriography. This may pertain equally as well to patients with single-vessel angiographic disease who exhibit a multivessel scintigraphy pattern due to variations in normal vascular supply.

INITIAL SIZE AND SEVERITY OF REVERSIBLE THALLIUM-201 DEFECTS

As measures of the amount of myocardium supplied by a stenotic vessel (myocardium at risk) and the degree of stenotic abnormality (potential for ischemia), the size and severity of reversible thallium defects (as variously defined by independent investigators) directly reflect the risk of future cardiac events. In 816 consecutive patients evaluated for chest pain, Iskandrian et al.[34] reported the size of thallium defects in the postexercise images to be their single most important predictor of subsequent events. This group also concluded that patients with large perfusion defects at exercise should be considered surgical candidates, regardless of their symptomatology, because of the attendant risk of adverse outcomes on medical therapy. Separately, a significantly elevated 1-year cardiac rate of 21 percent has been reported with severe thallium defects at exercise, designating this finding a high-risk predictor.[33]

REVERSIBLE DEFECTS IN THE LEFT MAIN CORONARY ARTERY DISTRIBUTION

Significant left main coronary artery (LMCA) stenosis is a well-defined category of high-risk CAD with a known poor prognosis with medical treatment. Noninvasive identification of these patients may take on added significance with recent advances in PTCA techniques. While the appearance of this high-risk perfusion pattern on ^{201}Tl stress images is a predictable reflection of decreased perfusion in the distribution of the left anterior descending (LAD) and circumflex arteries (the septum, free wall, and posterolateral wall of the left ventricle), it is in fact an uncommon finding in LMCA stenosis and may be seen in patients with multivessel disease with or without LMCA disease.[35] Thus, the LMCA pattern more frequently reflects the presence of stenoses in left coronary artery branches (LAD and circumflex arteries). Nevertheless, when identified, the pattern is indicative of high-risk coronary disease.

ABNORMAL LUNG ACCUMULATION OF THALLIUM-201

Abnormally increased lung activity at ^{201}Tl stress scintigraphy has consistently shown to be a marker of transient LV dysfunction at exercise.[36,37] In patients without noncoronary causes of resting LV dysfunction, such activity reflects a rise in left ventricular end-diastolic pressure (LVEDP) caused by significant stress-induced myocardial ischemia, resulting in transient interstitial pulmonary edema. Circulating ^{201}Tl present at the point of peak stress will serve as a marker of elevated pulmonary capillary pressure and interstitial lung fluid, manifested as increased lung activity on the immediate postexercise images. As pulmonary pressure returns to normal and pulmonary edema subsides, the scintigram approaches normal on the delayed images.

Whether determined by qualitative or quantitative methodology, abnormally increased thallium uptake in the lungs has been shown to correlate anatomically with multivessel CAD or single-vessel disease involving either a dominant left circumflex artery or a high-grade proximal LAD lesion and clinically with increased morbidity and mortality rates.[22,38] In an evaluation of 436 patients with known or suspected ischemic heart disease, Gill et al.[39] found that the presence of increased pulmonary thallium activity during exercise, as assessed by qualitative visual interpretation, exceeded the predictive value of other clinical, exercise, or thallium imaging variables for identifying patients at higher risk of adverse cardiac events during a 5-year follow-up period. This held true in the presence or absence of previous MI. Furthermore, patients exhibiting reversible thallium perfusion defects without increased lung activity were at intermediate risk, while those with normal scans demonstrated low risk of future events.

Exercise Radionuclide Ventriculography

Evaluation of LV function in the setting of CAD primarily provides a measure of fibrosis (lost myocardium) when ventriculography is performed at rest and is an indicator of both fibrosis and ischemia (myocardium at risk) when performed with adequate exercise stress. Attempts at risk stratification, using either gated or first-pass exercise ventriculography with or without consideration or resting LV function, have generally focused on the easily derived parameters of LVEF response to stress, absolute LVEF reached at peak exercise, induction or worsening of wall-motion abnormalities, and the level of stress accomplished during exercise. While the precise mapping of areas of stress-induced ischemia is not as practical with stress ventriculography as with ^{201}Tl perfusion imaging, the degree of functional impact of CAD on the heart derived from this technique can provide important predictors of future adverse events.

As with a normal exercise ^{201}Tl study, a low 1-year cardiac event rate can likewise be expected with normal LVEF and wall-motion responses to maximal stress.[40] Still, there remains a paucity of information regarding the prognostic value of exercise ventriculography in patients with known or suspected CAD and without a history of MI. However, the available data suggest an emerging role of exercise RNV in this setting.

In a population of 386 patients with stable angina pectoris (using upright radionuclide first-pass technique), Pryor et al.[41] reported that by both univariate and multivariate analysis, absolute exercise LVEF was the parameter most predictive of future adverse events. This was followed, respectively, by resting LVEF, wall-motion abnormalities, and exercise duration. While this study did not find LVEF response to stress to be a significant predictor, other investigators have found a direct relationship between exercise ejection fraction response and high-risk disease and survival. Phillips et al.[42] reported a decrease in normal resting LVEF values of 0.10 or more at exercise to be predictive of an approximate 50 percent likelihood of proximal left main or three-vessel disease. Bonow et al,[43] at the National Institutes of Health (NIH), confirmed the predictive value of decreasing LVEF during exercise for a significantly higher mortality in medically treated mildly symptomatic patients with three-vessel disease and preserved resting LV function.

Iskandrian et al.[44] evaluated risk stratification by exercise ventriculography in 604 patients with known or suspected CAD and by multivariate and univariate analysis identified the exercise LVEF ejection fraction as the most important predictor of deaths and of total adverse events. In this study, a predictive cutoff at an exercise LVEF of 0.50 was determined: patients with values at or above this level had significantly lower risk of future events, even among those with a history of previous coronary artery bypass grafts. Furthermore, risk was seen to increase progressively in a stepwise fashion as exercise LVEF decreased below the 0.50 cutoff. On the basis of these results, and earlier observations that maximum exercise heart rate had a significant predictive value, Iskandrian et al.[45] suggest that a simple clinical decision-making scheme may be valid. By segregating patients into high-risk, medium-risk, and low-risk groups, appropriate clinical decisions regarding conservative medical therapy, the need for arteriography, and surgical intervention may be facilitated:

High risk: Exercise LVEF less than 0.50 and exercise heart rate less than 120 bpm; event rate of 14 percent

Intermediate risk: Either exercise LVEF less than 0.50 or exercise heart rate (HR) less than 120 bpm; event rate of 7.7 percent

Low risk: Exercise LVEF greater than or equal to 0.50 and exercise HR greater than or equal to 120 bpm; event rate of 3.2 percent

Such evaluation in postcoronary bypass patients should provide valuable prognostic information in this setting as well.

The role of exercise radionuclide angiography in therapeutic decision-making has been explored in several nonrandomized studies. The largest of these includes the results of the Duke University data base relating to risk stratification of patients with known CAD and the identification of patients who may best benefit from surgical intervention with respect to pain relief, improvement of LV functional reserve, and prolongation of life. Using resting LVEF as a measure of permanent damage to the LV myocardium unlikely to be reversed by revascularization procedures and first-pass exercise LVEF response as an indicator of ischemic myocardium salvageable by such procedures, Jones[46] identified four subgroups in 857 patients with known CAD followed for 30 months: (1) 105 patients with normal rest and exercise left RNV (no fibrosis or ischemia) who exhibited excellent survival and equally variable pain relief with either medical or surgical treatment: (2) 413 patients with normal resting function but abnormal LV response to exercise (no fibrosis but evidence of ischemia) who experienced overall better long-term survival and pain relief when treated surgically rather than medically; (3) 103 patients with abnormal resting but normal stress ventriculograms (fibrosis with no evidence of ischemia) who showed better survival with medical therapy than with surgical treatment; and (4) 236 patients with abnormal resting LV function that further deteriorated during exercise (significant fibrosis and ischemia) who experienced poor survival and pain relief with medical therapy. However, long-term survival after surgical therapy was very good in this last group, and complete pain relief was common, even though there was a higher operative mortality. Significantly, both subgroups of patients without ischemia showed no benefit from revascularization surgery, whereas those subgroups with stress-induced ischemia did benefit.

While validation of these findings awaits randomized data, the potential for noninvasive functional information obtained through exercise left RNV for the risk stratification and prognostification of patients with CAD and the selection of appropriate treatment appears to be significant.

PREDICTION OF POST-PTCA RESTENOSIS

As experience with percutaneous transluminal coronary angioplasty (PTCA) has increased and as technologic improvements have been advanced, the success and complication rates of the procedure have significantly improved. Unfortunately, late restenosis, usually occurring within 6 months of dilation, remains a serious problem. While noninvasive radionuclide studies have been widely used to evaluate initial success after PTCA, data regarding their value as early prognosticators of future restenosis are less well established.

In general, it may be that the ability of exercise radionuclide studies performed during the early post-PTCA period (less than 1 month) to predict late restenosis depends in part on when those studies are performed, since such restenosis may occur as soon as 2 to 4 weeks postdilation. Using exercise thallium examinations performed 1 week post-PTCA, Stuckey et al.[47] concluded that exercise perfusion imaging was not useful as a predictor of late restenosis. However, using exercise thallium studies performed at 4 weeks post-PTCA, Wijns et al.[48] reported reversible perfusion defects to be approximately 75 percent accurate in predicting restenosis at 6 months.

More recently, O'Keefe et al.[49] showed the value of early post-PTCA exercise radionuclide angiography in segregating high- and low-risk groups for late restenosis. In their study, a normal exercise radionuclide angiogram within 1 month post-PTCA was highly predictive of a successful long-term dilation.

However, an abnormal examination was only 42 percent predictive in their population. Thus, in their experience, post-PTCA exercise radionuclide angiography seems to be most useful in identifying patients with low risk of restenosis.

REFERENCES

1. Ong L, Green S, Reiser P, et al: Early prediction of mortality in patients with acute myocardial infarction: A prospective study of clinical and radionuclide risk factors. Am J Cardiol 57:33, 1986
2. Shah PK, Pichler M, Berman OS, et al: Left ventricular ejection fraction determined by radionuclide ventriculography in early stages of first transmural myocardial infarction. Relation to short-term prognosis. Am J Cardiol 45:542, 1980
3. Dewhurst NG, Hannan WJ, Muir AL: Prognostic value of radionuclide ventriculography after myocardial infarction. Q J Med 49:479, 1981
4. Becker LC, Silverman KJ, Bulkley BH, et al: Comparison of early thallium-201 scintigraphy and gated blood pool imaging for predicting mortality in patients with acute myocardial infarction. Circulation 67:1272, 1983
5. Rude RE, Parkey RW, Bonte FJ, et al: Clinical implications of the technetium-99m stannous pyrophosphate myocardial scintigraphic "doughnut" pattern in patients with acute myocardial infarcts. Circulation 59:721, 1979
6. Ahmad M, Logan KW, Martin RH: Doughnut pattern of technetium-99m pyrophosphate myocardial uptake in patients with acute myocardial infarction: A sign of poor long-term prognosis. Am J Cardiol 44:13, 1979
7. Holman BL, Chisholm RJ, Braunwald E: The prognostic implications of acute myocardial infarct scintigraphy with 99m-Tc-pyrophosphate. Circulation 57:320, 1978
8. Buja LM, Poliner LR, Parkey RW, et al: Clinicopathologic study of persistently positive technetium-99m stannous pyrophosphate myocardial infarction. Circulation 56:1016, 1977

9. Shah PR, Maddahi J, Staniloff HM, et al: Variable spectrum and prognostic implications of left and right ventricular ejection fractions in patients with and without clinical heart failure after acute myocardial infarction. Am J Cardiol 58:387, 1986

10. Ong L, Valdellon B, Coromilas J, et al: Precordial S-T segment depression in inferior myocardial infarction. Evaluation by quantitative thallium-201 scintigraphy and technetium-99m ventriculography. Am J Cardiol 51:734, 1983

11. Silverman KJ, Becker LC, Bulkley BH, et al: Value of early thallium-201 scintigraphy for predicting mortality in patients with acute myocardial infarction. Circulation 61:996, 1980

12. The Multicenter Postinfarction Research Group: Risk stratification and survival after myocardial infarction. N Engl J Med 309:331, 1983

13. Meizlish JL, Berger HJ, Plankey M, et al: Functional left ventricular aneurysm formation after acute anterior transmural myocardial infarction. Incidence, natural history, and prognostic implication. N Engl J Med 311:1001, 1984

14. Corbett JR, Dehmer GJ, Lewis SE, et al: The prognostic value of submaximal exercise testing with radionuclide ventriculography before hospital discharge in patients with recent myocardial infarction. Circulation 64:535, 1981

15. Hung J, Goris ML, Nash E, et al: Comparative value of maximal treadmill testing, exercise thallium myocardial perfusion scintigraphy and exercise radionuclide ventriculography for distinguishing high- and low-risk patients soon after acute myocardial infarction. Am J Cardiol 53:1221, 1984

16. Borer JS, Miller D, Schreiber T, et al: Radionuclide cineangiography in acute myocardial infarction: Role in prognostication. Semin Nucl Med 17:89, 1987

17. Grodzinski E, Fentrop T, Scharf-Bornhofen E, et al: Bedeutung der auswurffraktion(EF) in ruhe und bei belastung mit hilfe der radionuklidventrikulographie (RNVA) fur die Prognose von herzinfarkt patienten. Z Kardiol 74(9):525, 1985

18. Morris KG, Palmeri St, Califf RM, et al: Vaue of radionuclide angiography for predicting specific cardiac events after acute myocardial infarction. Am J Cardiol 55:318, 1985

19. Morris DD, Rozanski A, Berman DS, et al: Noninvasive prediction of the angiographic extent of coronary artery disease after myocardial infarction: Comparison of clinical, bicycle exercise electrocardiographic, and ventriculographic parameters. Circulation 70:192, 1979

20. Brown KA et al: Prognostic value of exercise thallium-201 imaging in patients presenting for evaluation of chest pain. J Am Coll Cardiol 1:994, 1983

21. Staniloff HM, Diamond G, Forrester J, et al: Prediction of death, infarction and worsening chest pain with exercise electrocardiography and thallium scintigraphy, abstracted. Am J Cardiol 49:967, 1982

22. Gibson RS, Watson DD, Carabello BA, et al: Clinical implications of increased lung uptake of thallium-201 during exercise scintigraphy 2 weeks after myocardial infarction. Am J Cardiol 49:1586, 1982

23. Wackers FJT, Russo DJ, Russo D, et al: Prognostic significance of normal quantitative planar thallium-201 stress scintigraphy in patients with chest pain. J Am Coll Cardiol 6:27, 1985

24. Wahl JM, Hakki A, Iskandrian AS: Prognostic implications of normal exercise thallium-201 images. Arch Intern Med 145:253, 1985

25. Pamelia FX, Gibson RS, Watson DD, et al: Prognosis with chest pain and normal thallium-201 exercise scintigrams. Am J Cardiol 55:920, 1985

26. Gibson RS, Watson DD, Craddock GB, et al: Prediction of cardiac events after uncomplicated myocardial infarction: A prospective study comparing predischarge exercise thallium-201 scintigraphy and coronary angiography. Circulation 68:321, 1983

27. Gibson RS, Watson DD, Craddock GB, et al: Prediction of cardiac events after uncomplicated myocardial infarction: A prospective study comparing predischarge exercise thallium-201 scintigraphy and coronary angiography. Circulation 68:321, 1983

28. Patterson Re, Horowitz SF, Eng C, et al: Can noninvasive exercise test criteria identify patients with left main or 3-vessel coronary disease after a first myocardial infarction? Am J Cardiol 51:361, 1983

29. Leppo JA, O'Brien J, Rothendler JA, et al: Dipyridamole-thallium-201 scintigraphy in the prediction of future cardiac events after myocardial infarction. N Engl J Med 310:1014, 1984

30. Iskandrian AS, Heo J, Decoskey D, et al: Use of exercise thallium-201 imaging for risk stratification of elderly patients with coronary artery disease. Am J Cardiol 61:269, 1988

31. Beller GA, Gibson RS, Watson DD, et al: Prognosis of patients with chest pain and normal thallium-201 exercise scintigrams, abstr. Circulation 68:III-3, 1983

32. Landenheim ML, Pollack BH, Rozanski A, et al: Extent and severity of myocardial hypoperfusion as orthogonal indices of prognosis in patients with suspected coronary artery disease. J Am Coll Cardiol 7:464, 1986

33. Staniloff H, Diamond G, Forrester J, et al: Prediction of death, infarction, and worsening chest pain with exercise electrocardiography and thallium scintigraphy, abstr. Am J Cardiol 49:967, 1982

34. Iskandrian As, Hakki A-H, Kane SA: The use of exercise thallium-201 imaging in risk stratification in patients with suspected coronary heart disease. Am Heart J 138:135, 1985

35. Nygaard TW, Gibson RS, Ryan JM, et al: Prevalence of high-risk thallium-2301 scintigraphic findings in left main coronary artery stenosis: Comparison with patients with multi- and single-vessel coronary artery disease. Am J Cardiol 53:462, 1984

36. Bingham JB, McKusick KA, Strauss HW, et al: Influence of coronary artery disease on pulmonary uptake of thallium-201. Am J Cardiol 46:821, 1980

37. Boucher CA, Zir LM, Beller GA, et al: Increased lung uptake of thallium-201 during exercise myocardial imaging: clinical, hemodynamic and angiographic implications in patients with coronary artery disease. Am J Cardiol 46:189, 1980

38. Kushner FG, Okada RD, Kirshenbaum HD, et al: Lung thallium-201 uptake after stress testing in patients with coronary artery disease. Circulation 63:341, 1981

39. Gill JB, Ruddy TD, Newell JB, et al: Prognostic importance of thallium uptake by the lungs during exercise in coronary artery disease. N Engl J Med 317:1485, 1987

40. Kotler TS, Pollock BH, Work JW, et al: Prognostic stratification by thallium scintigraphy: Who needs it? J Am Coll Cardiol 6:232, 1986 (abst)

41. Pryor DB, Harrell FE Jr, Lee KL, et al: Prognostic indicators from radionuclide angiography in medically treated patients with coronary artery disease. Am J Cardiol 53:18, 1984

42. Phillips P, Borer JS, Jacobstein J, et al: Prognostically critical coronary stenoses: Identification by radionuclide cineangiography, abstr. Am J Cardiol 49:991, 1982

43. Bonow RO, Kent KM, Rosing DR, et al: Exercise-induced ischemia in mildly symptomatic patients with coronary artery disease and preserved left ventricular function: Identification of subgroups at high risk for death during medical therapy. N Engl J Med 311:1339, 1984

44. Iskandrian AS, Hakki A-H, Goel I, et al: The use of rest and exercise radionuclide ventriculography in risk stratification in patients with suspected coronary artery disease. Am Heart J 110:864, 1985

45. Iskandrian AS, Hakki A-H, Schwartz JS, et al: Prognostic implications of rest and exercise radionuclide ventriculography in patients with suspected or proven coronary heart disease. Int J Cardiol 6:707, 1984

46. Jones RH: Use of radionuclide measurements of left ventricular function for prognosis in patients with coronary artery disease. Semin Nucl Med 17:95, 1987

47. Stuckey TD, Burwell LR, Nygaard TW, et al: Value of quantitative exercise thallium-201 scintigraphy for predicting angina recurrence after percutaneous transluminal coronary angioplasty, abstr. J Am Coll Cardiol 5:531, 1985

48. Wijns W, Serruys PW, Reiber JH, et al: Early detection of restenosis after successful percutancous transluminal coronary angioplasty by exercise-redistribution thallium scintigraphy. Am J Cardiol 55:357, 1985

49. O'Keefe JH, Lapeyre AC, Holmes DR, et al: Usefulness of early radionuclide angiography for identifying low-risk patients for late restenosis after percutenous transluminal coronary angioplasty. Am J Cardiol 61:51, 1988

11

An Introduction to the Positron Camera

Nathaniel M. Alpert
John A. Correia

The evaluation of functionally impaired myocardium is crucial to the diagnosis and management of cardiac disease. There is now considerable clinical experience with myocardial applications of single photon emission tomography (SPECT) and, although these applications provide substantial benefit to the patient, they also have limitations. These limitations, both physical and physiological, have stimulated research on the myocardial applications of positron emission tomography (PET). The appeal of PET is attributable to (1) the unique physical properties associated with nuclear decay by positron emission, making is possible to achieve higher spatial resolution and higher photon sensitivity than does SPECT; (2) the fact that these same physical properties permit absolute measurements of radioactivity concentration, a measurement that is much more difficult with SPECT; and (3) the ease with which many of the positron–emitting isotopes can be incorporated into biologically active molecules without disturbing their fate in vivo.

Over the past several years, PET instrumentation, automation of radiopharmaceutical production, and imaging techniques have matured to the point where they may be considered for use in clinical applications. This chapter reviews the physical principles of positron imaging and discusses the general concepts of instrument development.

PHYSICAL PRINCIPLES OF POSITRON EMISSION TOMOGRAPHY

Some radioactive nuclei decay by emission of a positron, a particle having the same mass as the electron but an opposite charge. Positrons emitted in a tissue-like medium typically travel a short distance (1 to 3 mm)[1–3] and then undergo an annihilation reaction with an electron, such that their masses are converted to energy in the form of two 511-keV photons. The two annihilation photons are emitted at approximately 180 degrees to each other, so that their trajectories determine a straight line of flight. This is the basis of all positron imaging.

These paired photons are detected simultaneously by pairs of radiation detectors, thereby identifying a line of flight. Coincidence circuits that register the detection of a photon pair are incapable of simultaneous detection due to the limited response times of both detectors and electronics. Instead, all events occuring within a finite interval, called the *resolving time,* are registered as coincidence pairs. Since annihilation photons propagate at the speed of light, the time difference in their detection is small; however, this so-called time of flight can be used to further localize the position of the annihilation interaction along the line of flight if fast enough detectors are used. Theoretically, with infinitely fast detectors, the three-dimensional location of the event could be exactly determined, thereby obviating the need to reconstruct the data.

The simplest means for localizing the line of flight of a coincidence pair is to detect both annihilation photons. Knowledge of the location of the detector pair then determines the line of flight with an uncertainty (i.e., resolution) determined by the interaction volume of the detector for 511-keV photons (Fig. 11-1). Measurement of many of these coincidence lines is sufficient to calculate the underlying activity distribution, if certain criteria are met. Detection of the photon pair in time-coincidence is used to increase the probability that an event is a true coincidence. The term *true coincidence* refers to events involving two photons from the same annihilation reaction; the terms *random coincidence* and *accidental coincidence* refer to events involving two or more photons from different annhilation processes (Fig. 11-2). The accidental coincidence rate increases linearly with the coincidence resolving time and quadratically with the count rate of the individual detectors. This contribution can thus be estimated and subtracted from the total coincidence rate, if the individual detector rates and coincidence resolving time are measured.[4] When one or both of the annihilation photons undergoes Compton scattering, a true coincidence may still be registered, leading to an

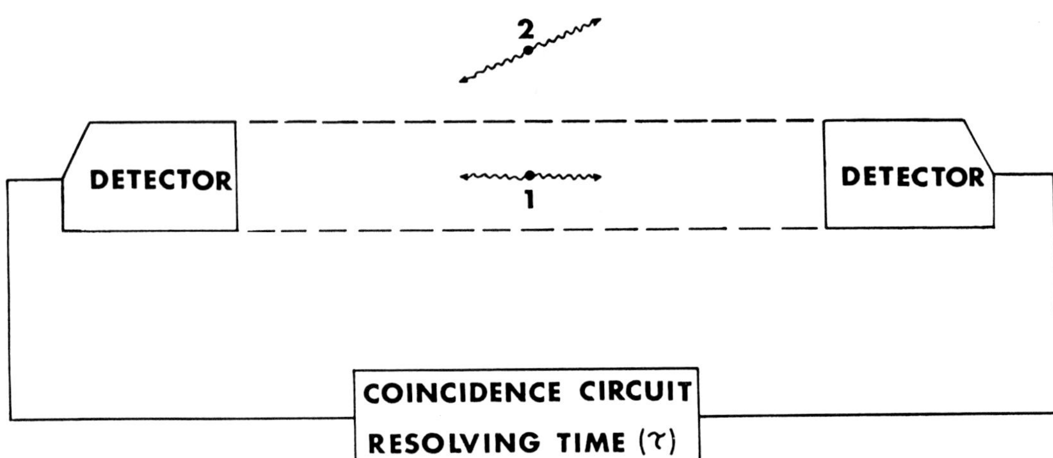

Fig. 11-1 Schematic representation of the principle of coincidence detection. Annihilation photons occurring in the sensitive volume denoted by the dashed lines, such as those labeled 1 in the figure, may give rise to true coincidence events. Those occurring outside the sensitive volume can only contribute to the accidental coincidence rate.

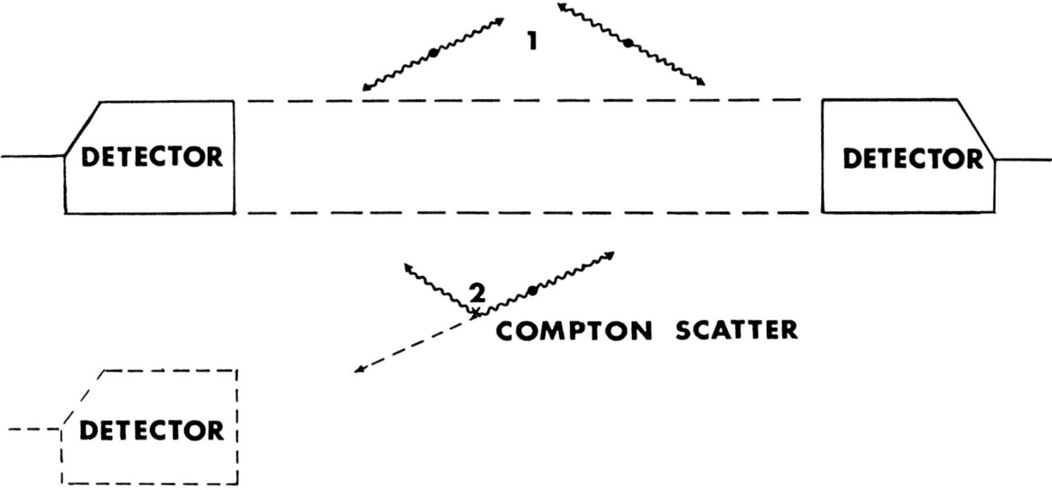

Fig. 11-2 Accidental and scatter coincidence events. Events labeled 1 may be recorded as an accidental coincidence if photons from both annihilation pairs are detected within the coincidence resolving time. Events labeled 2 may give rise to a scatter coincidence. These are true coincidences, since they arise from a single positron annihilation event. However, they may occur outside the sensitive volume and thereby degrade the spatial resolution.

incorrect determination of the line of flight (Fig. 11-2). Some of these scatter coincidences can be rejected electronically through the use of energy discrimination; some may be absorbed by collimators; in some instances, the effect of those remaining can be taken into account during image reconstruction.[5,6]

When compared with conventional single photon detection methods, the use of coincidence detection of annihilation radiation has a number of physical advantages that result in an ability to make quantitative measurements of radioactivity concentrations in vivo. With coincidence detection, all true coincidence events originate in the tubelike volume connecting the detector faces. True coincidences are registered with nearly equal sensitivity, independent of the source location between the detectors. The spatial resolution of a detector pair is largely determined by its cross-sectional dimensions (e.g., width and height) of the detector and this resolution is also nearly independent of source position along the line connecting the detectors. Colli-

mation is used to reduce scattered radiation and accidental coincidences rather than to improve spatial resolution as is the case with single photon systems; this leads to at least a 100-fold increase of sensitivity for PET relative to SPECT. The fact that photon absorption depends on the total attenuation length traversed by the photon pair (Fig. 11-3), rather than the specific location of the event (as it does for single photon applications), leads to simple and accurate methods for absorption correction, including absorption measurements with an external source or calculated corrections based on a knowledge of absorber boundary.[7–11]

INSTRUMENTATION

Positron emission tomography instruments are constructed by replication of elemental detector pairs, i.e. coincidence pairs. The physical size of an elemental detector, as well as the detector material, limit the spatial and temporal resolution of a complete instrument. The number of detectors, their

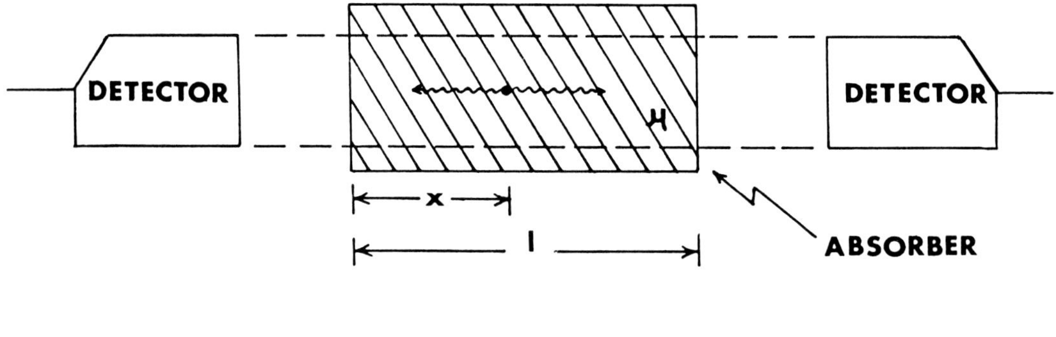

$$P\,(\text{COINCIDENCE}) \sim e^{-\mu x} \cdot e^{-\mu(l-x)} = e^{-\mu l}$$
$$\text{DETECTION}$$

Fig. 11-3 Principle of attenuation correction with PET. An event occurring within the sensitive volume gives rise to two annihilation photons, which together traverse the same thickness of absorber, independent of the origin of the event along the line of flight. Mathematically, the probability of coincidence detection is proportional to $e^{-\mu l}$. Since the attenuation is independent of source position along the line of flight, an external source can be used to measure $e^{-\mu l}$ for each detector channel.

geometric arrangement, and the stopping power and photofraction of the detector material play an important role in determining the overall sensitivity of a given instrument.

A positron camera usually consists of several interconnected modules, including the gantry and detector assembly, electronic processing modules, and associated computer hardware. Annihilation photons interact with the detector material, creating an electronic signal whose pulse height is proportional to the energy deposited in the detector and whose shape and duration depend on the detector material. These signals are amplified and fed to the electronic processing circuits, where a discriminator removes pulses whose amplitude are below a preselected energy (usually 200 to 300 keV). The signals are checked to determine whether additional events have occurred within the coincidence resolving time. Each potential coincidence is also checked against a list of valid detector pairs stored in programmable read only memory (PROM) circuitry. Once a valid coincidence has been identified, the position of its line of flight is digitally encoded. These data are buffered either as a histogram of the projections or as individual listmode events, which are subsequently transferred to magnetic disk storage.

Image reconstruction in non–time-of-flight instruments is usually performed with use of the now familiar filtered backprojection method.[12] Coincidence data from a given slice are first sorted into projections; corrected for physical effects such as random coincidences, photon attenuation, detector uniformity, and scatter coincidences, and then reconstructed. In time-of-flight tomographs, more complex and computationally demanding algorithms are used.[13–15] If care is taken in instrument calibration and in correcting for real-world effects, the reconstructed images of activity concentration can be accurate to about 5 percent.[4,6]

The spatial resolution of reconstructed images in recently designed positron tomographs ranges from about 3 to 6 mm full width at half-maximum (FWHM)[16–20] in the transverse plane with axial resolution of the same order, roughly a 100 percent improvement since 1985. The improvement in axial resolution emphasizes the growing realization that spatial resolution should be comparable in all three dimensions. It should also be noted that improvements in spatial resolution are usually accompanied by reductions in sensitivity. All else being equal, a twofold improvement in axial resolution is accompanied by a fourfold loss in sensitivity. However, the current generation of tomographs generally have increased sensitivity, by virtue of their geometry, which features closely packed (no shielding between detectors) arrays of small detectors. Some tomographs now achieve transverse-plane resolution of about 6 mm without the need for any mechanical motion of the detector assembly,[16,18,19] a feature that simplifies the collection of gated images.

Detector Systems

Detector systems may be built up from a large number of small detector elements. In this approach, a means is needed to identify which of the many detectors pairs registered a coincidence. A straightforward solution to this problem is to couple each detector to a photomultiplier tube (PMT) and coincidence logic; but, as the number of detector elements increases, the corresponding cost of the PMTs and the complexity of the coincidence logic, as well as the size of the available phototubes, become limiting. Over the past 5 years, several encoding schemes for identifying the detectors with a limited number of PMTs and coincidence logic have been developed.[17,21] In such schemes, an array of small closely packed detector elements is viewed by a smaller number of PMTs (Fig. 11-4). An event in an individual crystal is identified by computing the center of brightness of the light as "seen" by the phototube array in a fashion similar to that used in Anger-type scintillation cameras. The unique problems of dealing with photon depth of

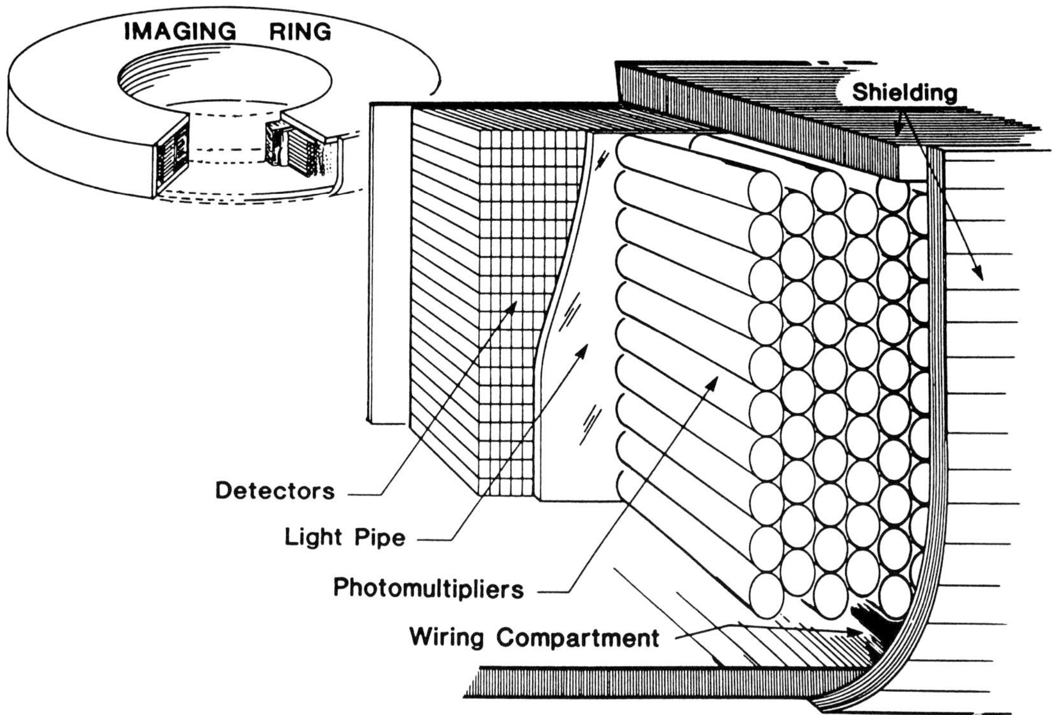

Fig. 11-4 Concept of detector coding using photomultiplier tubes (PMT) and individual small crystals. A detected event produces a flash of light that is spread out by the light pipe so that it may be "viewed" by several PMT. The output of the PMT is used to determine the center of brightness of the light flash, thereby identifying the struck crystal.

TABLE 11-1 Properties of Detector Materials for PET

Properties	Detector Material				
	NaI(Tl)	BGO	CsF	BaF$_2$	Plastic
Density (g/cm^3)	3.67	7.13	4.64	4.88	1.1
Decay time (nsec)	230	300	5	0.8	2–20
Relative stopping power	1.0	2.5	1.2	1.2	0.3

interaction effects and the large amount of light produced by 511-keV photons, however, require design details that are quite different from those for 150-keV photons. Detector systems of bismuth germanate (BGO) crystals can thus be fabricated with high coincidence detection efficiency for 511-keV photon pairs, with coincidence resolving times of 10 to 20 nsec and with one-fourth to one-sixteenth the number of PMTs, compared with a discrete detector system. Another approach to detector design is to employ a few large position-sensitive detectors, such as multiwire proportional chambers, operated in coincidence, but this approach has not yet achieved the high sensitivity and the short coincidence resolving times needed for most applications.

Detector systems can be characterized by their stopping power and speed of response. A variety of scintillation crystals have been studied for use in combination with photomultiplier tubes in positron cameras. These include sodium iodide (NaI), bismuth germanate (BGO), barium fluoride (BaF$_2$), cesium fluoride (CsF), and gadolinium silicate (Gd$_2$SiO$_5$). Table 11-1 lists and compares some of the relevant properties of detector materials that might be considered for use in positron cameras. When compared with NaI(Tl), detectors using BGO or Gd$_2$SiO$_5$ have the advantage of relatively high stopping power and photofraction, but their response is much slower than detectors using BaF$_2$ or CsF crystals.

Cameras using time-of-flight information require detector systems with a faster response

than can be obtained with BGO. Materials such as BaF$_2$ and CsF permit coincidence resolving times of 300 to 500 psec, sufficient to provide localization along the line of flight to about 7.5 cm (FWHM). In effect, this localization means that rather than determining line integrals through the object, as is done with conventional PET detectors, events are binned at 7.5-cm resolution along each line of flight. The addition of such time-of-flight information relaxes some of the constraints on the reconstruction process and this increases the statistical precision of the resulting reconstruction for a given number of detected photons.

However, it must be kept in mind that currently used time-of-flight detector materials are intrinsically less efficient than BGO, and thus some of the time-of-flight advantage is lost. Because of their shorter coincidence resolving times, time-of-flight systems are less susceptible to random coincidences and may be capable of functioning at higher count rates than are other systems.[22]

RADIOISOTOPES AND RADIOPHARMACEUTICALS

Conventional nuclear medicine depends primarily on the commercial distribution of radiopharmaceuticals based on [99m]Tc. The radiochemistry and design of Tc-labeled radiopharmaceuticals has been developed to a high level, but the incorporation of the ^{99m}Tc label (and other heavy metals for that matter) into biologically active compounds remains a difficult problem for many applications.

The use of PET is a great advantage in this regard, with the availability of several light short-lived biologically active atoms that decay by positron emission. Of particular interest are the isotopes ^{11}C, with a half-life ($t\frac{1}{2}$) of 20.3 minutes; ^{13}N, with a $t\frac{1}{2}$ of 10.4 minutes; ^{15}O, with a $t\frac{1}{2}$ of 2.04 minutes, and ^{18}F, with a $t\frac{1}{2}$ of 118 minutes. The short physical half-life of these isotopes usually leads to acceptable radiation dosimetry for human studies, but it is also a limitation in that an on-site cyclotron is usually required for production; also, radiochemistry and quality-control steps must be completed within a short time after the isotopes are produced. Small computer-controlled cyclotrons and automated radiochemistry facilities suitable for hospital installation are now available from several vendors, albeit at substantial cost. As there is little experience with such facilities, trained personnel are needed to ensure their satisfactory operation. Another appealing source of radioactive tracers for PET studies are the radionuclide generator systems, which offer a convenient source of isotopes at the expense of more limited possibilities in radiochemistry. The most widely used generators to date are those from the parent-daughter combinations ^{68}Ge-^{68}Ga and ^{82}Sr-^{82}Rb.

DISCUSSION AND CONCLUSIONS

Positron emission tomography instrumentation and radiopharmaceutical synthesis have continued to develop rapidly. The current generation of positron tomographs offers spatial resolution, both transverse and axial, of 5 to 6 mm FWHM, as well as the possibility of cardiac gating. Systems using BGO have reached a high level of development, with good stability, ease of operation, fully quantitative single-slice reconstruction times on the order of 20 seconds, and distributed processing work stations. Systems using time of flight have also been refined, but most require long image reconstruction times to achieve the advantage of improved signal to noise ratio.

Some prototype positron tomographs are approaching the theoretical resolution limit of 2 to 3 mm defined by the finite positron range in tissue, but further improvements in resolution will not be practical without corresponding increases in sensitivity and count rate capability. Another limitation of all currently available systems is that they acquire data in the form of transverse section slices. Images on sagittal and oblique planes are formed by reprojection of stacks of transverse images. Because the data are typically not sampled finely enough in the axial direction, some degradation of resolution is introduced by the reprojection procedure. It is not clear that the simple expedient of adding more, closer-spaced planes will suffice, since the requirements of interplane shielding are likely to lower the sensitivity per plane. Future designs employing cylindrical rather than ring geometries may offer improvements in both sensitivity and volume sampling.

The advent of fully developed commercially available PET scanners along with computer-controlled cyclotron operation and automated chemistry systems brings PET technology to the point at which it can be acquired and used by any large medical center for research applications. The feasibility of using PET for physiologic measurements in the myocardium has already been demonstrated by several groups, but further efforts to evaluate and understand this modality are necessary to demonstrate its clinical efficacy for particular applications before its introduction into routine clinical practice can be justified.

REFERENCES

1. Derenzo SE, Budinger TF: Resolution limit for positron imaging devices. J Nucl Med 18:491, 1977

2. Phelps ME, Hoffman EJ, Huang SC, et al: Effect of positron range on spatial resolution. J Nucl Med 16:649, 1975

3. Derenzo SE, Budinger TF, Huesman RH, Cahoon JL: Dynamic Positron Emission Tomography in Man Using Small Bismuth Germanate Crystals. North-Holland Publishing Company, Amsterdam, 1982

4. Litton J, Bergstrom M, Eriksson L, et al: Performance evaluation of the PC-384 camera system for emission tomography of the brain. J Comput Assist Tomogr 8:74, 1984

5. Bergstrom M, Litton J, Eriksson L, et al: Determination of object contour from projections for attenuation correction in cranial positron emission tomography. J Comput Assist Tomogr 6:365, 1982

6. Hoffman EJ, Phelps ME, Huang SC, Kuhl DE: Performance evaluation of a PET tomograph designed for brain imaging. J Nucl Med 24:249, 1983

7. Huang SC, Carson RE, Phelps ME, et al: A boundary method for attenuation correction in PET. J Nucl Med 22:627, 1979

8. Hoffman EJ, Huang SC, Phelps ME, Kuhl DE: Quantitation in PET 4: Effects of accidental coincidences. J Comput Asst Tomogr 5:391, 1981

9. Carrol LR, Kretz P, Orcutt G: The orbiting rod source: Improving performance in PET transmission correction scans. p. 235. In Emission Computed Tomography: Current Trends. Society of Nuclear Medicine, New York, 1983

10. Huesman RH, Derenzo SE, Cahoon JL, et al: Orbiting transmission source for positron tomography. IEEE Trans Nucl Sci NS-35:735, 1988

11. Daube-Witherspoon ME, Carson RE, Green MV: Post-injection transmission attenuation measurements for PET. IEEE Trans Nucl Sci NS-35:757, 1988

12. Brooks RA, DiChiro G: Theory of image reconstruction in computed tomography. Radiology 117:561, 1975

13. Shepp LA, Vardi Y: Maximum likelihood reconstruction for emission tomography. IEEE Trans Med Imaging 1:113, 1984

14. Lange K, Carson R: EM reconstruction algorithm for emission and transmission tomography. J Comput Assist Tomogr 8:306, 1984

15. Politte DG, Snyder DL: Results of a comparative study of a reconstruction procedure producing improved estimates of radioactivity distributions in time-of-flight emission tomography. IEEE Trans Nucl Sci NS-31:614, 1984

16. Burnham CA, Bradshaw J, Chesler DA, et al: A stationary positron emission ring tomograph using BGO detector and analog readout. IEEE Trans Nucl Sci NS-29:461, 1982

17. Burnham CA, Bradshaw J, Kaufman D, et al: A positron tomograph employing a one dimensional BGO scintillation camera. IEEE Trans Nucl Sci NS-30:652, 1983

18. Holte S, Eriksson L, Larsson JE, et al: A preliminary evaluation of a positron camera system using weighted decoding of individual crystals. IEEE Trans Nucl Sci NS-35:730, 1988

19. Spinks TJ, Jones T, Gilardi MC, Heather JD: Physical performance of the latest generation of commercial positron scanner. IEEE Trans Nucl Sci NS-35:721, 1988

20. Derenzo SE, Huseman RH, Cahoon JL, et al: A positron tomograph with 600 BGO crystals and 2.6 mm resolution. IEEE Trans Nucl Sci NS-35:659, 1988

21. Nutt R, Casey M, Carroll L: A new multicrystal two-dimensional detector block for PET. J Nucl Med 26:28, 1985

22. Ter-Pogossian MM, Ficke DC, M Yamamoto, et al: Super PET I: A positron emission tomograph utilizing time-of-flight information. IEEE Trans Med Imaging 1:179, 1983

12
Experience with Clinical Positron Imaging of the Heart

K. Lance Gould

Accurate noninvasive assessment of heart disease in symptomatic or asymptomatic subjects remains a major medical limitation for a number of reasons. Coronary heart disease continues to be the leading cause of death in most technologically advanced countries despite declining cardiovascular mortality since 1968. It is responsible for 640,000 deaths each year in the United States, including almost one-third of all deaths between the ages of 35 and 64 years.[1]

Most of this heart disease is asymptomatic. Typically, cardiomyopathy presents as pulmonary edema in advanced stages of dysfunction. Hypertensive heart disease presents similarly or as dyspnea in association with diastolic dysfunction and the stiff ventricle syndrome. Sixty percent of victims of sudden death or myocardial infarction present with no prior symptoms.[2-5] Up to 13 percent of middle-aged men in the general population have coronary artery disease (CAD),[6,7] apparently without symptoms. Silent ischemia is increasingly recognized in symptomatic

and asymptomatic patients[8,9] and may have a less favorable prognosis in the asymptomatic patient.[10] Finally, the community model of mass intervention for coronary atherosclerosis has been of questionable benefit compared with the medical model of intervention by risk-factor control in specific patients.[11] However, even assuming its effectiveness, the medical model of risk-factor control is limited by the low sensitivity and specificity with which risk factors identify patients who have significant CAD. For example, two-thirds of healthy adult men, aged 40 to 55, who have highest cholesterol and blood pressure risk factors remain well over the subsequent 25 years.[12]

Current noninvasive diagnostic techniques have limited accuracy for detecting or ruling out CAD in symptomatic, and particularly asymptomatic, patients. The sensitivity and specificity of exercise thallium imaging is about 80 to 90 percent in symptomatic patients but falls to significantly lower levels in asymptomatic patients. Yet routine yearly

203

treadmill testing is done commonly in asymptomatic patients, at great expense with little demonstrated efficacy for diagnosis in these circumstances and reasonable evidence that it provides limited diagnostic benefit. Consequently, an accurate method of assessing heart disease, particularly for reliably detecting or ruling out significant CAD in symptomatic or asymptomatic patients, in lieu of current widespread nondiagnostic testing would be useful.

Other important applications of noninvasive cardiac assessment that are now possible for the first time with positron emission tomography (PET) include quantitative assessment of the severity of physiologic stenosis for objective selection of patients for procedures; determination of myocardial viability, especially after thrombolysis when objective measures of viability provide a rational basis for a follow-up procedure in place of the current somewhat arbitrary practice of percutaneous transluminal coronary angioplasty (PTCA) or bypass surgery in most such patients; identification of significant collateral flow in CAD, thereby temporizing the need for mechanical interventions.

METHODS AND CLINICAL PROCEDURES

The concept of coronary flow reserve as a functional measure of stenosis severity was initially proposed in 1974 by Gould on the basis of empirical observations and was subsequently developed as a physiologic diagnostic method.[13–28] However, the application of this concept for clinical studies was limited by the lack of quantitative imaging techniques until positron imaging became fully developed for clinical applications. In the past, PET was a complicated expensive imaging technology that required a team of radiochemists, physicists, and physicians to carry out research studies providing important medical-scientific information but was limited in clinical applications because of its complexity. The development of current technology into routinely applicable clinical equipment and procedures has provided information not previously obtainable, with potentially significant impact on medical diagnosis, and therapy. Positron camera designs approaching the practical limits of resolution/speed and simplified, clinically oriented, dedicated software should enable a technologist to carry out routine clinical studies under the supervision of an appropriately trained clinical physician.

Although a cyclotron and radiochemist are necessary for the broad spectrum of metabolic studies for research purposes, the [82]Rb generator without a cyclotron provides a source of positron radionuclide, permitting routine clinical studies of cardiac perfusion, function, and viability. Positron imaging of the heart with either generator-produced [82]Rb or cyclotron-produced nitrogen-13 ammonia or fluorine-18 deoxyglucose is suitable for accurate noninvasive diagnosis of CAD in symptomatic or asymptomatic patients,[21,23,29–37] for assessing physiologic stenosis severity,[21,23,34–36] for imaging myocardial infarction[38–53] and viability,[39–49] for identifying the effects of interventions such as thrombolysis or PTCA on myocardial perfusion or coronary flow reserve[48,54] or of bypass surgery on function and metabolism,[42,48] for assessing three-dimensional regional left ventricular (LV) function,[23,55] for identifying collateral function noninvasively in humans,[56] and for diagnosing cardiomyopathy.[45,57,58] Positron imaging therefore provides the basis for specific therapeutic approaches toward preventing the sequelae of CAD in specific patients, thereby justifying the routine clinical use of PET in nuclear medicine.

Three characteristics of a positron camera are essential for routine clinical imaging, but particularly for routine cardiac imaging with [82]Rb. The first is a camera design with overlapping image planes such that sampling is uniform between detector rings.[23,55,59] If there is undersampling between image planes, anatomic structures lying parallel to the imaging plane may demonstrate significant artifactual defects, or real defects may be missed because of undersampling between banks of detectors.[23–25] Accordingly, a clinical camera should have significant overlap of the image planes to provide adequate sampling uniformly throughout the field of view and especially uniform z axis sampling. Recovery of activity data is also limited by the partial volume problem, which affects all positron tomography. However, in a camera with comparable resolution in the x, y, and z axes, the partial volume problems are minimized. The apparent greater sensitivity of PET for perfusion imaging in the diagnosis of CAD would appear to be due to technically better three-dimensional imaging and data recovery as compared with standard planar or SPECT imaging. Figure 12-1 shows the problem of undersampling. Figure 12-2 illustrates the limitation of smoothing or interpolation of data having undersampled regions. Figure 12-3 shows the importance of true three-dimensional imaging with uniform z-axis sampling.

The second important characteristic of a medical positron camera is high sensitivity in order to acquire high count rates[60–64] necessary for rapid patient throughput, for acquiring adequate counts using short half-lived radiopharmaceuticals such as ^{82}Rb, for first-pass gated blood-pool imaging, for measuring the arterial input function, and for first-pass extraction of various radiotracers.[65–68] For example, this capacity permits first-pass measurement of ejection fraction and the quantitative measurement of arterial input for calculating myocardial uptake of radiotracer at high coronary flow rates seen in stress imaging for the diagnosis of CAD. Practically speaking, the camera must accept

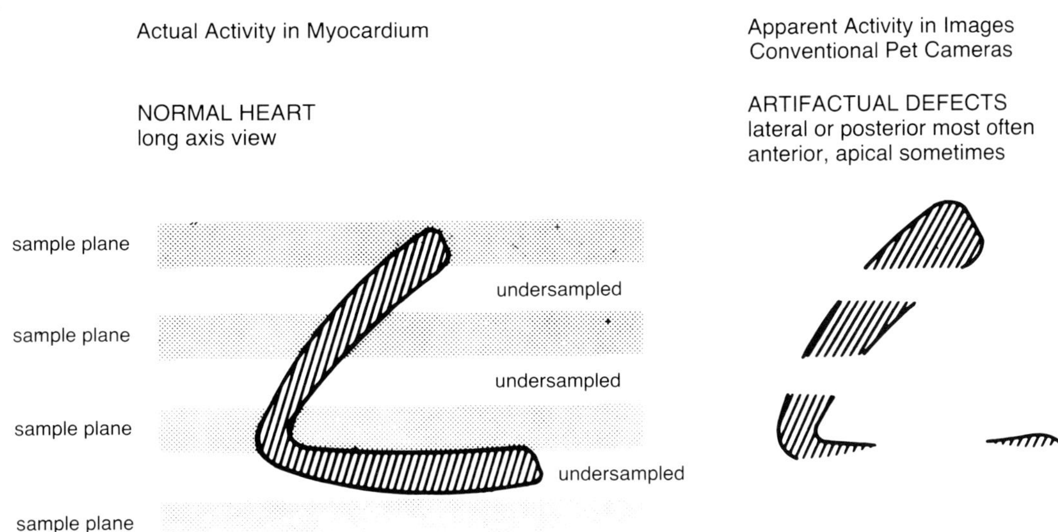

Fig. 12-1 Conventional positron cameras are constructed such that undersampled gaps occur in the z axis between image planes. This axial undersampling may result in artifactual defects or distortion seen on long-axis or axial views. Such artifacts are most likely to occur in the posterior-posterior lateral distribution of myocardium because of the orientation of the heart in the sample planes.

Actual Activity in Myocardium

Apparent Activity in Images
Conventional Pet — Smoothed

ANTERIOR OR POSTERIOR DEFECTS

FALSELY NORMAL OR EQUIVOCAL

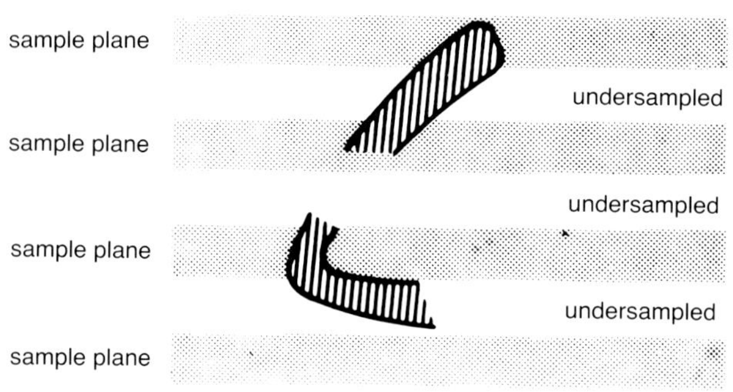

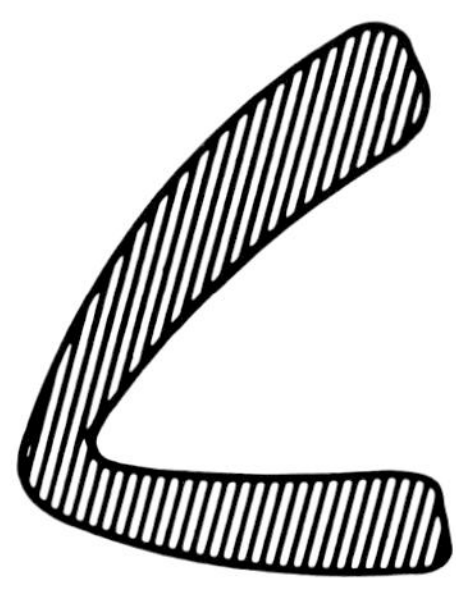

Fig. 12-2 Interpolation or smoothing of axial data from standard positron cameras may eliminate artifactual defects due to axial undersampling but may obscure or miss true defects in the undersampled planes.

Actual Activity in Myocardium

Apparent Activity in Images
3-D Uniform Sampling

REGIONAL DEFECT

ACCURATE IMAGING OF NORMAL AND ABNORMAL

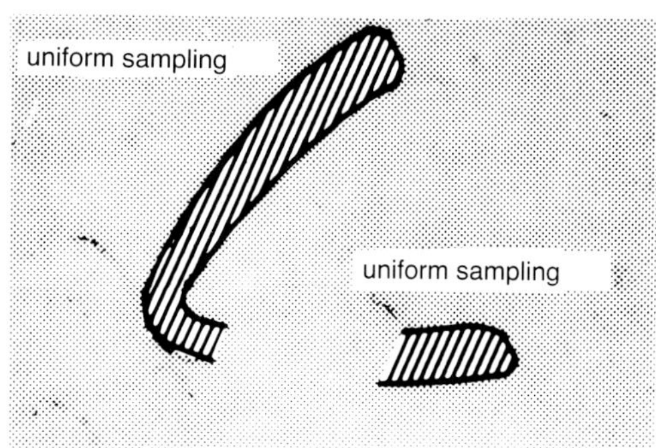

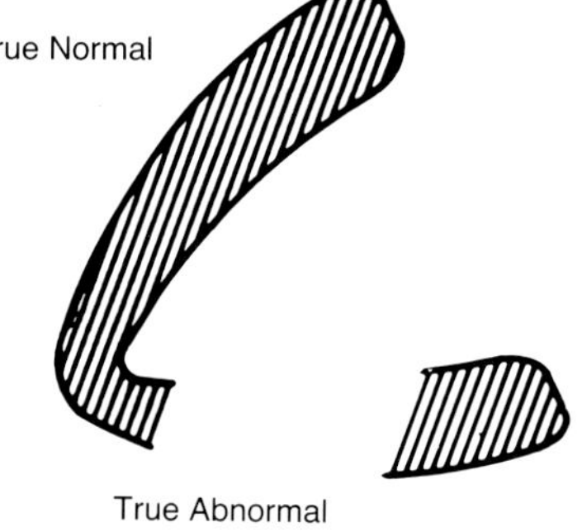

Fig. 12-3 True three-dimensional imaging with uniform axial sampling is necessary for a clinical positron camera. It is achieved by the staggered crystal design of the current University of Texas camera.

data without saturating with up to 30 mCi in the field of view.

The third characteristic essential for a clinical camera for routine cardiac work is complete user-friendly clinically oriented software that has been developed and validated in clinical applications. For example, most patients move slightly between the transmission, rest, and stress images. If marked, such motion may produce erroneous attenuation corrections. Artifactual defects may result, particularly of the left lateral free wall of the left ventricle. However, through the use of software that superimposes the transmission and emission images, translation between the transmission, rest, or stress images can be recognized and images corrected, permitting accurate interpretation.[23] The heavy technologic support usually needed for positron tomography can be eliminated by designing clinical software transparent to the user and validated for routine applications. Currently, a nurse and technician carry out clinical studies with the University of Texas camera, with the physician available to oversee patient management and safety.

Rubidium-82

For widespread routine cardiac practice, a simple-to-use radionuclide source is essential, such as the ^{82}Rb generator, which does not require a cyclotron[69-71] but permits all the major aspects of cardiac imaging for clinical purposes, as outlined below. Rubidium is an alkali metal analogue of potassium and is similar in its chemical and biologic properties. It is rapidly concentrated by the myocardium with a first-pass extraction of 60 percent at resting flow levels, which falls to 20 percent at high flows.[67] By comparison, first-pass myocardial extraction of nitrogen-13 ammonia is somewhat higher at 70 percent, falling to approximately 35 percent at high flows.[72,73] For equal millicurie doses, Rb images are inferior to ammonia images due to the short half-life of Rb. However, with ap-

propriately larger doses of ^{82}Rb (50 mCi), images are comparable to those with nitrogen-13 ammonia.[23,72,73]

Because of its short half-life (75 seconds), ^{82}Rb is an excellent agent for repeated or sequential myocardial imaging. It is particularly useful in acute clinical situations in which the patient's condition is changing rapidly or for studies before and after such interventions as dipyridamole stress or PTCA.

Rubidium-82 is eluted from the ^{82}Sr-^{82}Rb generator using a 50-ml syringe driven by a microprocessor-controlled motor connected to an on-line radiation monitor that provides preset volume, dose, and dose rate of ^{82}Rb to the patient. Typically, with a fresh generator, 30 to 50 mCi is injected in a 10 ml volume over 20 to 25 seconds. Toward the end of the useful life of the generator (5 weeks), volumes of 30 to 40 ml are required in order to deliver 30 to 50 mCi ^{82}Rb. With a half-life ($t^{1/2}$) of only 75 seconds, approximately one-half to two-thirds of this activity reaches the arterial circulation, with the balance decaying during the transit through the infusion tubing, the venous system, and the lungs.

Stress Imaging Protocol

After obtaining informed consent, the patients are brought to the positron imaging laboratory and positioned in the PET camera. After positioning, transmission images are obtained using a ^{68}Ga-filled Plexiglas ring containing 3 mCi gallium-68 EDTA in a ring space 12 cm wide, 1 cm deep, and 56 cm in diameter. Following the transmission image, intravenous ^{82}Rb (or ^{13}NH$_3$) is then injected followed by data acquisition for 5 to 8 minutes for ^{82}Rb (or 15 to 20 minutes for ^{13}NH$_3$). Ten minutes after the administration of the first dose of ^{82}Rb (or 40 minutes for ^{13}NH$_3$), dipyridamole is infused in a dose of 0.142 mg/kg/min for 4 minutes, followed by flushing in the residual dipyridamole in the tubing at the end of 4 minutes. Two minutes later (sixth minute after onset of dipyridamole infusion), unilateral handgrip at 25 to 30 percent of peak is begun on a hand dynamometer and held for 4 minutes. Four minutes after the end of dipyridamole infusion (and after 2 minutes of handgrip), ^{82}Rb (or ^{13}NH$_3$) is again injected with handgrip held for 2 more minutes. For patients in whom severe angina pectoris develops aminophylline, 125 mg, is injected intravenously over 20 to 30 seconds.

Transmission scans contain 200 to 400 million counts for the entire field, including all slices; emission images contain 10 to 20 million counts for ^{82}Rb (30- to 50-mCi dose) and 20 to 30 million counts for ^{13}NH$_3$ (20-mCi dose) for all slices. All tomographic slices are displayed simultaneously with optional magnification for any individual slice for examination of details.

Image Interpretation

The composite presentation of all slices showing the entire heart must be interpreted in toto for the entire heart on the rest and then stress studies. Slice-by-slice comparisons are not relied on because of the problem of translation of the heart along its long axis, or occasionally laterally, thereby causing a change in image planes or slice displacement between rest-stress studies.[23] Slice-by-slice comparisons are acceptable as long as any vertical displacement that has occurred on rest and stress studies is accounted for by shifting one image vertically until the image planes match.

For routine presentation, the range of count densities within all slices is scaled in 33 steps, each of which corresponds to 3 percent of maximum counts ranging in color from black for lowest counts (less than 20 percent of maximum), to blue (20 to 35 percent of maximum), to green (35 to 50 percent of maximum), to yellow (50 to 68 percent of maxi-

mum), to red (68 to 85 percent of maximum), to white (85 to 100 percent of maximum counts), with white representing maximum counts. Within each of the five basic colors, approximately five hues of color gradations reflect count density in steps of 3 percent of maximum counts. According to this scheme, a defect appears as a different color—blue or green—surrounded by yellow, red, or white; however, the gradation in colors reflects a continuum of changing count densities.

Figure 12-4 shows tomographic planes as if looking down from above on slices as the data are originally acquired where the long axis of the heart is at an angle to the long axis of the body (top panel). The data are then reoriented to provide true short axis (middle panel) and true long axis views (lower panel). Plate 12-1 shows the anatomic orientation of the coronary arteries on tomographic images. Plate 12-2 presents an example of a rest-stress study as if looking down on image planes from above as they are acquired (Plate 12-2A) in true short-axis (Plate 12-2B), and true long-axis views (Plate 12-2C). In this case, there is a severe stress defect in the distribution of the left anterior descending artery.

Coronary Arteriography as a Gold Standard

Visual interpretations of coronary arteriograms are marked by such great interobserver and intraobserver variability that comparison of arteriograms from different subjects, or at different times in the same subject, are of limited value in assessing severity, changes in severity, or the functional significance of coronary artery stenosis. The use of the relative percentage of diameter narrowing as a clinical measure of severity does not account for other important geometric characteristics of stenoses, such as length, absolute cross-sectional luminal area, multiple lesions in series, or eccentric narrowing, which may be

Color Plates

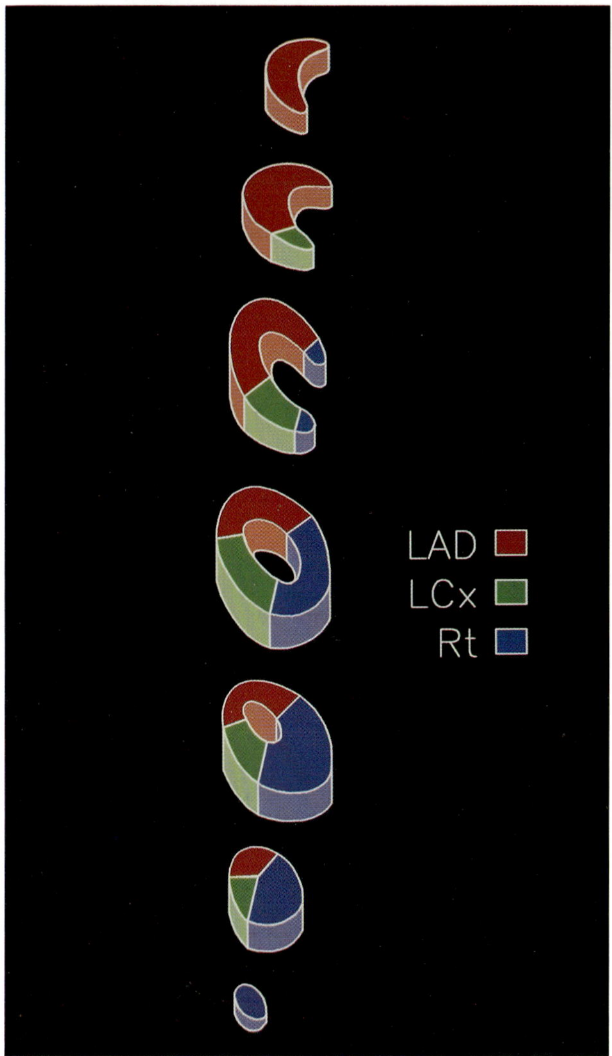

Plate 12-1

Plate 12-1 Orientation of coronary artery distributions in tomographic planes, as if looking down on the heart from above.

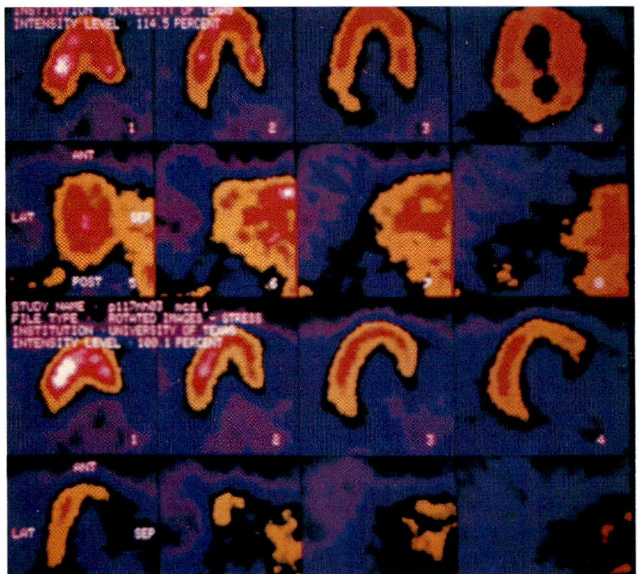

Plate 12-2A

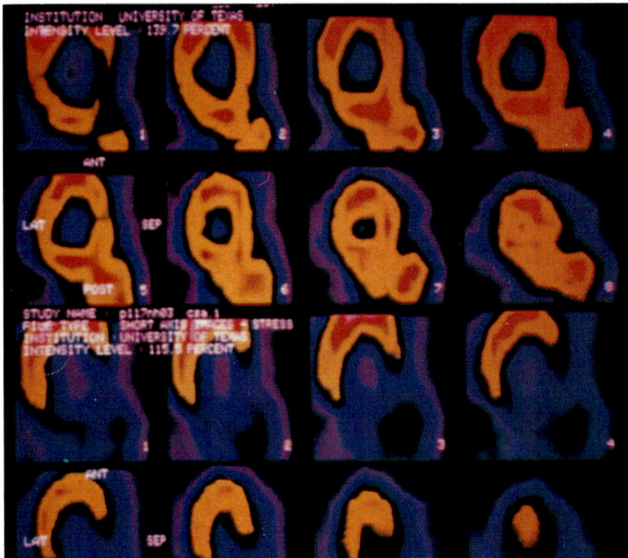

Plate 12-2B

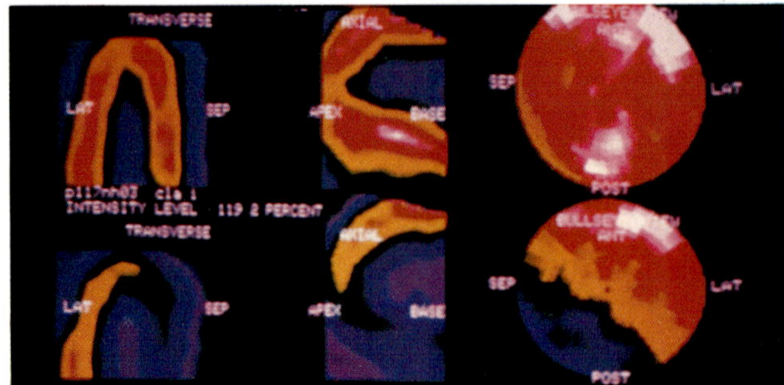

Plate 12-2C

Plate 12-2 (A) Acquisition views at rest in the two top rows and at stress in the two bottom rows. The apex is rotated to be at the top of each image with the left lateral wall of the left ventricle (LV) on the left, septum on the right, and posterior inferior at the bottom. **(B)** Short-axis views at rest in the upper two rows and at stress in the lower two rows. **(C)** (Top) Midline horizontal long-axis view at rest. (Bottom, left) At stress. (Top) Vertical midline long-axis views at rest and at stress (lower) are in the middle and polar maps at rest (upper) and at stress (lower) are on the right. The color code white indicates highest flow, red next highest with yellow intermediate; black indicates lowest flow, blue next lowest, green intermediate low flow. There is a large relative stress defect in the anterior septum and anterior and apical myocardium in this example.

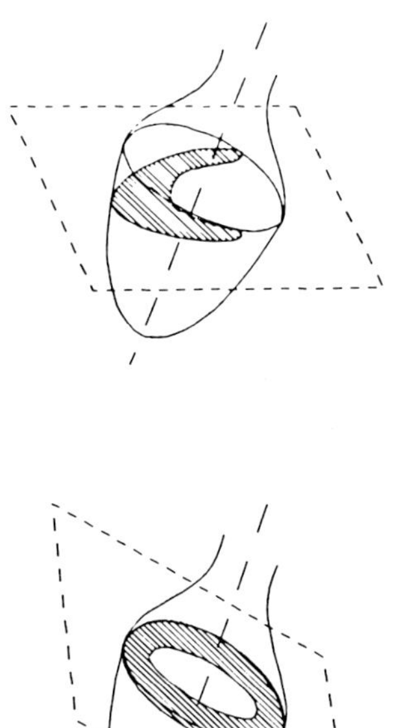

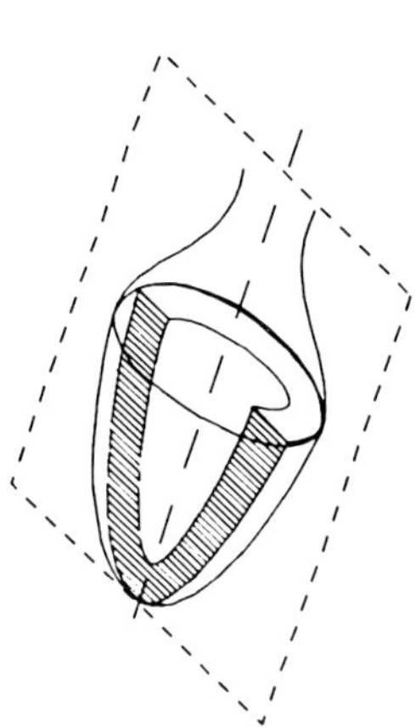

Fig. 12-4 Images are acquired as in the top panel looking down on the heart from above, called acquisition images (upper panel). Additional true short-axis (middle panel) and long-axis views (lower panel) are also obtained by software rotation in three dimensions.

worse in one view than in another. The validity of quantitative coronary arteriography for predicting the functional pressure-flow characteristics of stenoses has been demonstrated if all the dimensions of the lesion are taken into account, including the relative percentage of narrowing, absolute luminal area, and integrated length effects.[22,23,74,75] The percentage of narrowing alone or the absolute diameter alone is an inadequate measure of stenosis severity. In addition, optimal quantitative analysis does not depend on operator estimates of borders but is completely automated by a validated method correcting for the point-spread function of the radiographic system.[76,77]

Fluid dynamic equations demonstrate that stenosis flow reserve is derived from all stenosis geometric dimensions as a single integrated measure of its severity, reflecting all the combined effects of percentage of narrowing, absolute diameter, and length. Determination of stenosis flow reserve by this quantitative analysis of coronary arteriograms correlates well with directly measured flow reserve in animals and with perfusion effects in humans.[22,23]

RESULTS AND CURRENT CLINICAL INDICATIONS

The results of clinical and experimental studies document the following current clinical indications for cardiac PET:

Noninvasive diagnosis of coronary artery disease in either symptomatic or asymptomatic patients: The sensitivity of diagnosing CAD by PET using ^{82}Rb[23,30–33] or nitrogen-13 ammonia,[21,29] as compared with coronary arteriography, approximates 95 to 98 percent with comparable specificity, in symptomatic or asymptomatic patients with high risk factors for CAD.

Assessment of the physiologic severity of coronary artery stenosis: The quantitative severity of perfusion defects under stress conditions reflects the anatomic severity of the coronary artery stenosis as determined by automated quantitative coronary arteriography taking into account length, absolute dimensions, and the percentage of narrowing of the stenosis.[23,34–37] Therefore, noninvasive PET may be used to assess the physiologic severity of coronary stenoses as well as changes in severity after an intervention such as PTCA, vasodilator drugs, and regimens for cholesterol control, which may affect stenosis geometry.[48,54] Metabolic abnormalities resulting from transient ischemia may also be identified by positron imaging as an independent measure of the physiologic consequence of a stenosis, in addition to its anatomic geometry or effects on perfusion or flow reserve.[35–37]

Imaging myocardial ischemia, infarction and viability. The location and extent of myocardial infarction may be imaged by three-dimensional PET using ^{82}Rb, nitrogen-13 ammonia, and/or ^{18}F-deoxyglucose FDG and/or ^{11}C palmitate[38–53]; viability may also be evaluated.[39–49] Myocardial perfusion images using ^{82}Rb or ^{13}N ammonia indicate the underperfused area at risk of myocardial infarction. In the presence of injured or ischemic but viable myocardial cells, myocardial metabolism is shifted toward anaerobic glycolysis. FDG uptake then increases relative to the rest of the myocardium, thereby identifying ischemic viable tissue, since necrotic myocardium does not extract FDG. Patients with ischemic but viable myocardium demonstrate improved LV function after bypass surgery[42] or thrombolysis.[48] Viability may also be assessed by following kinetic changes of ^{82}Rb which, after initial myocardial extraction, leaks out of myocardium in the presence of irreversible injury.[53] By contrast, myocardium which is injured but viable retains rubidium with continuous redistribution or positive uptake during the period after IV injection.[53]

Accordingly, by assessing rubidium kinetics with two sequential PET images after a single IV injection of ^{82}Rb, injured but viable myocardium may be identified and separated from necrotic myocardium. The advantages of ^{82}Rb for assessing viability are that a cyclotron is not required, and only one injection of tracer is necessary with a standard 30-minute period for the entire study. The use of FDG/NH$_3$ for assessing viability requires two cyclotron produced radionuclides in sequence with 3 to 4 hours required for a complete study. However, FDG provides direct images of metabolic behavior; it is also better documented by clinical studies, whereas only experimental or preliminary clinical results have been published for the assessment of viability by rubidium.

Identification and assessment of significant collateral function in man by imaging coronary steal during dipyridamole-handgrip stress: Coronary steal occurs under conditions of near maximum coronary vasodilation if collaterals provide a significant proportion of resting myocardial perfusion. A fall in absolute myocardial uptake of activity after injection of a perfusion tracer during dipyridamole vasodilation as compared with rest indicates coronary steal and the presence of significant collaterals.[56]

Left ventricular function and wall thickening: By gating the PET with the electrocardiogram (ECG), left ventricular pumping function and wall thickening may be assessed regionally in three dimensions.[23,55]

Dilated cardiomyopathy: This condition, unrelated to CAD, may also be diagnosed by positron imaging as an enlarged poorly functioning heart with no resting or stress perfusion defects typical of ischemic cardiomyopathy due to CAD. Metabolic abnormalities are also typically found.[45,57,58]

The radiation burden to patients and staff by positron tracers of ^{82}Rb, nitrogen-13 ammonia, and fluorine-18 FDG are generally lower than standard cardiac nuclear tracers, such as ^{201}Tl because the half-lives of the positron tracers are short.[78-87]

Personnel and Facility Requirements

Two types of facilities for cardiac PET are appropriate. The first is a positron camera utilizing generator produced rubidium-82 in the absence of a cyclotron. The second includes a cyclotron-radiochemistry complex. For clinical studies, both facilities would require a room approximately 15 feet × 15 feet for the camera with an attached smaller space 10 feet × 10 feet as a computer room, control console, and reading center. Appropriate cardiac drugs and resuscitation equipment are required in the imaging room, including defibrillation, intubation facilities, and emergency cardiac drugs. Since the stress provided for the screening test uses IV dipyridamole, appropriate ECG monitoring should be available. Physician supervision is necessary for carrying out these studies due to the infusion of vasoactive drugs comparable to exercise stress. On occasion, patients with CAD who are undergoing dipyridamole-handgrip stress develop angina pectoris, which requires reversal with IV aminophylline. Aminophylline is effective in quickly reversing the effects of dipyridamole. Consequently, the test sequence may be well controlled. A physician is essential for evaluating the patient during the test in order to determine whether this reversal step is necessary.

Physicians with expertise in physiologic cardiovascular imaging are the appropriate persons to choose the appropriate patients and study to be done, to carry out the test protocol, to interpret the study results, and to supervise the program. Such physicians may be cardiologists, nuclear medicine physicians, or radiologists with experience in and active knowledge of functional cardiovascular imaging, cardiovascular physiology, cor-

onary arteriography, pharmacologic stress, and clinical management of cardiac disease, particularly cardiac emergencies, resuscitation, dysrhythmias, and cardiac arrest.

Status with Regulatory Agencies

PET cameras are now commercially distributed as a class II device registered with the FDA by filing form 510K under FDA guidelines USDHHS Section 21CFR 807, class II (Performance Standards), Premarket Notification for Medical Devices under a grandfather clause for pre-existing technology. Intravenous dipyridamole for stress perfusion imaging and the [82]Rb generator are both currently being reviewed by the Food and Drug Administration (FDA).

Comparison with Other High-Technology Cardiac Imaging

Some comparison to other high-technology imaging, particularly fast cine-computed tomography (CT) and magnetic resonance imaging (MRI), is appropriate. All advanced imaging systems provide some degree of anatomic and functional information. At one extreme, optimal quantitative coronary arteriography gives anatomic resolution to within ±0.1 mm but no directly measured functional data on flow, viability, function, or metabolism. At the other extreme, positron imaging provides the greatest breadth and depth of functional information with the least resolution, which, at 5 to 6 mm for current positron cameras, is appropriate for the functional process being imaged. Fast cine-CT and MRI lie between these extremes, as shown in Figure 12-5.

Although it provides some information on proton content and state, Paans et al.[88] pointed out the limited signal intensity of MRI for metabolic or perfusion imaging. This limitation is a particular problem for imaging myocardial perfusion during high

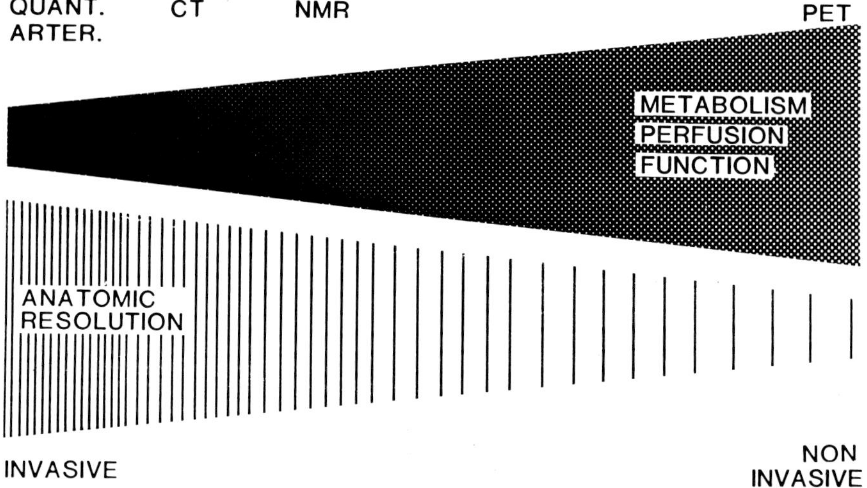

Fig. 12-5 Spectrum of anatomic and functional data from advanced imaging technology. The upper diagram indicates the spectrum of functional data, with PET best and high-resolution arteriography least useful for functional assessment. The lower diagram indicates the spectrum of anatomic data, with arteriography providing the maximal spatial resolution in terms of line pairs per millimeter. Computed tomography (CT) scanning and nuclear magnetic resonance (NMR) are intermediate between these extremes but fall toward anatomic end of the imaging spectrum.

coronary flow conditions necessary for diagnosis of coronary artery disease. Miller et al.[89] demonstrated a linear correlation between MRI signals from intravascular gadolinium and myocardial perfusion at coronary flow rates from resting down to ischemic conditions. However, at the high flows necessary to identify CAD, the MRI signal, even enhanced by gadolinium, does not increase appropriately. Consequently, significant regional differences in maximum myocardial perfusion due to coronary artery stenoses cannot be identified by MRI. Similarly, coronary flow measured by fast cine-CT after IV injection of contrast media parallels coronary flow from resting down to ischemic levels.[90] However, the density on CT images of myocardium does not increase appropriately as flow increases. As a result, regional abnormalities of maximum perfusion due to CAD cannot be identified reliably. Thus, MRI and fast cine-CT are primarily suited for high-resolution anatomic imaging, with less capacity for functional imaging, whereas positron imaging has the reverse characteris-

tic, with poorer anatomic resolution but more powerful functional imaging.

Finally, single photon computed emission tomography (SPECT) is frequently proposed as a less expensive tomographic substitute for positron imaging. However, the sensitivity and specificity of SPECT thallium perfusion imaging for the diagnosis of CAD have not been demonstrated to be significantly better than planar imaging,[91] except perhaps for the left circumflex coronary artery distribution,[92] and are not comparable to the sensitivity and specificity reported for positron imaging. This limitation is most likely due to inadequate atenuation correction and nonuniform resolution of SPECT. Figure 12-6 is a schematic calculated from reported data showing limitations of all these imaging modalities. The data for positron imaging in this schematic were derived from older camera designs, since extensive clinical or experimental data with new cameras designed to overcome these limitations are not yet available.

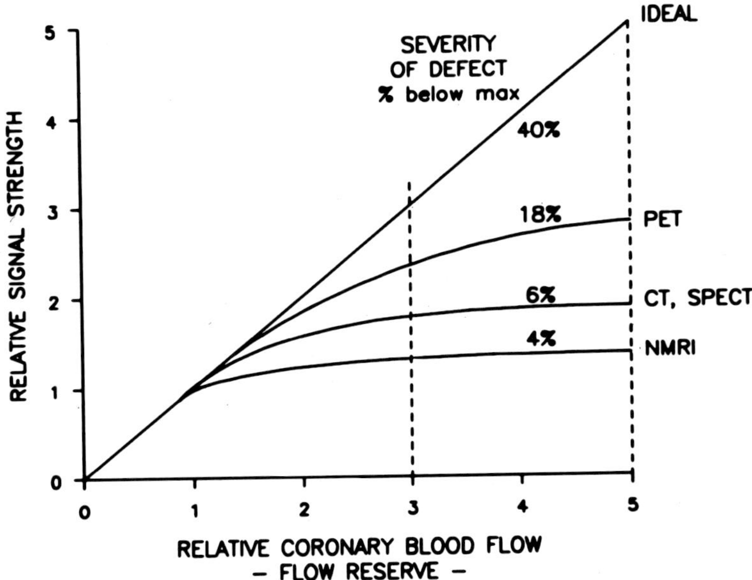

Fig. 12-6 Schematic showing the limits of various imaging modalities for detecting perfusion defects at high-flow states necessary in assessing coronary artery disease. Consider the example in which flow in a normally perfused segment of myocardium increases fivefold over resting levels versus a threefold increase in the distribution of a stenosed artery. Perfusion in the abnormal distribution is 40 percent below normal maximum (53/5 = 40 percent). The proportional signal from each of several imaging modalities is shown as coronary flow increases. These signals do not increase in proportion to flow for a variety of technical reasons. The data for positron imaging are better than for other modalities, even though obtained with our first prototype camera; with our new high-resolution high-speed camera, we anticipate a markedly improved proportionality with flow. However, this proportionality will always be limited by the nonlinear decrease in extraction of radiotracer as flow increases. The proportional change in signal with increasing flow is much worse for other imaging modalities.

It is also appropriate to compare relative costs of positron imaging. In our laboratory, for more than 1,000 cases per year over a 5-year period, the total costs of equipment, personnel, and radiotracer for rubidium positron imaging have been the same or less than for SPECT-thallium imaging because generator-produced rubidium appears to be less expensive than thallium.[93] For larger numbers of cases, rubidium-positron imaging is less costly than thallium. Patient throughput is potentially greater for rubidium–positron imaging, with 10 to 14 patients being studied per day, as compared with a maximum of 5 to 6 per day for SPECT. Since the cost of the rubidium generator is fixed with a relatively unlimited number of doses (every 10 minutes), the economy of positron imaging equals or surpasses that of SPECT *for larger numbers of studies* from the point of view *of both* radionuclide and equipment costs considered together.

CONCLUSIONS

Cardiac positron imaging should be considered an essential routine diagnostic tool of clinical cardiology. Cardiac PET provides accurate noninvasive assessment of the following:

Myocardial perfusion
    Symptomatic patients
    Silent ischemia
    Asymptomatic screening
Coronary stenosis severity
Myocardial infarct imaging
Myocardial viability
    Post-thrombolysis
    Pre- and post-PTCA bypass
Left ventricular function
Collateral function and cardiomyopathy
Therapy for CAD (medical, PTCA, surgical)

None of these evaluations can be carried out as well or at all by other imaging techniques.

Cardiac positron imaging may use cyclotron-produced agents or generator-produced ^{82}Rb as a substitute for current standard cardiac imaging agents, to obtain better data on myocardial perfusion, function, infarction, and viability, which currently requires three separate procedures and radionuclides:

Thallium-201 exercise testing
    Technetium-99m pyrophosphate-labeled RBC for gated blood-pool imaging
Technetium-99m, pyrophosphate for myocardial infarct imaging

For those centers that have a cyclotron, more complex metabolic studies may be carried out. Either asymptomatic or symptomatic patients may be studied on an outpatient or inpatient basis. A rest-stress cardiac PET study for the diagnosis of CAD using ^{82}Rb and dipyridamole-handgrip stress requires approximately 45 to 60 minutes, so that 8 to 10 patients may be studied per day.

Cardiac positron imaging may be carried out economically at costs similar to other high-technology diagnostic imaging. However, this technique provides functional information quantitatively for routine clinical studies.

REFERENCES

1. Exercise and Your Heart. Publication No. 83-1677. National Institutes of Health, Bethesda, MD, 1983
2. Midwall J, Ambrose J, Pichard A, et al: Angina pectoris before and after myocardial infarction. Chest 81:681, 1982
3. Reunanen A, Aromaa A, Pyörälä K, et al: The Social Insurance Institution's coronary heart disease study: Baseline data and 5-year mortality experience. Acta Med Scand 673(suppl):67, 1983
4. Kannel WB, Abbott RD: Incidence and prognosis of unrecognized myocardial infarction. An update on the Framingham Study. N Engl J Med 311:1144, 1984
5. Lown B: Sudden cardiac death: The major challenge confronting contemporary cardiology. Am J Cardiol 43:313, 1979
6. Langou RA, Huang EK, Kelley MJ, Cohen LS: Predictive accuracy of coronary artery calcification and abnormal exercise test for coronary artery disease in asymptomatic men. Circulation 62:1196, 1980
7. Olofsson BO, Bjerle P, Aberg T, et al: Prevalence of coronary artery disease in patients with valvular heart disease. Acta Med Scand 218:365, 1985
8. Campbell S, Barry J, Rebecca GS, et al: Active transient myocardial ischemia during daily life in asymptomatic patients with positive exercise tests and coronary artery disease. Am J Cardiol 57:1010, 1986
9. Resnekov L: Silent myocardial ischemia: Therapeutic implications. Am J Med 79(3A):30, 1985
10. Gottlieb SO, Weisfeldt ML, Ouyang P, et al: Silent ischemia as a marker for early unfavorable outcomes in patients with unstable angina. N Engl J Med 314:1214, 1986
11. Borhani NO: Prevention of Coronary Heart Disease in Practice. JAMA 254:257, 1985
12. Oliver MF: Strategies for preventing and

screening for coronary heart disease. Br Heart J 54:1, 1985

13. Gould KL, Lipscomb K, Hamilton GW: Physiologic basis for assessing critical coronary stenosis. Am J Cardiol 33:87, 1974

14. Gould KL, Hamilton GW, Lipscomb K, Kennedy JW: A method for assessing stress induced regional malperfusion during coronary arteriography: Experimental validation and clinical application. Am J Cardiol 34:557, 1974

15. Gould KL, Lipscomb K: Effects of coronary stenosis on coronary flow reserve and resistance. Am J Cardiol 34:48, 1974

16. Gould KL: Noninvasive assessment of coronary stenosis by myocardial perfusion imaging during pharmacologic coronary vasodilation. I. Physiologic principles and experimental validation. Am J Cardiol 41:267, 1978

17. Gould KL, Westcott RJ, Albro PC, Hamilton GW: Noninvasive assessment of coronary stenosis by myocardial imaging during pharmacologic vasodilation. II. Clinical Methodology and Feasibility. Am J Cardiol 41:41:279, 1978

18. Albro PC, Gould KL, Westcott RJ, et al: Noninvasive assessment of coronary stenosis by myocardial imaging during pharmacologic coronary vasodilation. III. Clinical trial. Am J Cardiol 42:751, 1978

19. Gould KL, et al: Assessment of coronary stenoses by myocardial perfusion imaging during pharmacologic coronary vasodilation. IV. Limits of stenosis detection by idealized experimental cross-sectional myocardial imaging. Am J Cardiol 42:761, 1978

20. Gould KL, Shelbert HR, Phelps ME, Hoffman EJ: Noninvasive assessment of coronary stenoses with myocardial perfusion imaging during pharmacologic coronary vasodilation. V. Detection of 47% diameter coronary stenosis with intravenous N-13 ammonia and positron emission tomography in intact dogs. Am J Cardiol 43:200, 1979

21. Schelbert HR, Wisenberg G, Phelps ME, et al: Noninvasive assessment of coronary stenosis by myocardial imaging during pharmacologic coronary vasodilation. VI. Detection of coronary artery disease in man with intravenous $^{13}NH_3$ and positron computed tomography. Am J Cardiol 49:119, 1982

22. Kirkeeide R, Gould KL, Parsel L: Assessment of coronary stenoses by myocardial imaging during coronary vasodilation. VII. Validation of coronary flow reserve as a single integrated measure of stenosis severity accounting for all its geometric dimensions. J Am Coll Cardiol 7:103, 1986

23. Gould KL, Goldstein RA, Mullani NA, et al: Noninvasive assessment of coronary stenoses by myocardial perfusion imaging during pharmacologic coronary vasodilation. VIII. Clinical feasibility of positron cardiac imaging without a cyclotron using generator-produced rubidium-82. J Am Coll Cardiol 7:775, 1986

24. Brown G, Josephson MA, Peterson RB, et al: Intravenous dipyridamole combined with isometric handgrip for near maximal acute increase in coronary flow in patients with coronary artery disease. Am J Cardiol 48:1077, 1981

25. Josephson MA, Brown BG, Hecht HS, et al: Noninvasive detection and localization of coronary stenoses in patients: Comparison of resting dipyridamole and exercise thallium-201 myocardial perfusion imaging. Am Heart J 103:1008, 1982

26. Leppo J, Boucher CA, Okada RD, et al: Serial thallium-201 myocardial imaging after dipyridamole infusion. Circulation 66:649, 1982

27. Bonaduce D, Muto P, Morgano G, et al: Effect of beta-blockade on thallium-201 dipyridamole myocardial scintigraphy. Acta Cardiol 34:399, 1984

28. Tavazzi L, et al: Dipyridamole test in angina pectoris: Diagnostic value and pathophysiologic implications. Cardiology 69:34, 1982

29. Tamaki N, Yonekura Y, Senda M, et al: Myocardial positron computed tomography with ^{13}N-ammonia at rest and during exercise. Eur J Nucl Med 11:246, 1985

30. Deanfield JE, Shea M, Ribiero P, et al: Transient ST-segment depression as a marker of myocardial ischemia during daily life. Am J Cardiol 54:1195, 1984

31. Deanfield JE, Kensett M, Wilson RA, et al: Silent myocardial ischaemia due to mental stress. Lancet 2:1001, 1984

32. Deanfield JE, Shea MJ, Wilson RA, et al: Direct effects of smoking on the heart: Silent ischemic disturbances of coronary flow. Am J Cardiol 57:1005, 1986

33. Selwyn AP, Allan RM, L'Abbate AL, et al:

Relation between regional myocardial uptake of rubidium-82 and perfusion: Absolute reduction of cation uptake in ischemia. Am J Cardiol 50:112, 1982

34. Goldstein RA, Kirkeeide R, Demer L, et al: Assessment of coronary flow reserve with positron tomography: A comparison with quantitative coronary arteriography. J Nucl Med 27:943, 1986 (abst)

35. Camici P, Araujo LI, Spinks T, et al: Increased uptake of 18-F-fluorodeoxyglucose in postischemic myocardium of patients with exercise-induced angina. Circulation 74:81, 1986

36. Grover-McKay M, Schelbert HR, Schwaiger M, et al: Identification of impaired metabolic reserve by atrial pacing in patients with significant coronary artery stenosis. Circulation 74:281, 1986

37. Selwyn AP, Shea M, Deanfield J, et al: The character of transient myocardial ischemia: Clinical studies and progress using positron emission tomography. Int J Cardiac Imaging 1:61, 1985

38. Goldstein RA, Mullani NA, Wong WH, et al: Positron imaging of myocardial infarction with rubidium-82. J Nucl Med 27:1824, 1986

39. Geltman EM, Biello D, Wlech MJ, et al: Characterization of transmural myocardial infarction by positron-emission tomography. Circulation 65:747, 1982

40. Schwaiger M, Brunken R, Grover-McKay M, et al: Regional myocardial metabolism in patients with acute myocardial infarction assessed by positron emission tomography. J Am Coll Cardiol 8:800, 1986

41. Marshal RC, Tillisch JH, Phelps ME, et al: Identification and differentiation of resting myocardial ischemia and infarction in man with positron computed tomography, ^{18}F-labeled fluorodeoxyglucose and N-13 ammonia. Circulation 67:766, 1983

42. Tillisch J, Brunken R, Marshall R, et al: Reversibility of cardiac wall-motion abnormalities predicted by positron tomography. N Engl J Med 314:884, 1986

43. Brunken R, Tillisch J, Schwaiger M, et al: Regional perfusion, glucose metabolism, and wall motion in patients with chronic electrocardiographic Q wave infarctions: Evidence for persistence of viable tissue in some infarct regions by positron emission tomography. Circulation 73:951, 1986

44. Schelbert HR, Henze E, Phelps ME, Kuhl DE: Assessment of regional myocardial ischemia by positron-emission computed tomography. Am Heart J 103:588, 1982

45. Jaffee AS, Spadaro JJ, Schechtman K, et al: Increased congestive heart failure after infarction of modest extent in patients with diabetes mellitus. Am Heart J 108:31, 1984

46. Schelbert HR, Henze E, Schon HR, et al: C-11 palmitic acid for the noninvasive evaluation of regional myocardial fatty acid metabolism with positron computed tomography. IV. In vivo demonstration of impaired fatty acid oxidation in acute myocardial ischemia. Am Heart J 106:736, 1983

47. Schelbert HR, Henze E, Sochor H, et al: Effects of substrate availability on myocardial C-11 palmitate kinetics by positron emission tomography in normal subjects and patients with ventricular dysfunction. Am Heart J 111:1055, 1986

48. Sobel BE, Geltman EM, Tiefenbrunn AJ, et al: Improvement of regional myocardial metabolism after coronary thrombolysis induced with tissue-type plasminogen activator or streptokinase. Circulation 69:983, 1984

49. Ter-Pogossian MM, Klein MS, Markham J, et al: Regional assessment of myocardial metabolic integrity in vivo by positron-emission tomography with ^{11}C-labeled palmitate. Circulation 61:242, 1980

50. Sobel BE, Weiss ES, Welch MJ, et al: Detection of remote myocardial infarction in patients with positron emission transaxial tomography and intravenous ^{11}C-palmitate. Circulation 55:853, 1977

51. Walsh WF, Harper PV, Resnekov L, Fill H: Noninvasive evaluation of regional myocardial perfusion in 112 patients using a mobile scintillation camera and intravenous nitrogen-13 labelled ammonia. Circulation 54:266, 1976

52. Harper PV, Schwartz J, Beck RN, et al: Clinical myocardial imaging with nitrogen-13 ammonia. Radiology 108:613, 1973

53. Goldstein RA: Kinetics of rubidium-82 after coronary occlusion and reperfusion. J Clin Invest 75:1131, 1985

54. Goldstein RA, Kirkeeide R, Nishikawa A, et al: Improvement in coronary flow reserve after coronary angioplasty as assessed with positron tomography. J Nucl Med 27:977, 1986 (abst)

55. Kehtarnavaz N, DeFigueiredo RJP: A novel surface reconstruction and display method for

cardiac PET imaging. IEEE Trans Med Imaging MI-3(3):108, 1984

56. Demer LL, Goldstein R, Mullani N, et al: Coronary steal by non-invasive PET identifies collateralized myocardium. J Nucl Med 27:977, 1986 (abst)

57. Geltman EM, Smith JL, Beecher D, et al: Altered regional myocardial metabolism in congestive cardiomyopathy detected by positron tomography. Am J Med 74:773, 1983

58. Perloff JK, Henze E, Schelbert HR: Alterations in regional myocardial metabolism, perfusion and wall motion in Duchenne's muscular dystrophy studied by radionuclide imaging. Circulation 69:33, 1984

59. Senda M, Yonekura Y, Tamaki N, et al: Axial resolution and the value of interpolating scan in multislice positron computed tomography. IEEE Trans Med Imaging MI-4(1):44, 1985

60. Mullani NA, Ficke DC, Hartz R, et al: System design of fast PET scanners utilizing time-of-flight. IEEE Trans Nucl Sci NS-28(1):104, 1981

61. Mullani N, Wong W, Hartz R, et al: Sensitivity improvement of TOFPET by the utilization of the interslice coincidences. IEEE Trans Nucl Sci NS-29(1):479, 1982

62. Wong WH, Mullani NA, Phillipe EA, et al: Image improvement and design optimization of the time-of-flight PET. J Nucl Med 24:52, 1983

63. Mullani NA, Gaeta J, Yerian K, et al: Dynamic Imaging with high resolution time-of-flight PET camera—TOFPET I. IEEE Trans Nucl Sci NS-31(1):609, 1984

64. Wong WH, Mullani NA, Wardworth G, et al: Characteristics of small barium fluoride (BaF$_2$) scintillator for high intrinsic resolution time-of-flight positron emission tomography. IEEE Trans Nucl Sci NS-31(1)381, 1984

65. Mullani NA, Gould KL: First pass regional blood flow measurements with external detectors. J Nucl Med 24:577, 1983

66. Mullani NA, Goldstein RA, Gould KL, et al: Myocardial perfusion with rubidium-82. I. Measurement of extraction fraction and flow with external detectors. J Nucl Med 24:898, 1983

67. Goldstein RA, Mullani NA, Fisher D, et al: Myocardial perfusion with rubidium-82. II. The effects of metabolic and pharmacologic interventions. J Nucl Med 24:907, 1983

68. Mullani NA: Myocardial perfusion with Rb-82. III. Theory relating severity of coronary stenosis to perfusion defect. J Nucl Med 25:1190, 1984

69. Yano Y, Chu P, Budinger TF, et al: Rubidium-82 generators for imaging studies. J Nucl Med 18:46, 1977

70. Yano Y, Budinger TF, Chiang G, et al: Evaluation and application of alumina-based Rb-82 generators charged with high levels of Sr-82/85. J Nucl Med 20:961, 1979

71. Yano Y, Cahoon JL, Budinger TF: A precision flow-controlled Rb-82 generator for bolus or constant-infusion studies of the heart and brain. J Nucl Med 22:1006, 1981

72. Schelbert HR, et al: Regional myocardial perfusion assessed with N-13 labeled ammonia and positron emission computerized axial tomography. Am J Cardiol 43:209, 1979

73. Schelbert HR, Phelps ME, Huang SC, et al: N-13 ammonia as an indicator of myocardial blood flow. Circulation 63:1259, 1981

74. Gould KL, Kelley KO: Experimental validation of quantitative coronary arteriography for determining pressure-flow characteristics of coronary stenoses. Circulation 66:930, 1982

75. Gould KL, Kelley KO: Significance of coronary flow velocity and changing stenosis geometry during coronary vasodilation in awake dogs. Circ Res 50:695, 1982

76. Kirkeeide RL, Fung P, Smalling RW, Gould KL: Automated evaluation of vessel diameter from arteriograms. Computers in cardiology. Proc IEEE Computer Soc 00:215, 1982

77. Kirkeeide RL, Smalling RW, Gould KL: Automated measurement of artery diameter from arteriograms. Circulation 66:II–325, 1982

78. Atkins HL, Budinger TF, Lebowitz E, et al: Thallium-201 for medical use. 3. Human distribution and physical imaging properties. J Nucl Med 18:133, 1977

79. Feller PA, Sodd VJ: Dosimetry of four heart-imaging radionuclides: ^{43}K, ^{81}Rb, ^{129}Cs, and ^{201}Tl. J Nucl Med 16:1070, 1975

80. Lockwood AH: Absorbed doses of radiation after an intravenous injection of N-13 ammonia in man. (Concise communication.) J Nucl Med 21:276, 1980

81. Jones SC, Alava A, Christman O, et al: The radiation dosimetry of 2-[F-18]fluoro-2-deoxy-D-glucose in man. J Nucl Med 23:613, 1982

82. Smith T. The radiation dosimetry of 2-[F-

18]fluoro-2-deoxy-D-glucose in man. J Nucl Med 24:447, 1983

83. Reivich M, Kuhl D, Wolf A, et al: The [^{18}F]fluorodeoxyglucose method for the measurement of local cerebral glucose utilization in man. Circ Res 44:127, 1979

84. Kearfott KJ: Radiation absorbed dose estimates for positron emission tomography (PET): K-38, Rb-81, Rb-82, and Cs-130. J Nucl Med 23:1128, 1982

85. Budinger TF, Rolio D: Physics and Instrumentation. Prog Cardiovasc Dis 20:19, 1977

86. Squibb Investigators Brochure, April 1983

87. Kearfott KJ: Absorbed dose estimates for positron emission tomography (PET): C^{15}O, ^{11}CO, and CO^{15}O. J Nucl Med 23:1031, 1982

88. Paans AMJ, Vaalburg W, Woldring MG: A comparison of the sensitivity of PET and NMR for in vivo quantitative metabolic imaging. Eur J Nucl Med 11:73, 1985

89. Miller DD, Holmbang G, Gill JB, et al: Detection of coronary stenoses by continuous paramagnetic contrast infusion during dipyridamole-induced hyperemia: The nuclear magnetic resonance imaging "stress test." Circulation 74:II-319, 1986 (abst)

90. Wolfkiel CJ, Ferguson JL, Chomka EV, et al: Myocardial blood flow determined by ultrafast computed tomography. Circulation 74:II-122, 1986 (abst)

91. Smalling RW: The SPECTrum of thallium-201 imaging in coronary artery disease. J Nucl Med 24:854, 1983

92. Maddahi J, Van Train KF, Rozanski A, et al: Is Tl-201 single photon emission computerized tomography (SPECT) superior to planar imaging for evaluation of coronary artery disease? Circulation 74:II-61, 1986 (abst)

93. Mullani N: SPECT imaging: a question of ethics and economics. J Nucl Med 27:145, 1986

13
Radionuclide Venography

Warren H. Moore

Radionuclide venography (RNV) is a valuable tool that is used frequently in some institutions but rarely in others. At centers that take advantage of this procedure, one form of the technique usually predominates. The purpose of this chapter is to describe the techniques, interpretation, and applications of various radionuclide venous studies. Emphasis is placed on procedures in more widespread use, but new and less common techniques are also included.

Evaluation of the venous system and particularly the veins of the lower extremities is most commonly undertaken due to the known or suspected presence of pulmonary emboli (PE), deep venous thrombosis (DVT), or thrombophlebitis (TP). Any or all of these concerns may be present in a given patient. Thrombi form in response to vascular damage, alteration of blood coagulability, and/or venous stasis, and conditions predisposing to any of these factors will predispose to DVT and subsequent embolization.

It is generally agreed that almost all clinically significant PE arise in the deep veins of the pelvis or lower extremities.[1,2] Although the actual incidence of thrombi is probably much higher in the smaller veins of the calf than in the iliofemoral system, the clinical consequences of smaller thromboemboli are less, and they usually go undetected.[3-5]

The real incidence of TP, DVT, and PE is unknown, largely due to the problem of clinical diagnosis, which is less than 50 percent accurate for the diagnosis of DVT. Autopsy studies have shown prevalences of 20 to 90 percent for DVT of the lower extremities in hospitalized patients, depending on the patient population and the method of diagnosis; studies with careful postmortem examinations revealed prevalences of 60 to 70 percent in general acute care facilities.[6,7] Similarly, while clinical diagnoses of PE are less than 200,000 cases per year in the United States, estimates based on autopsy surveys suggest that more than 600,000 symptomatic pulmonary emboli occur annually, with a fatality rate of at least 30 percent.[8,9] Although autopsy studies may overestimate the importance of small in situ thrombi and thromboemboli, the disparity between clinical and autopsy series underscores the insensitivity of clinical diagnosis and the need for further diagnostic measures, if reasonable accuracy is to be attained.

Evaluation of the venous system can be performed by several different isotopic methods. Choosing the best procedure depends on knowledge of the alternative forms, the clinical situation, the equipment available, and the capabilities of the individual laboratory's technical and professional staff. Specific questions include the following:

Is a perfusion lung scan also desirable or necessary?

Is analysis of flow important?

Is assessment of activity (age) of venous disease important?

What degree of sensitivity and specificity are necessary?

Are there special instrumentation or clinical limitations?

After these questions have been defined, an appropriate test can be initiated. In general, these procedures may be divided into four major categories, which have some overlap: flow studies, blood pool studies, markers of active thrombogenesis, and markers of inflammation.

FLOW STUDIES: ALBUMIN VENOGRAPHY

Almost any ^{99m}Tc-labeled compound can be used to evaluate venous flow. Most simply, a 5- to 10-mCi dose of pertechnetate can be injected intravenously (IV) to assess a particular region using a rapid imaging sequence (1–3 seconds/frame). Smaller doses can be injected sequentially, but recirculation of the tracer as well as its appearance in the urinary tract limit the usefulness of this technique. Other technetium-99m compounds that are rapidly removed from the bloodstream or that are concentrated outside the region of interest (ROI), including sulfur colloid (SC), and most commonly macroaggre-

gated albumin (MAA), are preferred if more than one injection is to be made. Commonly available radiopharmaceuticals labeled with other isotopes rarely have count rates approaching those of ^{99m}Tc and have little to offer for evaluation of flow.

RNV with albumin particles was first described by Webber et al.,[10] in 1969. These and subsequent investigators used ^{99m}Tc-labeled MAA or human albumin microspheres (HAM) to evaluate the inferior vena cava (IVC), iliofemoral and popliteal veins, and to some extent the deep veins of the calf.

In addition to being adequate for flow imaging, albumin compounds have added advantages. First, because these (10- to 90-μm) particles are normally cleared from the blood by passive trapping in the first arteriolar bed they encounter, almost all the particles are removed in the first pass through the lungs, and there is minimal recirculation to complicate subsequent injections. The particles may also accumulate in areas of actively forming venous thrombi. This process has been postulated to occur both by means of entrapment in the fibrinoprotein mesh and by an electrostatic attraction between the albumin and components at the surface of the clot.[11,12] The ultimate fate of this compound is leaching and decay of technetium and proteolysis of the albumin particles, until they are small enough to pass into the systemic circulation from which they are sequestered and further metabolized within the reticuloendothelial system.

Technique

LOWER EXTREMITIES

A typical venous blood flow procedure includes dynamic and static imaging.[11] For the lower extremities, tourniquets are placed at the ankles and knees. A 23- or 25-gauge scalp vein needle is inserted into a dorsal pedal vein of each foot and, with the camera positioned over the pelvis, 1-mCi doses are injected and followed by a heparinized flush solution. Camera acquisition is begun when the bolus reaches the field of view, and three to five 15-second images are obtained. Similar series are repeated with the detector positioned over the thighs and then over the calves. (Fig. 13-1A). After walking or other leg exercise, 50,000-count static images are obtained in the same fields of view (Fig. 13-1B).

Alternative protocols use a whole body technique in which the patient is placed on a moving table/camera system.[13] A set of paired injections is made, acquisition is started, and the table is set in motion. By coordinating table speed with venous flow, a single image defines the venous system (Fig. 13-2). Resolution with this technique is less than that seen with multiple spot images; difficulties result when there is great disparity between the rates of ascent of the tracer in different legs.

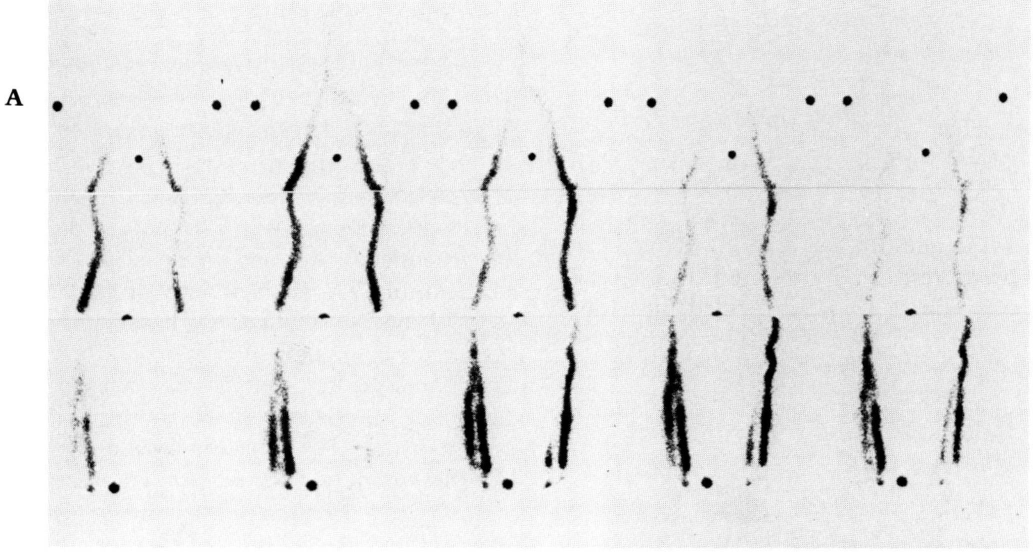

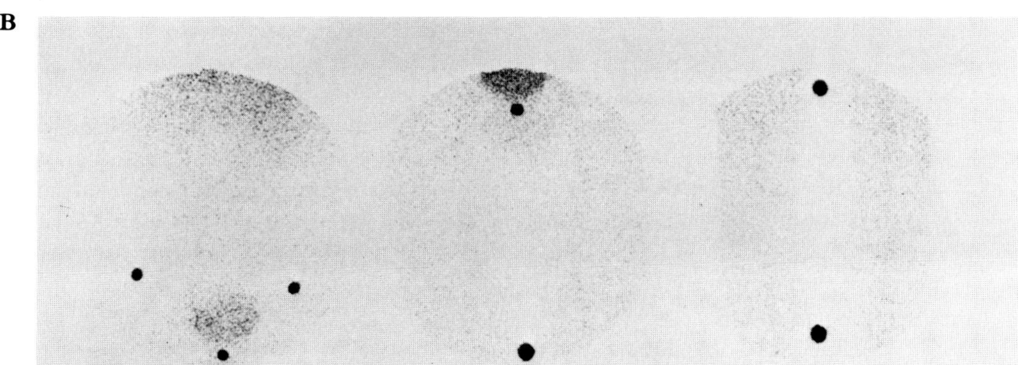

Fig. 13-1 Normal albumin RNV, anterior view. **(A)** Composite of 15-sec flow images showing pelvis, thigh, and calf fields of view. **(B)** Static delayed images of same regions. Spot markers indicate iliac crests, pubis, knees, and ankles.

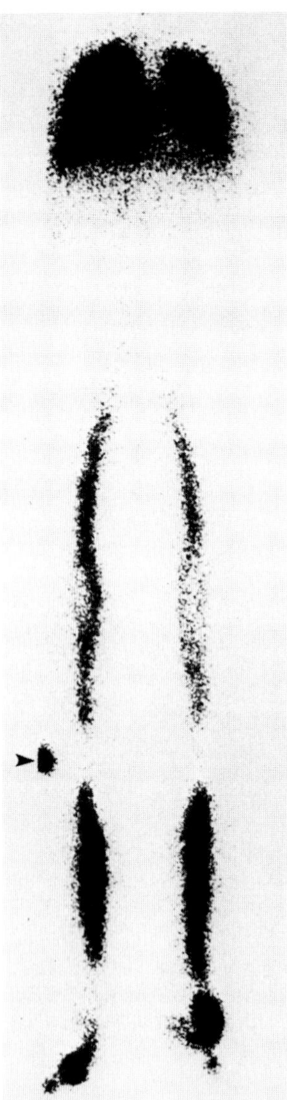

Fig. 13-2 Normal albumin RNV, single-pass technique. Arrow marks location of tourniquet at right knee. (From Magoun et al.,[13] with permission.)

If these techniques are to be optimally useful, attention to details of the injection process is important. Tourniquets must be tight, but occlusion of the superficial veins can generally be accomplished with minimal discomfort. Tourniquets at the knees are less critical but reinforce the effect of those at the ankle. If visualization of the saphenous veins is de-

sired, the tourniquets may be omitted. For contrast venography (CV), it has been suggested that the injection needle be directed retrograde for better filling of the deep veins. This technique offers no advantage in routine RNV. Blood should not enter the syringe with the albumin particles. When this occurs, small thrombi may be formed and labeled with the high specific activity dose material, resulting in injection of "hot emboli." The radiolabeled clots may simulate in vivo thrombogenesis or may entrap so many of the particles that venous and pulmonary imaging is compromised.

UPPER EXTREMITIES

Upper extremity venography can be performed in a similar manner. With the patient supine and the detector positioned over the upper arm and central chest, a 1-mCi bolus is injected into the basilic vein. Sequential 15- to 20-second images are obtained, and the series may be repeated from the other arm (Fig. 13-3A,B). Alternatively, the camera may be positioned centrally and injections made simultaneously in each arm. Although the large-field-of-view (LFOV) scintillation camera is the most convenient instrument for performing RNV, standard-field-of-view (SFOV) instruments may be used. If only a SFOV camera is available, separate injections using technetium-99m SC will permit better definition of the origin of collateral vessels if they are present (Fig. 13-3C). If a parallel hole collimator is used with the SFOV camera, each extremity may be imaged separately. This problem can be avoided by the use of a diverging collimator. Although resolution suffers somewhat with this modification of the technique, the ability to image very ill patients at the bedside is a substantial advantage.

Interpretation

Interpretation of albumin venography is straightforward. The simple physiologic behavior of the radiopharmaceuticals, the lim-

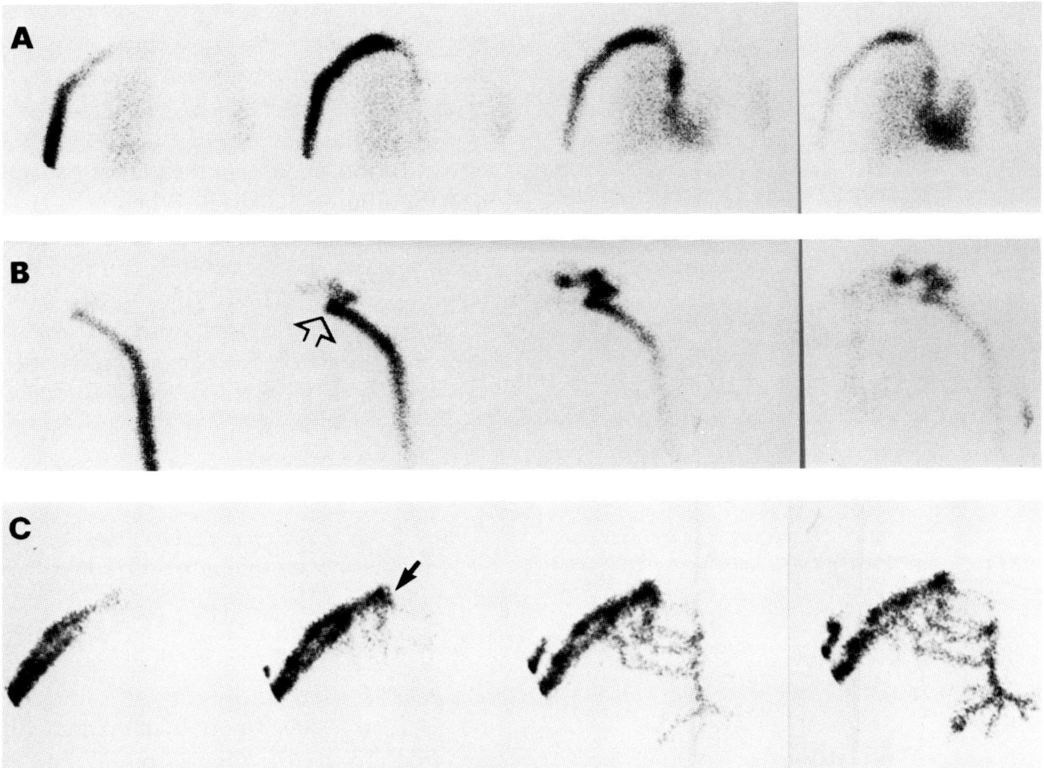

Fig. 13-3 **(A)** Normal right upper extremity RNV with technetium-99m SC, showing unobstructed flow. **(B)** Left arm RNV in the same patient with subclavian vein obstruction (arrowhead) and collateral vessels. **(C)** Right arm RNV with subclavian obstruction (arrowhead) and extensive chest wall collaterals.

ited number of anatomic structures that may appear on normal or abnormal studies, and the relatively small number of normal variations all contribute to this ease. A normal RNV is shown in Figure 13-1A. The most cephalad component is an inverted **Y** representing the IVC and the common and external iliac veins. The internal iliac veins are usually not visualized. The only vessel to be seen in the thigh is the superficial femoral vein. This channel may be duplicated in part or rarely in its entirety. The popliteal vein is formed in the upper calf by the confluence of the three major deep veins of the calf: the anterior and posterior tibial and the peroneal veins. One, two, or occasionally all three of these may be seen. Each major tributary

regularly consists of two or more branches, but these subunits are never separately resolved. Other deep veins of the calf include the sural veins, the soleal and gastrocnemius plexuses, and many small muscle veins. These vessels are rarely demonstrated by albumin venography.

It is important to be aware of several areas of normal decrease in tracer activity (Fig. 13-4). Proximally, the IVC is compressed as it passes behind the liver, attenuating emissions. There may be focal diminution or irregularity of the tracer column at the level of the renal veins due to crossing defects of the right renal vessels or dilution by nonradioactive blood from the renal veins, as is

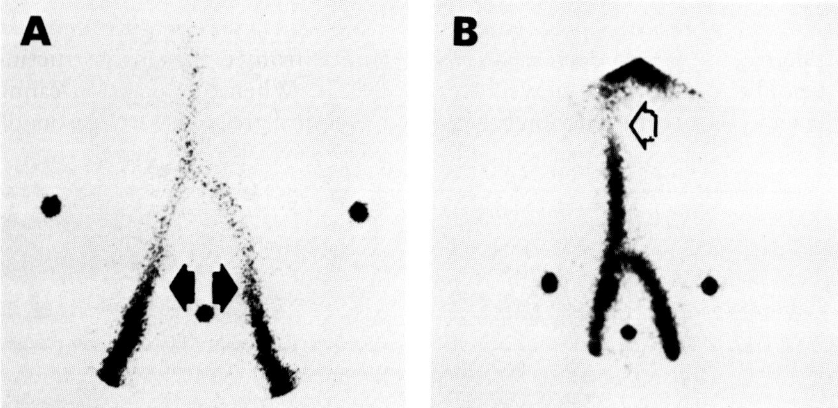

Fig. 13-4 Albumin venogram. Closed arrows **(A)** Indicate normal decrease in activity at the inguinal ligament. Open arrow **(B)** denotes normal attenuation of the hepatic portion of the IVC in a child.

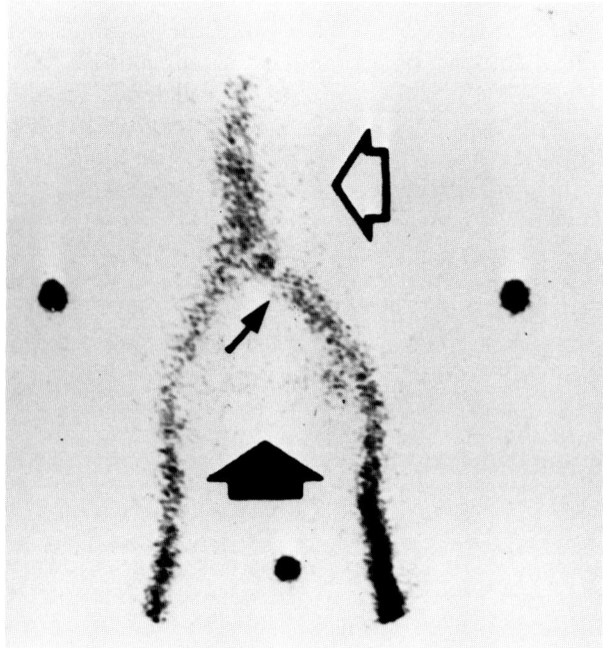

Fig. 13-5 Anterior view of albumin RNV. Iliac compression syndrome in an asymptomatic patient. Arrow indicates decreased activity due to crossing right common iliac artery. Open and closed arrowheads indicate faint visualization of ascending lumbar and sacral collateral vessels, respectively.

seen routinely on contrast cavagrams. Another area of decreased activity is cephalad to the inguinal ligament, where the external iliac veins course posteriorly away from the detector. There is frequently decreased activity in the popliteal fossa, as viewed from the anterior view, due to attenuation by bone and soft tissues and/or compression of the vein by the posterior aspect of the femur when the knee is extended. Special mention should be made of a common anatomic relationship in the pelvis. Indentation of the left common iliac vein by the right common iliac artery is seen in a sizeable minority of patients referred for RNV. This partial obstruction is usually asymptomatic, but the degree of obstruction is variable and in the extreme may be total.[14,15] This iliac compression syndrome is shown in Figure 13-5 and is typically seen as an area of the left common iliac vein, which is persistently decreased in intensity on all parts of a dynamic sequence. Occasionally, there is minimal collateralization in the ascending lumbar or pelvic channels.

True abnormalities may be manifested by (1) obstruction to flow, (seen as cutoff, attenuation, or focal delay), (2) collateral flow, (3) generalized delay in tracer appearance, or (4) persistence of tracer activity on later static images. The most specific criterion is a cutoff, as demonstrated in Figure 13-6A. RNV does not permit differentiation of intrinsic from extrinsic obstruction (Fig. 13-6A,B). When this decision cannot be made on clinical grounds with reasonable certainty, cross-sectional anatomic imaging may be useful.

Collateral flow may occur with or without evidence of discrete obstruction and may have a number of patterns. Obstruction of the IVC or iliac veins leads immediately to visualization of collaterals. These vessels can be grouped into four main categories, as demonstrated in Figure 13-7A-D. The most striking collaterals are those of the anterior abdominal wall. These arise at the level of the inguinal ligament and proceed in a branching pattern in the wall and subcutaneous tissues. This flow may re-enter the IVC above the obstruction or may proceed cephalad to enter the SVC. The most commonly seen collaterals are those of the pelvic and sacral plexuses. These vessels cross from one iliac vein to the other at or below the level of the internal iliac veins. Less often seen with RNV are vertically oriented deep central vessels, including the ascending lumbar/

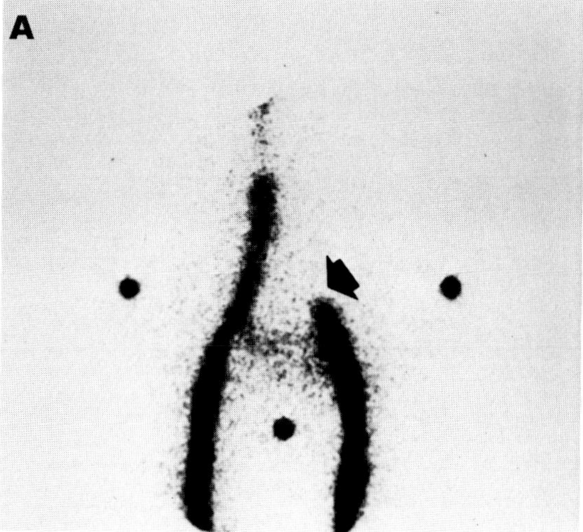
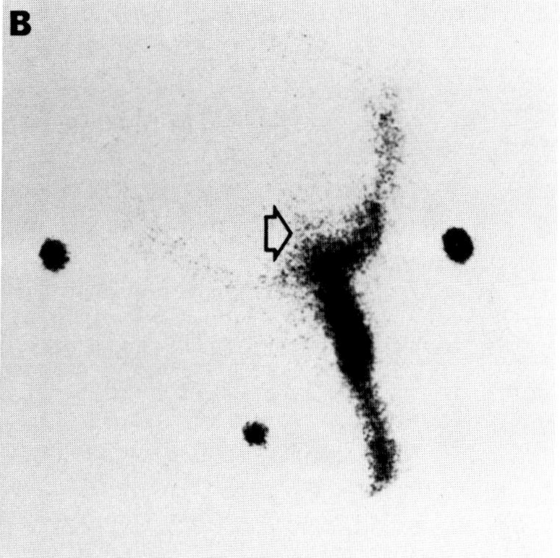

Fig. 13-6 (A) Pelvic image in a patient with thrombotic obstruction of the left common iliac vein (closed arrow). **(B)** Pelvic image following left foot injection of HAM in a patient with extrinsic obstruction (open arrow) due to uterus at 36 weeks gestation.

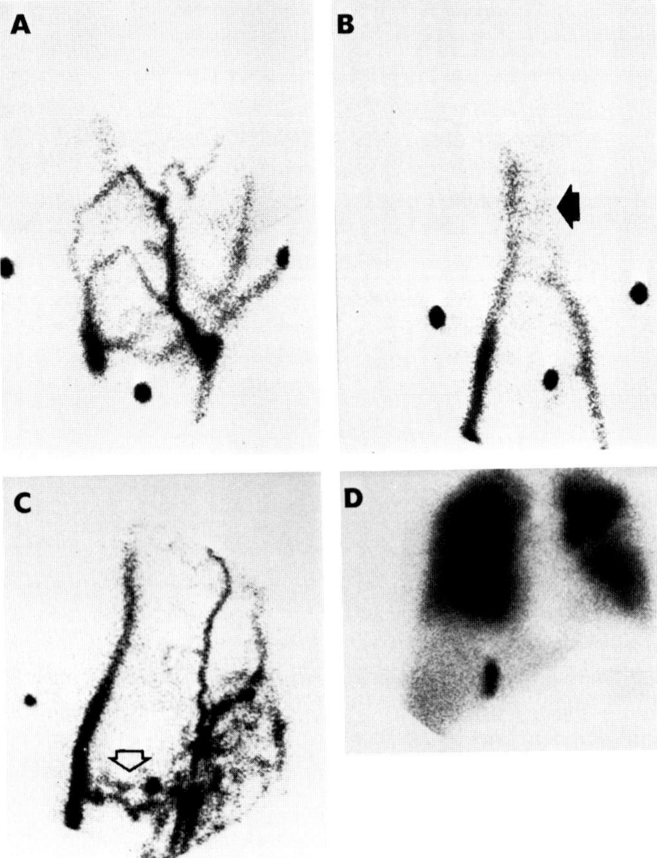

Fig. 13-7 Collateral channels demonstrated by albumin venography. **(A)** Superficial anterior vessels. **(B)** Central paravertebral collaterals (arrow). **(C)** Pelvic vessels (arrow). **(D)** Diffuse and focal hepatic uptake due to systemic-portal communication in a patient with IVC obstruction and PE.

hemiazygos system and other parallel and perpendicular branches of the paravertebral system. The fourth major collateral system is systemic-portal communication. These vessels arise in the pelvis, or occasionally at the level of the renal veins, and flow into the portal vein or its branches in the liver, accounting for diffuse or focal tracer activity in the liver. This pattern has also been reported from upper-extremity collaterals in SVC obstruction. Collateral flow in the lower extremities is quite variable in course and involves large and small superficial channels that reconstitute the deep system down-stream from the obstruction.

Despite early reports indicating that delay in ascent of tracer from one pedal injection with respect to the other was a sign of abnormality, this finding is often related to normal anatomic variation or differences in the injection technique.[16-18] Looser tourniquets, larger injection needles, larger pedal veins, or a more forceful flush may each cause a bolus to ascend faster on a given side. When disparity is seen in ascent, one should look carefully for abnormality on the slow side but, if no other abnormality is seen, this pattern is best disregarded or the injection repeated after attention to the details mentioned above.

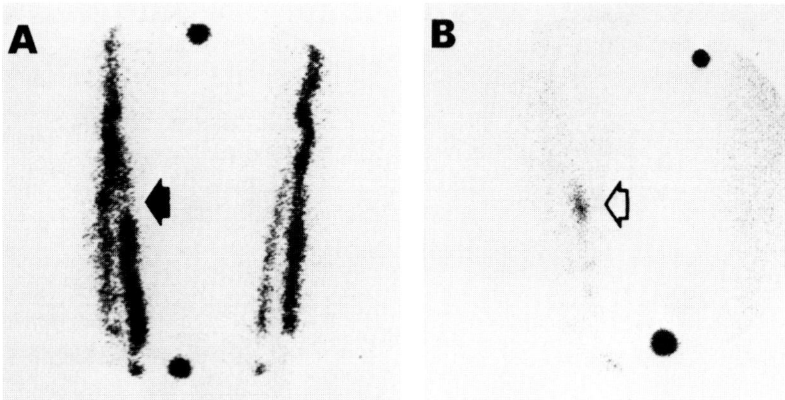

Fig. 13-8 (A) Anterior calf image from albumin RNV demonstrating partial obstruction of a right calf vein (arrow) but no collateral vessels. **(B)** Delayed image in the same patient. Arrow indicates focal radioparticle entrapment consistent with thrombophlebitis at the site of partial obstruction.

Webber et al.[10] suggested that delayed images obtained after flow imaging could detect active thrombogenesis. Abnormal results are indicated by focal persistence of activity in the veins (Fig. 13-8). These images are particularly useful when TP or nonocclusive thrombi are present. However, veins that are nearly totally occluded may not have sufficient flow to permit detectable entrapment, creating a false-negative scan. False-positive results also occur due to persistence of tracer around valves and other areas of slow flow. This inability to distinguish passive persistence from active entrapment can be improved if the patient performs leg exercise, helping to clear nonspecific activity. This maneuver is especially important in patients with pre-existing venous disease. However, many patients needing venography are not able to perform such exercise, and the reliability of this portion of the procedure is questionable.[19]

BLOOD-POOL STUDIES: RBC VENOGRAPHY

Radionuclide venography can also be performed with technetium-labeled red blood cells (RBC).[20–23]

Technique

Cells are labeled by in vivo, or preferably semi-in vitro, technique as for equilibrium cardiac imaging. Following cell labeling and tracer injection, images of the pelvis and thighs are obtained in the anterior view with the patient in the supine position; images of the popliteal and calf regions are obtained in the posterior view with the patient prone (Fig. 13-9). Instrumentation is the same as for albumin venography. Technique is critically important for proper imaging. The patient should avoid pressure and constriction on the ROI. For the anterior images, slight bending of the knees with pillow support may be useful to avoid excessive tensing of thigh muscles. This muscle contraction, whether subconscious or purposeful, can alter blood-pool volume and create artifactual asymmetry suggesting DVT. Symmetry of position is likewise important to avoid interpretive errors. Optimal imaging of the popliteal and calf regions requires that images be collected in the prone position, again to minimize compression of the blood pool. Images of each region of interest may be obtained with an all purpose, high resolution, or diverging collimator. Images should be collected for 0.8 to 2.0 million counts (depend-

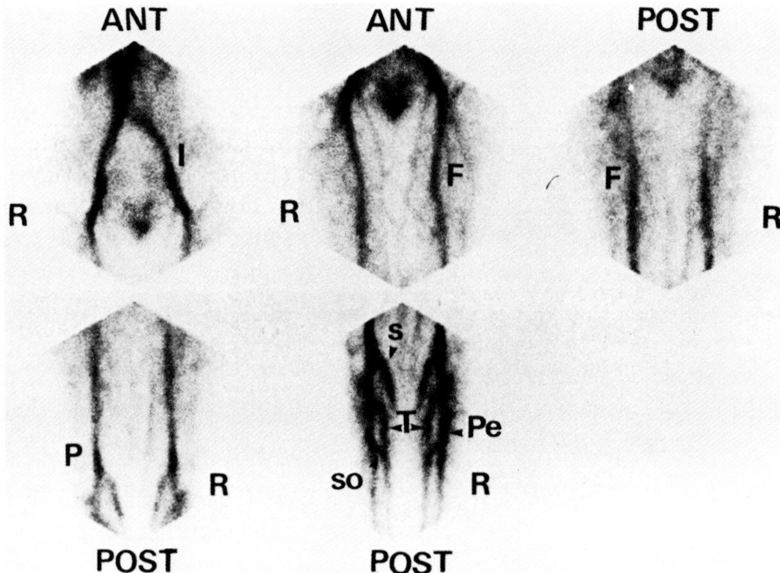

Fig. 13-9 Normal RBC venogram. Note symmetry of vascular appearance and faint visualization of multiple other vessels. R, right side; I, left iliac vessels; F, left superficial femoral vein; P, left popliteal vein; s, medial sural vein; so, soleal vein; Pe, peroneal vein; T, posterior tibial vein. (From Lisbona et al.,[21] with permission.)

ing on the field of view and the collimator). A similar technique can be used for upper extremity/chest venography.[24]

Interpretation

As with albumin venography, knowledge of the normal and variant anatomy is essential to interpretation of RBC venography. Because the entire blood pool is labeled, many more vascular structures are present to be evaluated. These include sural and other deep veins of the calves; the profunda femoris vein in the thigh; superficial veins, in general; abdominal mesenteric, visceral, and portal vessels; and the abdominal organs. Despite this increase in complexity of interpretation, RBC has certain advantages over the albumin technique.

Red blood cell venography may be considered abnormal by the same criteria as those used for albumin venography. Differences in technique should be considered, however. Although an absolute cutoff of activity is the most specific finding in obstruction, it is less likely to be perceived with RBC due to the proximity of arteries and a higher general background (Fig. 13-10). Collaterals may be less distinct but more numerous, owing to the fact that this is an equilibrium technique and the entire blood pool is labeled. Some difficulty may exist due to normal visualization of vessels other than the iliofemoral trunk, but extensive collaterals strongly suggest venous disease. Similarly, a diffuse increase in background activity suggests underlying venous obliteration. Albumin RNV or CV may be used to evaluate equivocal RBC studies.

MARKERS OF ACTIVE THROMBOGENESIS

Radioiodinated Fibrinogen Venography

As suggested by Hobbs and Davies in 1960, and reported for humans in 1964, ^{131}I-labeled fibrinogen, in theory, combined venous im-

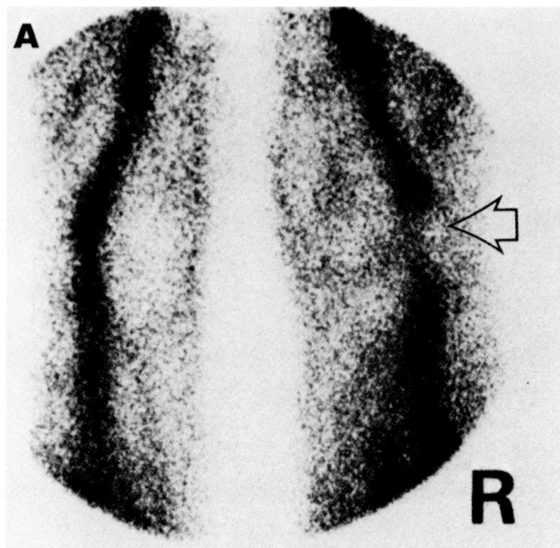

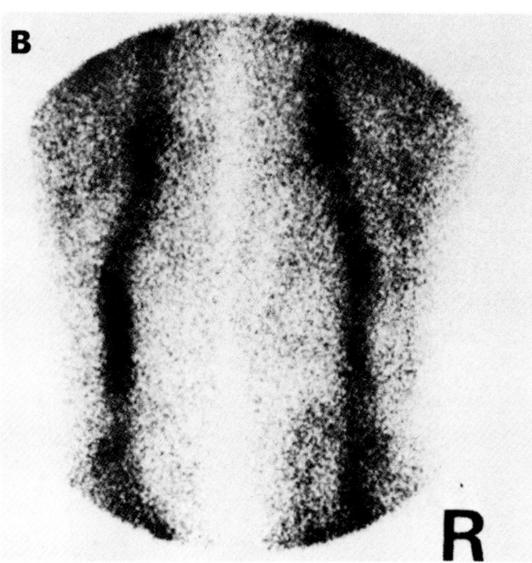

Fig. 13-10 RBC venogram with posterior view of knee region. **(A)** Arrow denotes popliteal vein obstruction. **(B)** Flow through this region is normal in a follow-up study after removal of a popliteal cyst. (From Lisbona et al.,[21] with permission.)

aging with the physiologic advantages of incorporation of labeled fibrinogen into actively forming thrombi.[25,26] Imaging was suboptimal, however, and iodine-131-fibrinogen is now not commercially available for this use in the United States.[27]

The imaging successor to iodine-131-fibrinogen is iodine-123-fibrinogen.[28] This com-

pound, which is also not commercially available in the United States, retains the physiologic advantage of fibrinogen but substitutes an isotope with more optimal photon yield and energy. The shorter half-life ($t\frac{1}{2}$) of ^{123}I (13 hours versus 8 days) also reduces radiation dose to the patient. Preparation of the compound, however, is not a trivial radiochemical problem, because of the need for a relatively large number of iodine atoms on each fibrinogen molecule.[29] After dose preparation and injection, images of the venous system are obtained at 4 to 6 hours and 24 hours later. Abnormal tracer activity is seen as irregular and/or increased tracer accumulation or abnormal lack of activity in proximal vessels (Fig. 13-11A,B).

Fibrinogen Uptake Test

The only radioiodinated fibrinogen compound that is readily available in the United States is iodine-125-fibrinogen. Its low photon energy (35 keV) effectively prohibits imaging with ordinary gamma cameras, but it is used for the fibrinogen uptake test (FUT), a nonimaging procedure.[30]

Following injection of 100 μCi of iodine-125-fibrinogen a probe counter is used to measure activity at carefully marked points on the patient's legs (Fig. 13-12). These counts are expressed as a percentage of cardiac counts and are recorded graphically. Preparation for counting requires the bladder to be as empty as possible and the patient's legs to be elevated just prior to imaging. Counting is begun 4 hours after injection and continued for 7 to 10 days, or until the study becomes positive.

Although the use of homologous fibrinogen entails a concern for transmission of hepatitis and other infectious diseases, this potential risk is, in fact, less than that of a blood transfusion, because of the small amount of protein used and the extensive testing of these donors. An additional concern with the use of the iodinated compounds is the presence of free iodine. Lugol's solution (10 to 20

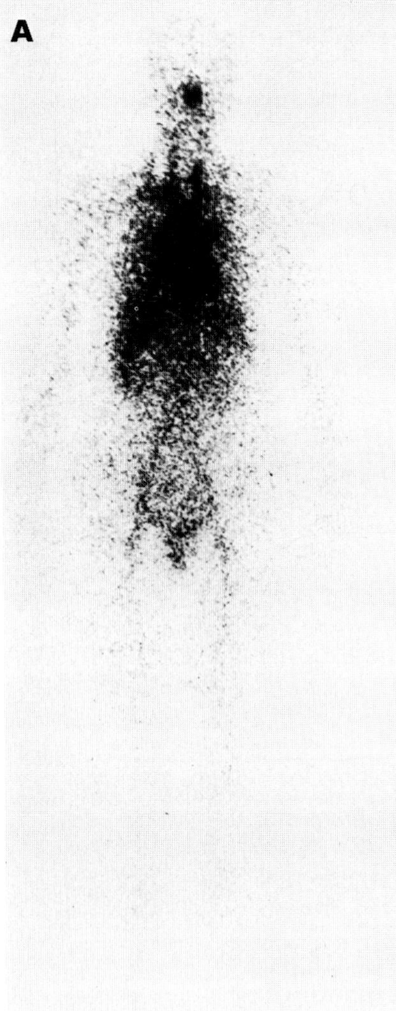
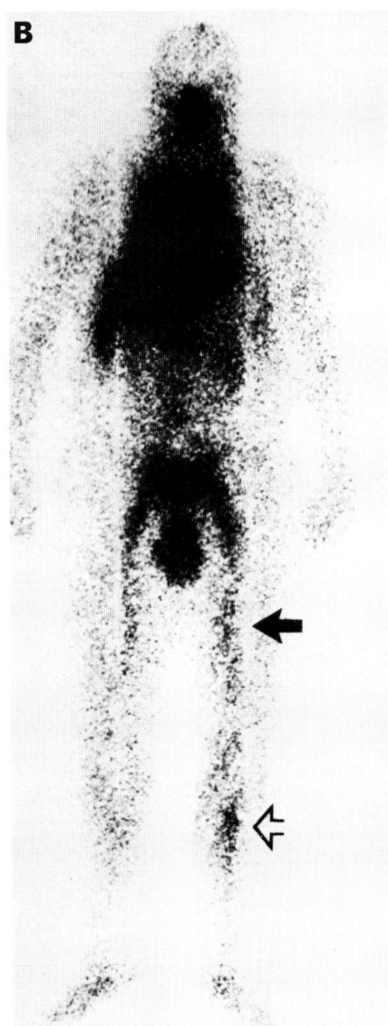

Fig. 13-11 (A) Anterior whole-body view of normal iodine-123-fibrinogen venogram. **(B)** Abnormal iodine-123-fibrinogen venogram. Note focal increase in activity distally (open arrow) and proximally (closed arrow) in a patient with thrombophlebitis. (From DeNardo and DeNardo,[28] with permission.)

drops daily for 10 days) will block thyroid uptake. Free iodine crosses the placenta and, despite the small proportion of the injected dose, these studies are relatively contraindicated in pregnant women.

The FUT is interpreted as positive if any of three criteria are met. The criteria are a 20 percentage point increase in tracer activity (1) between corresponding points on different legs at the same time, and (2) between adjacent points on the same leg at the same time, and (3) at a particular point from one day to the next[30,31] (Fig. 13-13).

Other Tests of Active Thrombogenesis

Other tests of active thrombogenesis include venography and/or FUT-like procedures with Tc-labeled fibrinogen, as well as labeled streptokinase, urokinase, plasmin, and other

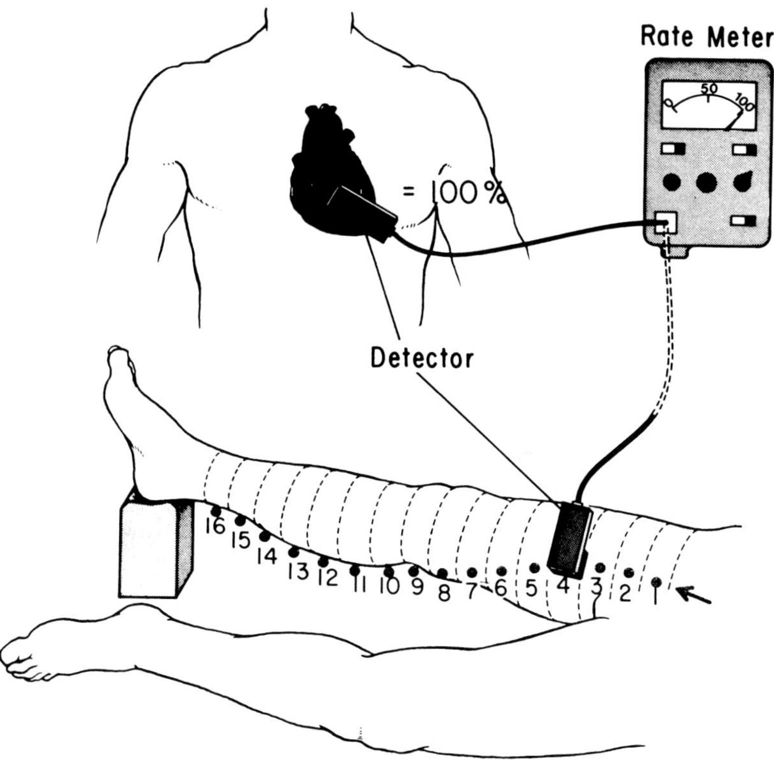

Fig. 13-12 Marking and counting arrangement for iodine-125-fibrinogen FUT. Note course of marks over the deep vessels and elevation of the leg. Activity is expressed as a percent of cardiac activity. (From DeNardo and DeNardo,[31] with permission.)

proteins of the coagulation or fibrinolytic pathways. Autologous platelets labeled with ^{111}In have recently been used as well. None of these techniques has had sufficient clinical testing to be adequately evaluated, and most of these radiopharmaceuticals are not generally available.[32–34]

INFLAMMATORY MARKERS

Several agents have been used to assess venous inflammation, phlebitis, and thrombophlebitis. Gallium citrate, ^{111}In-labeled white blood cells (WBC), and SC, as well as several other compounds may accumulate in areas of venous inflammation.[35–37] Although theoretically pleasing, clinical experi-

ence with these agents is also too small to assess their accuracy.

APPLICATIONS

Thromboembolic Disease

The most common use of any type of RNV is for the detection and evaluation of deep venous disease of the lower extremities. In comparison with CV, albumin venography has been demonstrated to be effective for assessment of clinically significant venous disease. Its accuracy varies from 65 percent to 98 percent, depending on the site, criteria for interpretation, and method of comparison with CV. Where site-by-site analysis has

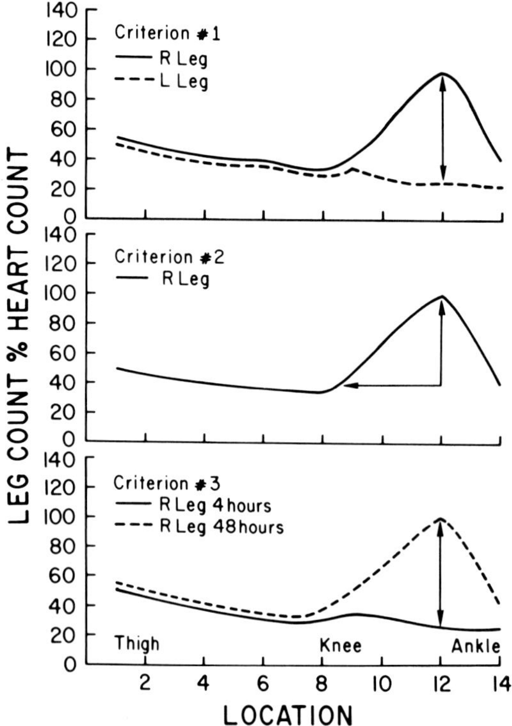

Fig. 13-13 Graphic display of activity profiles from an abnormal FUT. Activity is abnormally increased by all three criteria in the right mid-calf region. (From DeNardo et al.,[45] with permission.)

been done, this technique is at least 90 percent accurate in the iliac veins and infrarenal IVC as well as the femoral and popliteal veins, but only approximately 65% accurate below the popliteal vein.[38–41] Accuracy in this region is a consequence of both false-negative tests, where nonocclusive disease is not detected on flow images, and false-positive tests due to nonspecific persistence. Overall accuracy is related to the degree of disease present. If the test is to be used for screening, and sensitivity is desired, all components of the test should be used. Radionuclide venography with labeled RBC compares similarly to albumin venography.[20,21] Although its accuracy in the pelvis is slightly less, its more extensive calf visualization compensates.

Nonetheless, differences in the techniques and images between flow and blood-pool studies are important in choosing one or the other for a particular clinical situation. Because of the greater flexibility of injection, the RBC technique is rarely hampered by an inability to find a suitable venous access point. It is thus particularly useful when the feet or hands, due to edema, inflammation, injury (casts, burns), or amputation, are not accessible for venipuncture. Inexperience on the part of the technical staff with pedal injection is a remediable limitation of the albumin technique, but the additional time and personnel required for optimal performance of the albumin test is a further advantage for the RBC procedure. From an imaging standpoint, advantages of the RBC study include visualization of the superficial veins without compromise of deep venous filling and visualization of more deep venous structures, such as the sural and soleal veins in the calves.

While there are relative contraindications to albumin venography in patients with severe pulmonary hypertension, right-to-left circulatory shunts, and pregnancy, only the warning with respect to pregnancy applies to the RBC technique. The albumin method is objectionable to some members of certain religious groups (e.g., Jehovah's Witnesses), whereas the RBC technique, with in vivo labeling, eliminates this concern.

Advantages of the albumin technique include better definition of the deep venous system from the popliteal vein proximally due to the lower background, lack of visualization of the adjacent overlapping artery, and the availability of dynamic flow imaging. The previously mentioned property of uptake in active thrombi is at least a theoretical advantage, and the ability to perform pulmonary perfusion imaging in association with RNV is a major argument for using albumin. Neither form of RNV shares the potential complications of CV, such as iodine allergy, induction of TP, and significant skin damage from dose extravasation. Fortunately, venous disease is much less common in children but, other than occasional technical difficulties in finding suitable veins, RNV can be performed equally as well in children as in adults, using a decreased dose (based on weight or body surface area).

To keep radiation exposures as low as reasonably achievable, requests for radionuclide studies in pregnancy must be considered on a case-by-case basis. However, given the prevalence of extremity swelling and dyspnea in pregnant women, the difficulty of clinical diagnosis, and the complications of medical treatment of TP and PE in this population, RNV with ^{99m}Tc-labeled agents and ventilation-perfusion lung scanning are safe and effective tests in pregnant women. Because the weight of the gravid uterus may significantly obstruct pelvic venous flow, abnormal studies obtained with the patient supine should be repeated with the patient in the lateral decubitus position.

The usefulness of either form of RNV in the evaluation of chronic venous disease is much less clear. While both may show evidence of partial or complete venous obstruction, with or without well-developed collateral channels, neither can conclusively exclude the presence of active disease superimposed on a setting of chronic venous insufficiency. Neither study is useful in the routine assessment of patients with varicosities or in decision-making concerning vascular surgery.

Upper Extremity and Thoracic Disorders

Assessment of TP in the upper extremities is similar in principle to that in the lower extremities. Diagnosis of disorders of the cephalic and basilic veins in the upper arm is fairly reliable, and assessment of the axillary, subclavian, and brachiocephalic veins is very accurate. Furthermore, RNV is an excellent screening technique for SVC obstruction.[42,43] It is also useful in patients with indwelling venous catheters; at our institution, RNV is used to assess potential sites of vascular access in patients with chemotherapy or hyperalimentation catheters who must have new catheters placed due to infection or thrombosis.

A separate but useful indication for upper extremity RNV is the evaluation of patients with thoracic outlet obstruction. By obtaining images with the arm in a relaxed (anatomic) position and subsequent images with the arm abducted and externally rotated, differences in flow can be observed.

Assessment of Active Thrombogenesis

If the primary clinical question relates to activity of venous disease, one of the fibrinogen studies should be considered. On theoretical grounds, iodine-123-fibrinogen would seem to be the current procedure of choice, but its limitations in terms of expertise in preparation, cost, and availability make it impractical for most laboratories.[44] Iodine-125-fibrinogen, however, does have a limited but definite place in the evaluation of active venous disease. The FUT is recognized as a legitimate gold standard for the presence or absence of thrombosis in many studies, such as most of those designed to test the efficacy of anticoagulant regimens in operative or debilitated patients.[3,45,46] As such, a negative FUT is a very good indication of the absence of active thrombogenesis. The limitation of this study lies in the fact that many of the disorders in the differential diagnosis of a tender, swollen, and/or reddened leg will cause physiologically (true) positive tests. Such conditions as cellulitis, superficial venous disease, ruptured popliteal cyst, muscle hematoma, and skeletal fracture may all result in a positive FUT. Although many of these conditions can rapidly be excluded on the basis of clinical data, a definitive diagnosis of DVT may not be aided much by a positive FUT in patients with these coexistent problems. To be most effective, the FUT should be used prospectively with serial follow-up studies. Such an approach is to inject the fibrinogen the day before hip surgery and monitor the patient for the next 7 to 10 days.[3] In this manner, anticoagulation can be postponed until the test shows signs of conversion, that is, postoperative onset of thrombogenesis. However, because of the very high sensitivity of the test and its ability to detect physiologically true-positive but clinically inconsequential thrombi, conversion to a positive test, while it does indicate an increased risk of thromboembolic events, is not necessarily an absolute indication for full anticoagulant therapy.[19] A further limitation of the FUT is that, despite its sensitivity in the calf and popliteal regions, its accuracy decreases considerably in the upper thigh. Increased intervening tissue and bladder activity account for this decrease and make the study worthless in the pelvis.

The use of inflammatory cell labels such as gallium citrate and indium-oxine has not received the same degree of clinical and radiologic testing as have other RNV techniques. Whereas, in principle, inflamed veins are not different from inflammation of other body tissues, the relatively small degree and extent of inflammation present in most types of phlebitis compared with the degree of infection present in an abscess hampers these agents in the evaluation of venous disorders. In this regard, and particularly in cases of recent inflammation, ^{111}In-labeled WBC will probably prove superior to gallium due primarily to the lower background activity. Platelets, which have been labeled with ^{75}Se, ^{51}Cr, ^{99m}Tc, or more successfully with ^{111}In, are accurate in the diagnosis of arterial and vascular graft thrombosis.[34,47,48] While their current application to venous imaging is limited by relatively small numbers of clinical cases, this technique has considerable potential.

CONCLUSION

A number of radionuclide techniques are useful in the evaluation of venous disease. Careful attention to the specific clinical question to be addressed, and knowledge of the various imaging and nonimaging isotope techniques that are available can usually lead the practitioner to the most effective choice. Overall, RNV by any of several techniques is an acceptable option for the diagnosis of venous thromboembolic disease, and the FUT is a sensitive detector of active thrombogenesis with reasonable clinical value when used in the appropriate setting. The accuracy, mobility, relative ease of performance, and patient acceptance make isotopic techniques reasonable alternatives to CV both for patient screening and for more definitive diagnostic testing.

REFERENCES

1. Mavor GE, Galloway JMD: Iliofemoral venous thrombosis: Pathological considerations and surgical management. Br J Surg 56:45, 1969
2. Mahaffy RG, Mavor GE, Galloway JMD: Iliofemoral phlebography in pulmonary embolism. Br J Radiol 44:172, 1971
3. Kakkar VV, Field S, Nicolaides AN: Low doses of heparin in prevention of deep-vein thrombosis. Lancet 2:669, 1971
4. Lea Thomas M, O'Dwyer JA: Site of origin of deep vein thrombosis in the calf. Acta Radiol Diagn 18:418, 1977
5. Nicolaides AN, Kakkar VV, Field ES, et al: The origin of deep vein thrombosis: A venographic study. Br J Radiol 44:653, 1971
6. Havig O: Deep vein thrombosis and pulmonary embolism: An autopsy study with multiple regression analysis of possible risk factors. Acta Chir Scand 478(suppl):1, 1977
7. Sevitt S, Gallagher N: Venous thrombosis and pulmonary embolism: A clinico-pathological study in injured and burned patients. Br J Surg 48:475, 1961
8. Dalen JE, Alpert JS: Natural history of pulmonary embolism. Prog Cardiovasc Dis 17:259, 1975
9. Gibbs NM: Venous thrombosis of the lower limbs with particular reference to bed-rest. Br J Surg 45:209, 1957
10. Webber MM, Bennett LR, Cragin M, et al: Thrombophlebitis—Demonstration by scintiscanning. Radiology 92:620, 1969
11. Henkin RE, Yao JST, Quinn JL, et al: Radionuclide venography (RNV) in lower extremity venous disease. J Nucl Med 15:171, 1974
12. Webber MM, Victery W, Cragin MD: Demonstration of thrombophlebitis and endothelial damage by scintiscanning. Radiology 100:93, 1971
13. Magoun S, Shih L-J, DeLand FH, et al: Advantages of applying the LFOV camera with a moving imaging table to lower extremity venography. J Nucl Med Technol 14:59, 1986
14. Cockett FB, Lea Thomas M: The iliac compression syndrome. Br J Surg 52:816, 1965
15. Negus D, Fletcher EWL, Cockett FB, et al: Compression and band formation at the mouth of the left common iliac vein. Br J Surg 55:369, 1968
16. Yao JST, Henkin RE, Conn J, et al: Combined isotope venography and lung scanning: A new diagnostic approach to thromboembolism. Arch Surg 107:146, 1973
17. Nillius AS, Lindvall R, Nylander G: Dynamic radionuclide phlebography: A clinical study in patients with total hip replacement. Eur J Nucl Med 3:161, 1978
18. Johnson W, Patten D, Widrich W, et al: Technetium 99m venography. Am J Surg 127:424, 1974
19. Yao JST, Henkin RE, Bergan JJ: Venous thromboembolic disease: evaluation of new methodology in treatment. Arch Surg 109:664, 1974
20. Lisbona R, Stern J, Derbekyan V: 99m-Tc red blood cell venography in deep vein thrombosis of the leg: A correlation with contrast venography. Radiology 143:771, 1982
21. Lisbona R, Derbekyan V, Novales-Diaz JA: Tc-99m red blood cell venography in deep venous thrombosis of the lower limb: An overview. Clin Nucl Med 10:208, 1985
22. Zorba J, Schier D, Posmituck G: Clinical value of blood pool radionuclide venography. AJR 146:1051, 1986
23. McCalley MG, Braunstein P: Diagnosing iliofemoral vein occlusion from radionuclide blood pool venography. Clin Nucl Med 12:180, 1987
24. Silverstein AM, Turbiner EH: Technetium-99m red blood cell venography in upper extremity deep venous thrombosis. Clin Nucl Med 12:421, 1987
25. Hobbs JT, Davies JWL: Detection of venous thrombosis with 131-I-labelled fibrinogen in the rabbit. Lancet 2:134, 1960
26. Palko PD, Nanson EM, Fedoruk SO: The early detection of deep venous thrombosis using I-131 tagged human fibrinogen. Can J Surg 7:215, 1964
27. Prescott SM, Tikoff G, Coleman RE, et al: 131-I-labeled fibrinogen in the diagnosis of deep vein thrombosis of the lower extremities. AJR 131:451, 1978
28. DeNardo SJ, DeNardo GL: Iodine-123-fibrinogen scintigraphy. Semin Nucl Med 7:245, 1977
29. DeNardo SJ: Role of nuclear medicine in the

detection of venous thrombosis. p. 341. In Freeman LM, Weissmann HS (eds): Nuclear Medicine Annual 1980. Raven Press, New York, 1980

30. Kakkar V: 125-Iodine-fibrinogen uptake test. Semin Nucl Med 7:229, 1977

31. DeNardo GL, DeNardo SJ: Diagnosis of Thrombophlebitis: Medical Monograph. Amersham Corporation, Arlington Heights, IL: 1978

32. Hale TI, Jucker A: Tc-fibrinogen as a thrombus-imaging agent. Eur J Nucl Med 3:267, 1978

33. Edenbrandt CM, Hedner U, Nilsson J, et al: Return to normal of 99m-Tc-plasmin test after deep venous thrombosis and its relationship to vessel wall fibrinolysis. Eur J Nucl Med 12:197, 1986

34. Davis HH, Siegel BA, Sherman LA, et al: Scintigraphy with 111-In-labeled autologous platelets in venous thromboembolism. Radiology 136:203, 1980

35. Miller JH: Detection of deep venous thrombophlebitis by gallium 67 scintigraphy. Radiology 140:183, 1981

36. D'Alonzo WA, Alavi A: Detection of deep venous thrombosis by indium-111 leukocyte scintigraphy. J Nucl Med 27:631, 1986

37. Bardfeld PA, Rand J, Goldsmith SJ: The use of technetium-99m sulfur colloid as a marker for experimental venous thrombosis. (Concise communication.) J Nucl Med 22:598, 1981

38. Hayt DB, Blatt CJ, Freeman LM: Radionuclide venography: Its place as a modality for the investigation of thromboembolic phenomena. Semin Nucl Med 7:263, 1977

39. Ryo UY, Qazi M, Srikantaswamy S, et al: Radionuclide venography: Correlation with contrast venography. J Nucl Med 18:11, 1977

40. Ennis JT, Elmes RJ: Radionuclide venography in the diagnosis of deep vein thrombosis. Radiology 125:441, 1977

41. Gomes AS, Webber MM, Buffkin D: Contrast venography vs. radionuclide venography: A study of discrepancies and their possible significance. Radiology 142:719, 1982

42. Houtte PV, Fruhling J: Radionuclide venography in the evaluation of superior vena cava syndrome. Clin Nucl Med 6:177, 1981

43. Coltart RS, Wraight EP: The value of radionuclide venography in superior vena caval obstruction. Clin Radiol 36:415, 1985

44. DeNardo SJ, Bogren HG, DeNardo GL: Detection of thrombophlebitis in the lower extremities: A regional comparison of 123-I fibrinogen scintigraphy and contrast venography. AJR 145:1045, 1985

45. DeNardo GL, DeNardo SJ, Barnett CA, et al: Assessment of conventional criteria for the early diagnosis of thrombophlebitis with 125-I-fibrinogen. Radiology 125:765, 1977

46. Nicolaides AN, DuPont PA, Desai S, et al: Small doses of subcutaneous sodium heparin in preventing deep venous thrombosis after major surgery. Lancet 2:890, 1972

47. Goodwin DA, Bushberg JT, Doherty PW, et al: Indium-111-labeled autologous platelets for location of vascular thrombi in humans. J Nucl Med 19:626, 1978

48. Ezekowitz MD, Pope CF, Sostman HD, et al: Indium-111 platelet scintigraphy for the diagnosis of acute venous thrombosis. Circulation 73:668, 1986

Index

Page numbers followed by t *represent tables; those followed by* f *represent figures.*